AF555929

HEALTH CARE AND MEDICAL TOURISM IN INDIA AND ASIAN COUNTRIES
Development of Medical Cities

HEALTH CARE AND MEDICAL TOURISM IN INDIA AND ASIAN COUNTRIES

Development of Medical Cities

DR. R. KUMAR

MBBS, MS, Ex. PGI, Eye Specialist
Author of Books on Health Care, Hospitals, Women Empowerment, NGOs, Social Sciences, Health, Fiction, Biography, etc.
Columnist on Health Education, Medical Tourism and Management.

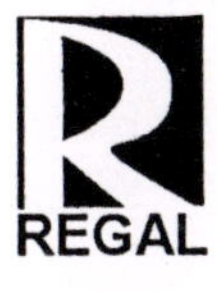

REGAL PUBLICATIONS
New Delhi

HEALTH CARE AND MEDICAL TOURISM IN INDIA AND ASIAN COUNTRIES
Development of Medical Cities

ISBN 978-81-8484-239-5

Typeset by
S.S. COMPOSERS
3190, Mohindra Park, Shakur Basti,
Delhi-110034.

Printed in India at
MAYUR ENTERPRISES
WZ Plot No. 3, Gujjar Market, Tihar Village,
New Delhi-110018.

Published by
REGAL PUBLICATIONS
F-159, Rajouri Garden, New Delhi-110027.
Phone: +91-11-45546396, 25435369
E-mail: regalbookspub@yahoo.com, regaldeepbooks@yahoo.com

Contents

Preface

Modern technologies and outlook have transformed the globe's vast population into a "Global village." From a 'consumer' point of view, it is now possible to take advantage of both cheap airfares and often higher standards or more affordable medical treatment in foreign countries, than those available in their own countries. From a patient perspective, the benefits of global health care are numerous. The Asian nations are facing an unprecedented surge in demand for health care products and services and the same is going to increase in the next few years. Socio-economic development, characterized by increasing income and access to modern amenities and services, has led to changes in the population's nutritional and lifestyle habits, increasing the prevalence of lifestyle-related medical conditions such as obesity, heart disease and diabetes. The expectations of better care, together with growing populations and better-informed patients, are driving investment in hospitals and medical facilities, and pushing up demand for health care services, innovative drugs and the latest medical technologies. With the tightening of immigration rules and security checks, the US has seen a decline in the number of foreign patient visits. More patients, especially those from the Middle-East, are moving towards alternatives like India, Thailand and Singapore.

Medical Cities in the SAARC

India is a leader among the SAARC nations in the field of health tourism. Other seven countries of the region have relatively weaker health care infrastructure because of lack of resources or lack of thrust for health care. Medical tourists come to India from these SAARC countries as well as from the west Asia and central Asia. A good number of medical tourists also come from US, Canada, Europe and other countries. Many of them are attracted by wellness tourism, Yoga, Aurveda and Spirituality. As mentioned in the text, India has set-up several Medical cities to improve tertiary health care for its citizens as well as medical tourists. The benefits of medical city model of health care are also mentioned.

While looking beyond SAARC one finds centers of excellence in several countries, viz. Singapore, Thailand, Malaysia, Philippines, China and several others. One may look at these places to complement the efforts of global community in providing health care and not destinations of competition.

Why should the Medical Tourist come to SAARC?

In the past 30 years or so, the costs of health care have soared in developed countries, especially the United States. Americans and, to some extent, the British, Canadians, Australians began to look for ways to reduce these expenses. Certain services and procedures in American hospitals are now being contracted out to Third World countries, from transcriptions of medical records to the reading of X-rays. Medical tourism presents an opportunity for hospitals to fuel economic growth by tapping the potential of the international patient market. To attract foreign patients, health care providers may consider leveraging on both business and clinical considerations. Though cost is the over-riding factor, the wait for surgeries in some developed nations can also be annoying. USA, Canada and Great Britain have reported a surge in the number of people traveling outside the country to avoid long queues in the National Health Service, which can often be for a year or more for some surgical procedures. The South-East Asian countries such as Thailand, Malaysia, Singapore, Korea and Philippines are the popular destinations for medical treatment. India is also positioning itself as the primary destination for advanced medical procedures in the SAARC region. Some of Indian hospitals are also competing with their South-East Asian peers to get a slice of the cake in the booming health tourism market for international patients. Medical cities being raised in the Middle East have a potential for the people of the world from the East and West, to have a look at them, because huge 'Oil money' is being ploughed for improving health care infrastructure.

Medical City Model of Health Care

Medical cities would not only provide world class medical treatment to the citizens of India but would also attract a large number of health tourists from the globe, far and near. The medical city will not limit its activity to administering only medical and surgical treatment. It will provide, administer and supervise primary health care as well. It will train and educate the necessary medical, paramedical and nursing personnel to fulfil the needs of other hospitals in the region. In addition, it will be a centre of research for generic medicines and pharmaceuticals, biotechnology and stem cell research and an epicenter of medical and health conventions. It will also interact with the community to make them aware and to provide services for prevention of disease and development of health and fitness of the community. Since India is short of 30 lakh hospital beds as per CII study, setting up of large medical cities with 5000-10000 beds would be a good beginning to meet the demands and to make the cost affordable. For this involvement of corporate houses and foreign collaboration will be required. This entails making the health care sector an attractive avenue of investment. Since procurement of land has become the most ticklish issue all over the country, this has to be facilitated. The role of Government is paramount in these two matters. The government has also to act as a regulator and supervisor and oversee the process of accreditation and implementation of quality control and fair delivery of the committed facilities.

A chain of Medicare cities all over the country can improve the health care for countrymen, provided a balance is reached viz. well managed cluster of hospitals but with a motto of service for the people of India/ world.

Chandigarh Health Care City (CHCC)

The name CHCC was coined on the pattern of Dubai Health Care City (DHCC). The author studied the model of DHCC and advised to adopt a modified, enhanced and improved model of DHCC, in setting up the CHCC. Mr. Vivek Atray, the then director, tourism, union territory of Chandigarh took keen interest in the proposed project, but the project remained on the paper.

Dubai took monumental step towards becoming a regional center of excellence for health care delivery. The DHCC has Harvard medical International (HMI) and Mayo clinic as its partners, besides others. The example of Bumrungrad hospital, Thailand, the best hospital from Medical tourism point of view, as a management-model for the proposed Medicare city was also cited while making recommendations. However, this will also require modification as per local needs, resources and to showcase India's best before the world.

This book has been designed to help doctors, nurses, midwives, health administrators and planners to better comprehend the needs and preferences of the modern day patients/clients of SAARC or visiting these countries. The political leaders and bureaucrats also need to comprehend the benefits of medical city model of comprehensive health care. The health care professionals from SAARC countries who reside/visit other regions of the world would also find this book useful in meeting with the aspirations of their patients. It has deep implications to improve health care for the people of India as well.

We have dealt with various issues in the following chapters:

1. Health Care in SAARC and Beyond
2. India's Health Care Sector
3. Will the Indian Medical Cities Deliver Health Care and Promote Tourism?
4. The Advent of Medical and Health Cities in South India
5. Medical and Health Cities can Boost Biotechnology
6. Foreign Collaboration in Health and Medical Cities
7. Health Tourism on the Rise in Indian Medical Cities
8. Health Tourism: Medical Cities in Philippines, Korea
9. Proposed Model of Medical City in India: A Dream or Reality

   Appendices

Chandigarh DR. R. KUMAR

1

Health Care in SAARC and Beyond

Asia is the world's largest and most populous continent, located primarily in the eastern and northern hemispheres. It covers 8.6% of the Earth's total surface area (or 29.9% of its land area) and with approximately 4 billion people, it hosts 60% of the world's current human population. During the 20th century Asia's population nearly quadrupled. Asia is traditionally defined as part of the landmass of Eurasia—with the western portion of the latter occupied by Europe—located to the east of the Suez Canal, east of the Ural Mountains and south of the Caucasus Mountains and the Caspian and Black Seas. It is bounded on the east by the Pacific Ocean, on the south by the Indian Ocean and on the north by the Arctic Ocean. Given its size and diversity, Asia—a topo-nym dating back to classical antiquity—is more a cultural concept incorporating a number of regions and peoples than a homogeneous physical entity. The wealth of Asia differs very widely among and within its regions, due to its vast size and huge range of different cultures, environments, historical ties and government systems. In terms of nominal GDP, Japan has the largest economy on the continent and the second largest in the world. In purchasing power parity terms, however, China has the largest economy in Asia and the second largest in the world. We will focus on some aspects of health care of a limited area of Asia here, i.e. SAARC. India is one of the 8 SAARC countries and is the largest by geographical area and population. Other 7 countries are Pakistan, Afghanistan, Nepal, Bhutan, Bangladesh, Maldives and Sri Lanka. India is the largest and most populous country of this region and is the epicenter of health care facilities for its neighbours as well.

REGIONAL COOPERATION HOLDS THE KEY TO HEALTH CARE

Overall Indian health care is not something to be proud of; it has several big and good hospitals in the public and private domains, both. As mentioned elsewhere several health care groups viz. Medanta, Apollo, fortis, Max, Wockhard, Global, Tatas, Ambanis and many more are setting up islands of excellence in the form of world class hospitals. While there is a large scale internal health tourism by the Indian population to seek medical treatment. Indian hospitals are receiving many patients from the neighbouring SAARC countries as well as from the Gulf and western countries. Excepting India no other country is able to set-up a Mega hospital or health city for want of resources and technical knowhow. Even to provide primary health care and secondary health care there is a great need for regional co-operation. The results of such a co-operation will be more rewarding than in any other sector.

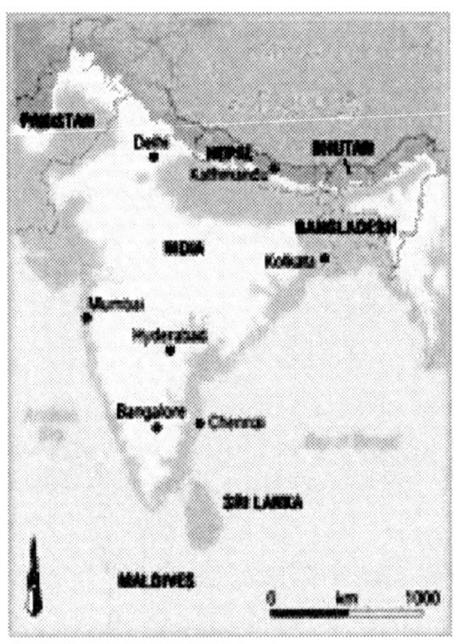

HISTORY OF SAARC FORMATION

SAARC was created in 1985 to promote economic development and social progress in South Asia. India was the Chair of the SAARC Summit in 2007 and this was arguably the most productive summit that SAARC ever witnessed. The launching of negotiations to bring services into the South Asia Free Trade Area (SAFTA), the unilateral granting of zero duty access by India to SAARC Least Developed Countries (LDCs), the formal induction of Afghanistan into SAARC as the eighth member, the setting up of the South Asian University, the establishment of the SAARC Food Bank and the SAARC Development Fund, the signing of the Convention on Mutual Assistance on Criminal Matters were significant steps. Bilateral agreements between countries of South Asia are mutually beneficial. The Indo-Sri Lanka Free Trade Agreement became operational in 2000 and has produced good results within a short time. The Indo-Nepal Trade Treaty is also a good example of bilateral cooperation. India has now bilateral agreements with Nepal, Bhutan, Sri Lanka and Bangladesh. There are problems sometimes and stumbling blocks on the way to economic cooperation but they should be removed in the larger interests of all the countries.

Though the governments of SAARC nations have made efforts since independence to improve the condition of their people, these attempts are often thwarted by multifarious religious, ethnic and linguistic problems. Discontent and frustration among the masses, faced with such tribulations, emboldens subversive forces both within and outside to exploit national inadequacies. It is sometimes claimed that unless economic cooperation between India and Pakistan is normalized, South Asian economic cooperation will not succeed. A regional block provides a stabilizing cushion from the destabilizing fluctuations in the global economy. Regional cooperation is pivotal for prosperity in South Asia. Economic synergy often leads to solutions of disputes including political differences. However, intra-regional trade among SAARC countries is at present less than 5 per cent, whilst it is 62 per cent in the European Union, 55 per cent in the North American Free Trade Area and 35 per cent in the Association of Southeast Asian Nations. SAFTA is the first step towards a more intense synergy which should ultimately lead to a South Asian Union and a single currency.

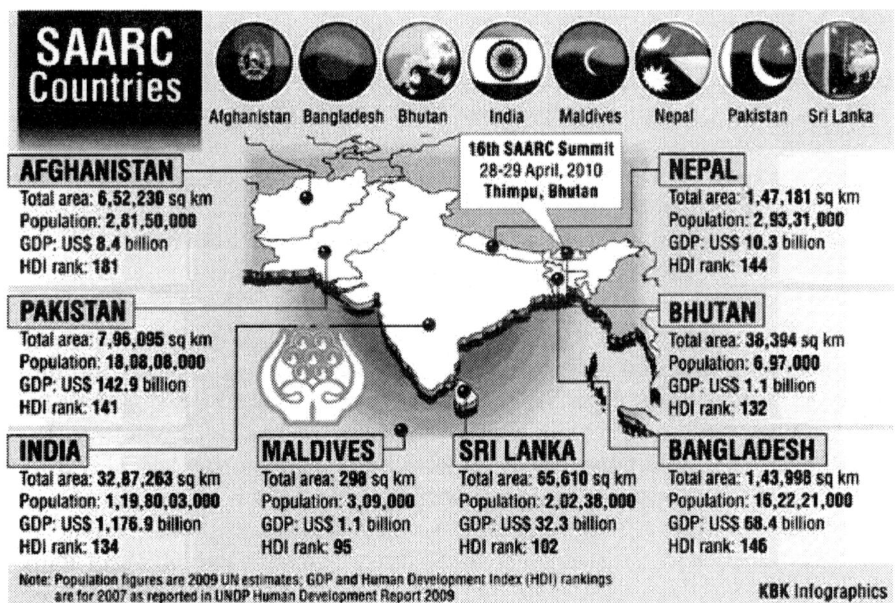

INDIA AND PAKISTAN HAVE TO MOVE FORWARD FOR MUTUAL DEVELOPMENT

India, Pakistan and other SAARC members ought to join hands

across national borders and religious differences, agree on zero tolerance towards every form of extremism and terrorism and redress the grievances of the disaffected and marginalized. They must beware of the machinations of neo-imperialism and its strategy to divide and rule. South Asia continues to have the highest number of people in the world living below the poverty line, outstripping sub-Saharan Africa in this regard. According to the United Nations Educational, Scientific and Cultural Organization (UNESCO), among the 154 countries for which data are available, 28 are not expected to attain any of the three objectives which the international community gathered at the World Education Forum had agreed should be achieved by all nations by 2015. The three goals are: universal primary education, free schooling of acceptable quality, and the removal of gender disparities in education. All the countries of South Asia with the exception of Sri Lanka are among these 28 countries.

THIMPU CONFERENCE 2010, SUCCESSFUL?

Addressing the SAARC (Pakistan, Afghanistan, Sri Lanka, Nepal, Maldives, Bangladesh and Bhutan) Standing Committee meeting in Thimphu, India's Foreign Secretary Nirupama Rao said that SAARC has evolved into a service provider for the economic and development needs of the people of the region. "At the same time, this milestone also provides us with an opportunity to introspect on the experience of the last 25 years and the course we need to chart in the future not only to maintain, but to accelerate, the momentum SAARC has achieved in the recent past," she said. "Let us derive impetus from this to work towards a Summit Declaration that is focused, incisive, visionary, and future-oriented as a lasting outcome of our Summit," Rao said. "Each of the areas of cooperation under SAARC has a direct bearing on the lives and livelihoods of the people of our region. Our leaders have correctly identified the focus of SAARC as being development-oriented," the foreign secretary said.

Two important SAARC agreements on environment and trade in services will be signed during the summit. The pact on trade in services will enable the realisation of the region's immense potential in service areas such as health, hospitality, communications, computer and information services and air transport. The SAARC Convention on Environment is expected to promote cooperation among member-countries in the field of environment and sustainable development. The Indian side is expected to draw the attention of SAARC on the need to improve regional connectivity through the development of new trade, transport and tele-communication links.

Rao said SAARC has facilitated slow but sure steps towards greater cooperation in the security sector and in the prevention of trafficking of women and child development. She said valuable progress has been achieved in developing a regional framework of cooperation in areas such as environment, energy, agriculture and rural development, food security, health, trade and transportation.

GLOBALIZATION AND HEALTH CARE OPPORTUNITIES

The new globalization environment has driven several developing countries with a sizeable public sector to adopt policy reforms including macroeconomic and financial stabilization policies, creation of market-oriented environment and more space for the private sector. This goes hand in hand with increasing internationalization of goods, services, labour and capital, and exchange and exposure of human beings for development-oriented programmes. However, such a process is likely to have far reaching effect on health—both direct and indirect—particularly in developing countries, where health attainments are low and majority of population lacks resources to finance their health care needs. The dynamics, mechanism and pathways through which the process of globalization effects the health sector is not yet clear as their linkages are complex and influenced by several key set of endogenous and exogenous factors.

The rising health care cost is a matter of great concern. The issues are further discussed in the light of accessibility, efficiency, and quality of health care delivery, geographical inequalities, heavy burden of private health care financing, and fiscal stress faced by governments in these countries. This analysis assumes importance if health objectives set forth in the Millennium Development Goals (MDG) have to be realized in the SAARC region.

WHAT DETERMINES HEALTH CARE?

Determinants of health range widely to include income and wealth, education, peace and security, and environmental conditions are likely to be influenced during the globalization process especially in public sector dependent economies. In addition, globalization induced policies, as stated above, are in question due to their likely adverse effect on the poor, the domestic industry and economy, and burdening the health systems with infectious diseases associated with international travel and migration particularly if the existing problems with respect to accessibility, efficiency, quality of health care delivery and inter-regional inequalities in health care financing continue to persist.

This region continues to suffer from many health problems, and in the global context, lags behind all other regions of the world, both in its income and in human development levels. South Asia is by now the poorest region in the world—its per capita income of US$ 309 is much below the US$ 555 of Sub-Saharan Africa and is only one-third of the average of US$ 970 for all developing countries. In terms of composite human development index (HDI), the rank was as low as 142nd (out of a list of 177 countries) for Pakistan, 140th for Nepal, 138th for Bangladesh, 134th for Bhutan, 127th for India with Sri Lanka and Maldives were placed much better at 96th and 84th position, respectively

HEALTH CARE SYSTEMS IN SAARC COUNTRIES

Over time the health care system in SAARC countries has expanded considerably with both public and private sectors playing critical role in delivery of primary and secondary health care. With some exceptions the major health needs of the public are catered for by the public sector. The major boost in infrastructure of the public health care system in SAARC region took place after they endorsed the Alma Ata declaration of 1978—"health for all by 2000" initiative launched by the World Health Organization. Three-tier public health infrastructure were created—'primary health care centers' at village level with first referral unit, community hospital at sub-divisional headquarter as secondary units, and district hospitals and teaching and referral units representing tertiary care.

Along with this a significant public health campaign was launched for the first time, keeping in view local needs and WHO guidelines to meet the target. These included the expanded immunization programme to eradicate the prevalent infectious diseases; malaria, tuberculosis, diarrhea and pneumonia control programmes; family planning programme, and many others such disease control programmes. Due to various socio-economic and political reasons, most SAARC countries (Sri Lanka is an exception) have failed to achieve desired health targets by 2000. Nevertheless under every government the "health for all by 2000" remained an official policy for the state-owned health system, which despite poor resources and mismanagement provided a big relief to the people of SAARC region.

THE PUBLIC HEALTH CARE

The public health care system in SAARC countries is financed through tax revenues. There is a mixed pattern in government health spending in the region. The share of public spending in India, Pakistan and Nepal is very low (ranging between 18 and 30% of total health expenditure) whereas for Bangladesh and Sri Lanka, it is about half; and for Bhutan and Maldives as high as 90%. Both in terms of budgetary allocation and as percentage of GDP, the share of public spending has not been stepped up in India and Pakistan. Over time, fiscal crunch and mismanagement in the public sector contributed to a worsening of the health service provided. In the meantime a vibrant private health care sector flourished in South Asia. No doubt, it is efficient and equals Western standards, but unfortunately, it is run on purely business lines with no ethical values. It is totally unaffordable for the general public and has become one of the most successful businesses in India and Pakistan. The policies of successive governments failed to improve the public health care system.

Traditionally, it had been the policy of the government to provide free health care. Health Care utilization data for India for 1986-87 and 1995-96 indicate a considerable decline in the provision of free health services by the public sector agencies (Gumber 2002). This all changed when SAARC countries officially endorsed the free trade WTO treaties. Over the last decade, these countries have been undertaking economic reforms to pursue privatization, liberalization and globalization. And health sector is not an exception as large-scale inefficiencies and mismanagement have been pointed out in the public sector hospitals. As a first step to check this mismanagement, hospitals have been given more autonomy and allowed to maintain their budgets. Consequently, there was an increase in the cost of treatment as free diagnostic tests were withdrawn and service charges were imposed, making the equity issue more serious (Gumber, 2000).

A high income nation can provide better health infrastructures for its people, who in turn can afford not only to pay for their health care directly or indirectly through taxation, but they can also afford to spend more on better and healthy living. However, health also affects income levels. With improved overall health of the community, the ability of individuals to earn more also improves, their medical expenditures decline, and the income of the nation improves, as the country has to spend less on providing health care infrastructure to unproductive population. It is equally important to note that both these are influenced by the forces of globalization.

It needs to be kept in mind that the public systems for health care arose in most countries because private systems proved inadequate and inequitable. Globalization affects global health through changes in economic growth, poverty, inequality and the sustainability of our environment, although the extent of this effect is yet unclear. Globalized tourism industry which is inseparable from the sexual exploitation of children, adolescents, and adults in third world countries (Buss, 2002), has aggravated the infectious diseases. Even the child health is endangered (indirectly at least) by the growth in economic activity by women if it is not accompanied by the development of adequate childcare infrastructure and nutrition levels (Cornia, 2001). The population-level health influence of tobacco marketing is another important example. China—the most quoted success story of economic reforms have shown that sexually transmitted diseases that were nearly eliminated in the 1960s have spread rapidly in recent times (Dollar, 2001).

RISE OF AGEING POPULATION: A BANE

Health care problems are still dominated by communicable, respiratory and diarrheal diseases, and the high maternal, perinatal and neo-natal morbidity rates. Under-nutrition, micronutrient deficiencies and associated health problems coexist with obesity and non-communicable diseases. In India, during the 1990s, while mortality rates reached a plateau, there emerged a challenging dual disease burden. Communicable diseases have become more difficult to encounter because of the development of insecticide resistant strains of vectors, antibiotics resistant strains of bacteria; and the emergence of HIV infection for which there is no therapy (Government of India, 2002, Tenth Five Year Plan, Part II, p. 82). Two, with increased flow of information through print and electronic media, the active role of NGOs and campaigns led by grassroots organizations, the rising awareness and expectations of the people, stress on international health security, technological advances and improvements in access to health care infrastructure, people have become more right conscious and both the demand and supply side perspectives are changed now. In addition to infections, lifestyle diseases have also invaded the region in a big way, with the advent of ageing population.

FOREIGN INVESTMENTS ARE NOW MORE LIBERAL

Globalization and changes in national policies together with global markets created by the spread of MNCs and global governance affect health attainments by affecting health care system, and individual level health risks. Health outcomes (physical, social and mental well being; ill health; and mortality, morbidity, disability, violence and social maladjustment) determine human development, which in turn can explain the health of the economy.

The diffusion of new knowledge and technology and easing of the trade restrictions while enhancing disease surveillance, treatment and prevention, foreign investment in health services and even the medical tourism have exposed the developing world including the SAARC region to serious health risks. Having sustained an average annual growth rate of above 5 per cent over the last two decades, this region still suffers from many serious health problems, and lags behind all other regions of the world while displaying wide range of variations in their health outcomes.

BEYOND SAARC

India's neighbouring countries constitute another region called : South-East Asia Region. It presents a vibrant and diverse socioeconomic and cultural picture. With more than 1.5 billion people, the Region, comprising Bangladesh, Bhutan, Democratic People's Republic of Korea, India, Indonesia, Maldives, Myanmar, Nepal, Sri Lanka, Thailand, Malaysia, Singapore, and Timor-Leste, accounts for 25% of the world's population. Philippines is another country in the same region and is struggling to establish as a destination of health tourism. The population increased by 61% from 1975 to 2000 and is estimated to exceed two billion by 2025. An interesting demographic change in the Region is the decline in the proportion of the population who are less than 15 years of age. From 41% in 1975, the percentage declined to 33% in 2000, and is likely to drop to less than 23% by 2025. At the same time, the proportion of those aged 65 years and above increased from 3.7% in 1975 to 4.8% in 2000, and is expected to reach 8.4% by 2025. The widespread poverty in some countries of the Region poses a serious threat to health. This is evident from the high percentage of low-birth-weight infants and malnourished children. More than 400 million people are estimated to go hungry every day and the deprivation of human capabilities and access to opportunities affect more than 510 million people. Poverty is also a major contributor to disabilities and to shorter life expectancies in the Region.

The Region carries the largest portion of the global burden of many communicable diseases. A new dimension is the rising trend of non-communicable diseases, such as cardiovascular and cerebro-vascular diseases, cancer and diabetes mellitus as well as accidents and injuries. High maternal mortality ratios (40% of the world's maternal deaths occur in this Region) are also a cause for concern, as are the low literacy levels for women and girls.

Every year, more than 600,000 adults in the Region die of TB and 250,000 children die of measles. More than six million people are living with HIV/AIDS and 250 million are at risk of contracting a severe form of malaria. In addition, the Region has faced epidemics of emerging infectious diseases, adding to the burden of the health systems. Severe acute respiratory syndrome (SARS) and avian influenza are recent examples of such diseases which have caused enormous health and socio-economic hardship and posed a major threat to health security across countries, and beyond national borders. Dengue/DHF, the Nipah virus and the new strain of cholera are spreading to new areas, while age-old diseases like leprosy, kala-azar and lymphatic filariasis continue to cause considerable suffering and psychosocial disruption.

RISE OF LIFESTYLE DISEASES

With increasing life expectancies and marked changes in lifestyles, the past two decades have seen a sharp increase in cardiovascular diseases, diabetes mellitus, hypertension and cancers. For example, 10-15% of the adult population is already affected by hypertension in countries such as India, Indonesia and Thailand. Violence, traffic and work-related accidents, and mental disorders, as well as problems related to substance abuse, are also increasing. Diseases and deaths attributable to tobacco use are a cause of serious concern.

The estimated prevalence of diabetes mellitus in adults in countries of the Region ranges from 2% to 4%. Contrary to trends in developed countries, where the majority of diabetics are 65 years or older, most diabetics in the South-East Asia Region are between 45 and 64 years of age—an economically productive age group. By 2020, according to some estimates, non-communicable diseases are expected to account for seven out of every ten deaths, compared with less than half today—from 47% of the total mortality burden to almost 70%. The situation is compounded by the unprecedented earthquakes and tsunamis, which severely affected six of the Region's 11 Member-States (India, Indonesia, Maldives, Myanmar, Sri Lanka and Thailand). It caused an estimated 280,000 deaths, with thousands still missing.

Life expectancies have risen and infant mortality rates have decreased. This is especially so in Singapore, Malaysia and Thailand where the health care facilities are much better than the rest. The Region is close to eliminating leprosy and eradicating poliomyelitis. It was certified free of guinea-worm disease in February 2000. Efforts for the prevention and control of TB, HIV/AIDS, malaria and other communicable diseases are being scaled up. With more resources, many more challenges can be met.

HEALTH CARE FACILITIES

Over the past few years, Member-States in the Region have strengthened their primary health services considerably. The recognition that functional access is more important than physical access to the basic health needs of the people has encouraged the development of district health systems to provide maximum coverage. Millions of health personnel and volunteers have been trained and deployed in the Region's rural areas. Noteworthy progress has been made in countries with social welfare-oriented policies. The District Health System has proven to be a successful approach for health delivery in an integrated, cost-effective way in countries of the Region. Hospitals play an important role in health care in the Region and are considered the backbone of the health services. With the public health facilities already stretched to the limit, many have little option but to turn to the private sector for their needs even if it is beyond their means. In fact, out-of-pocket expenditure on health care has landed many poor families in dire catastrophic expenses. Some studies however also have shown that people generally prefer private health care facilities and there is little or no difference between the costs of care in either public or private facilities, especially for paying services. The number of hospitals, especially in the private sector, has increased significantly during the last few decades. The growth has been facilitated by the shift in financing policy in health care. Currently, the most common for-profit private service providers in all countries are private practitioners. Therefore, private health care in the Region is also growing rapidly. In some cases, the growth in the health sector is more than what the national economy can handle. Private hospitals in India and Thailand are attracting patients from neighbouring countries and are also extending their services to other countries in the form of offshore activities. (See Appendix to this chapter for Asian Medical Cities in Health Tourism).

GLOBALIZATION PRESENTS OPPORTUNITIES

It is impossible to extend public health services to the entire population through hospitals since they take up a disproportionately high share of resources.

More investments need to be made on first-referral facilities and preventive and promotive care. Policy-making and policy-related budgeting is therefore required for systems that are most responsive to the prevailing needs and conditions.

The rapidly escalating costs of health care in both the private and public sectors seem to be influenced by use of high technology in areas of specialization and super specialization. The main challenge is to curb costs. There is a need to provide care and cure. Public hospitals pose major challenges. Their configuration often reflects the practice of health care in a by-gone era in many of the countries. Their incompatibility with present needs ranges from major problems, such as scarcity of operating theatres, to shortcomings such as the lack of power sockets for the ever-expanding amount of electronic equipment. The majority are also poorly designed to cater to the needs of the elderly. It is not only the physical structure that is difficult to change. An emerging factor that further aggravates the situation is the increasing competition between the public and the private sectors. Concerted and sustained efforts are required to strike a balance between the primary health care approach and tertiary hospital-based care. It is in this context that it is important for hospitals, whether they are public or private, to have a mix of functions incorporating primary care, outpatient services and screening programmes and not be restricted to offering only inpatient care. Hospitals should be responsible and accountable. Health Care systems, therefore, need to be properly reoriented towards the provision of holistic, integrated and continuous health care. More attention needs to be paid to health promotion and protection rather than cures.

Demographic changes, particularly the increase in the percentage of elderly people in the Region's population are exerting serious pressure on health services in the countries. Health facilities everywhere are crowded and the need for long-term and chronic care is becoming increasingly evident.

SAARC HEALTH INDICATORS DISMAL

The SAARC region has one of the poorest health indicators in the world—it houses the largest number of people with micronutrient deficiencies and diabetes; carries 40% of the world's tuberculosis burden, and has a high burden of cardiovascular diseases and one of the worst indicators for reproductive health in the world. In addition, issues of rural health, risks posed by close contact with animal population and high prevalence of zoonotic diseases, highlight issues of a regional nature that could be amenable to locally tailored public health strategies.

HEALTH IS ONE OF THE FIVE AREAS OF CO-OPERATION

Health and Population Activities was one of the original five areas of cooperation identified by member-states. Important activities undertaken by TC05 include the setting up of the SAARC Tuberculosis Centre (STC), in Kathmandu in 1992, devising a standard Format for preparing the Annual

Review of the Situation of Children in the SAARC region; establishment of networking arrangements for training, research and eradication of malaria and regional approach for combating major diseases in the region. A Directory of training programmes in six priority areas, i.e. malaria, tuberculosis, leprosy, diarrheal diseases, human rabies and maternal and child health have been prepared and circulated. In addition, several status papers on important subjects relating to health have been circulated among member-states.

The Second SAARC Summit (Bangalore, 1986) decided that the survival, protection and development of Children should be given highest priority and directed that annual reviews be undertaken on the situation of children in SAARC countries. Such annual reviews for the years 1993 and 1994 have been completed by TC05 based on annual country reports submitted by member-states. These annual reviews have indicated, *inter-alia,* reduction of infant mortality and significant progress in the immunization programme for children in the region.

HIV/AIDS

The Regional Strategic Framework for the Protection, Care and Support of Children Affected by HIV/AIDS provides guidance to the eight member-States of the South Asian Association for Regional Cooperation (SAARC) on a consistent approach across South Asia to the protection, care and support of children affected by HIV/AIDS. It locates children affected by HIV/AIDS within the broader group of children in difficult circumstances, and focuses on delivering an integrated response to children's medical, nutritional, educational, legal and psychosocial needs, within the context of the UN Convention on the Rights of the Child, which all Member-States have ratified. The Regional Framework promotes a universal approach to ensure children affected by HIV/AIDS have access to the same public and social support systems which are available to other children, rather than being separated or singled out. However, within this universal approach the Regional Framework calls for additional and specific measures in relation to overcoming the stigma that surrounds HIV/AIDS and to intervene on behalf of children who are discriminated against as a result of this stigma. The Regional Framework recommends that the response be age- and gender-sensitive, take into account the specific situation and location in which affected children live, and that prioritise legal, policy and practical action to reduce the stigma and discrimination around HIV/AIDS. It recognises that many of the threats to the rights of children affected by HIV/AIDS relate to the health and survival of their parents, and in this light encourages action to ensure expanded access to HIV testing and counselling, and to appropriate treatment and care for those infected. The Regional Framework takes into account that many of the children affected by HIV/AIDS are also at risk of HIV infection and some may be HIV-positive, and promotes strong intervention-level linkages to essential HIV/AIDS prevention and treatment services for children and their families, including prevention of mother-to-child transmission.

Between 2.3 and 3.7 million people in the SAARC region are estimated to be HIV positive. UNAIDS and UNICEF estimated that in 2004 there were nearly 1.3 million children who have lost one or both parents to AIDS in South Asia. A significantly larger number of children—estimated upto 10 million—are living in families where one or both parents is HIV positive. Whilst these numbers are large, the children affected by HIV/AIDS are still a small proportion of the large number of children who are living in vulnerable households where their rights are not protected.

TRAFFICKING IN WOMEN AND CHILDREN FOR PROSTITUTION

EMPHASISING that the evil of trafficking in women and children for the purpose of prostitution is incompatible with the dignity and honor of human beings and is a violation of basic human rights;

RECALLING the decision of the Ninth SAARC Summit (May, 1997) that the feasibility of a regional Convention to combat the grave crime of trafficking in women and children for prostitution should be explored;

RECALLING ALSO the relevant international legal instruments relating to prevention of trafficking in women and children, including the Convention for the Suppression of Trafficking in Persons and of the Exploitation of Prostitution of Others, 1949; Convention on the Elimination of all Forms of Discrimination against Women.

NOTING with concern the increasing exploitation by traffickers of women and children from SAARC countries and their increasing use of these countries as sending, receiving and transit points; RECOGNISING in this regard the importance of establishing effective regional cooperation for preventing trafficking for prostitution and for investigation, detection, interdiction, prosecution and punishment of those responsible for such trafficking; EMPHASISING the need to strengthen cooperation in providing assistance, rehabilitation and repatriation to victims of trafficking for prostitution.

Article I

For the purpose of this Convention:

"Child" means a person who has not attained the age of 18 years;

"Prostitution" means the sexual exploitation or abuse of persons for commercial purposes;

"Trafficking" means the moving, selling or buying of women and children for prostitution within and outside a country for monetary or other considerations with or without the consent of the person subjected to trafficking;

"Traffickers" means persons, agencies or institutions engaged in any form of trafficking;

"Persons subjected to trafficking" means women and children victimized or forced into prostitution by the traffickers by deception, threat, coercion, kidnapping, sale, fraudulent marriage, child marriage, or any other unlawful means;

"Protective home" means a home established or recognized by a Government of a Member-State for the reception, care, treatment and rehabilitation of rescued or arrested persons subjected to trafficking.

"Repatriation" means return to the country of origin of the person subjected to trafficking across international frontiers.

Article II

SCOPE OF THE CONVENTION

The purpose of this Convention is to promote cooperation amongst Member-States so that they may effectively deal with the various aspects of prevention, interdiction and suppression of trafficking in women and children; the repatriation and rehabilitation of victims of trafficking and prevent the use of women and children in international prostitution networks, particularly where the countries of the SAARC region are the countries of origin, transit and destination.

Article III

The State Parties to the Convention shall take effective measures to ensure that trafficking in any form is an offence under their respective criminal law and shall make such an offence punishable by appropriate penalties which take into account its grave nature.

The State Parties to the Convention, in their respective territories, shall provide for punishment of any person who keeps, maintains or manages or knowingly finances or takes part in the financing of a place used for the purpose of trafficking and knowingly lets or rents a building or other place or any part thereof for the purpose of trafficking.

Any attempt or abetment to commit any crime mentioned in paras 1 and 2 above or their financing shall also be punishable.

Article IV

The State Parties to the Convention shall ensure that their courts having jurisdiction over the offences committed under this Convention, can take into account factual circumstances which make the commission of such offences particularly grave, viz. the involvement in the offences of an organized criminal group to which the offender belongs; the involvement of the offender in other international organized criminal activities; the use of violence or arms by the offender; the fact that the offender holds a public office and that the offence is committed in misuse of that office; the victimization or trafficking of children; the fact that the offence is committed in a custodial institution or in an educational institution or social facility or in their immediate vicinity or in other places to which children and students visit for educational, sports, social and cultural activities; previous conviction, particularly for similar offences, whether in a Member-State or any other country.

Article V

In trying offences under this Convention, judicial authorities in Member-States shall ensure that the confidentiality of the child and women victims is maintained and that they are provided appropriate counselling and legal assistance.

Article VI

The State Parties to the Convention shall grant to each other the widest measure of mutual legal assistance in respect of investigations, inquiries, trials or other proceedings in the requesting State in respect of offences under this Convention. Such assistance shall include: taking of evidence and obtaining of statements of persons; provision of information, documents and other records including criminal and judicial records; location of persons and objects including their identification; search and seizures; delivery of property including lending of exhibits; making detained persons and others available to give evidence or assist investigations; service of documents including documents seeking attendance of persons; and any other assistance consistent with the objectives of this Convention.

Requests for assistance shall be executed promptly in accordance with their national laws and in the manner requested by the Requesting State. In the event that the Requested State is not able to comply in whole or in part with a request for assistance or decides to postpone execution it shall promptly inform the Requesting State and shall give reasons for the same.

Article VII

The offences referred to in the present Convention shall be regarded as extraditable offences in any extradition treaty which has been or may hereinafter be concluded, between any of the Parties to the Convention.

If a State Party which makes extradition conditional on the existence of a treaty, receives a request for extradition from another State Party with which it has no extradition treaty, the Requested State shall, if so permitted by its laws, consider this Convention as the basis for extradition in respect of the offences set forth.

Extradition shall be granted in accordance with the laws of the State to which the request is made.

The State Party in whose territory the alleged offender is present shall, if it does not extradite him or her, submit, without exception whatsoever and without undue delay, the case to its competent authorities for the purpose of prosecution in accordance with the laws of that State.

In States where extradition of their nationals is not permitted under their law, nationals who have committed offences under the present Convention shall be prosecuted and punished by their courts.

Article VIII

The State Parties to the Convention shall provide sufficient means, training and assistance to their respective authorities to enable them to effectively conduct inquiries, investigations and prosecution of offences under this Convention.

The State Parties to the Convention shall sensitize their law enforcement agencies and the judiciary in respect of the offences under this Convention and other related factors that encourage trafficking in women.

The State Parties to the Convention shall establish a Regional Task Force consisting of officials of the Member-States to facilitate implementation of the provisions of this Convention and to undertake periodic checking.

The State Parties to the Convention may also, by mutual agreement, set-up bilateral mechanisms to effectively implement the provisions of the Convention, including appropriate mechanisms for cooperation to interdict trafficking in women and children for prostitution.

The State Parties to the Convention shall exchange, on a regular basis, information in respect of agencies, institutions and individuals who are involved in trafficking in the region and also identify methods and routes used by the traffickers through land, water or air. The information so furnished shall include information of the offenders, their fingerprints, photographs, methods of operation, police records and records of conviction.

The State Parties to the Convention may consider taking necessary measures for the supervision of employment agencies in order to prevent trafficking in women and children under the guise of recruitment.

The State Parties to the Convention shall endeavour to focus preventive and development efforts on areas which are known to be source areas for trafficking.

The State Parties to the Convention shall promote awareness, *inter-alia*, through the use of the media, of the problem of trafficking in women and children and its underlying causes including the projection of negative images of women.

Article IX

The State Parties to the Convention shall work out modalities for repatriation of the victims to the country of origin.

Pending the completion of arrangements for the repatriation of victims of cross-border trafficking, the State Parties to the Convention shall make suitable provisions for their care and maintenance. The provision of legal advice and health care facilities shall also be made available to such victims.

The State Parties to the Convention shall establish protective homes or shelters for rehabilitation of victims of trafficking. Suitable provisions shall also be made for granting legal advice, counselling, job training and health care facilities for the victims.

The State Parties to the Convention may also authorize the recognized non-governmental organizations to establish such protective homes or shelters for providing suitable care and maintenance for the victims of the State Parties to the Convention shall encourage recognized non-governmental organizations in efforts aimed at prevention, intervention and rehabilitation, including through the establishment of such protective homes or shelters for providing suitable care and maintenance for the victims of trafficking.

Article X

The State Parties to the Convention shall adopt, in accordance with their respective Constitutions, the legislative and other measures necessary to ensure the implementation of the Convention.

Article XI

The measures provided for in the Convention are without prejudice to higher measures of enforcement and protection accorded by relevant national laws and international agreements.

Article XII

The Convention shall be open for signature by the Member-States of SAARC at the Eleventh SAARC Summit at Kathmandu and thereafter, at the SAARC Secretariat at Kathmandu. It shall be subject to ratification.

The instruments of Ratification shall be deposited with the Secretary-General.

Article XIII

This Convention shall enter into force on the fifteenth day following the day of the deposit of the seventh Instrument of Ratification with the Secretary General.

Article XIV

The Secretary-General shall be the depository of this Convention and shall notify the Member-States of signatures to this Convention and all deposits of Instruments of Ratification. The Secretary-General shall transmit certified copies of such instruments to each Member-State. The Secretary-General shall also inform Member-States of the date on which this Convention will have entered into force in accordance with Article XIII.

DONE at Kathmandu on this Fifth Day of January Two Thousand and Two.

—Sd/- Ministers for Foreign Affairs, all SAARC countries

MILLENNIUM DEVELOPMENT GOAL (MDG) 5

With less than seven years to go in the countdown to 2015, the target date set by the United Nations Millennium Declaration, for achieving various development goals and targets, countries in the South Asian Region are concerned with the slow progress on reducing maternal mortality. The Millennium Development Goal (MDG) 5, for improving maternal health, with targets for reducing maternal mortality (target 5A) and achieving universal access to reproductive health (target 5B) provides an opportunity to review key policy and operational constraints and advocate for actions to accelerate progress. Key considerations are to ensure that good quality reproductive health services and commodities are accessible to all.

CURRENT STATUS AND ACHIEVEMENTS ON MDG 5 IN THE REGION

Although some progress has been made, in many countries in our region, coverage for family planning and access to comprehensive reproductive health services and commodities is still inadequate. A number of countries experience a high unmet need for family planning, low facility-based deliveries and deaths or disabilities associated with pregnancy or childbirth. Overall, women continue to experience an unacceptably high rate of sexual and reproductive health problems from preventable causes and issues associated with gender and social status. Significant inequities and disparities remain in achieving universal access to services within countries.

RECOGNIZING that the attainment of the MDGs and other international goals and targets require, as a priority, a strong investment and political commitment to, and advocacy for, improving sexual and reproductive;

ACCEPTING that as legislators, parliamentarians, policy-makers, representatives of national organizations, religious leaders, civil society and media professionals, we have a responsibility, together with our governments, to ensure the health of our women, men and young people in our countries by providing high quality, accessible, affordable and sustainable reproductive health care at all levels;

NOTING, with concern, that the impact of the HIV pandemic in our countries puts at risk some of our health gains, particularly those that pertain to women, young people, and children and threatens to overwhelm the resources needed to improve reproductive health services;

RECALLING and recognizing the Programme of Action of the International Conference on Population and Development (ICPD Cairo, 1994) and key actions for the further implementation of the Programme of Action of the ICPD, adopted by the twenty-first special session of the United Nations General Assembly;

ACKNOWLEDGING the importance of achieving universal access to reproductive health services and commodity security in meeting international goals for reducing maternal mortality and morbidity;

FURTHER RECALLING the Global reproductive health strategy to accelerate progress towards the attainment of international development goals and targets adopted in 2004 by Health Ministers at the World Health Assembly;

RECOGNIZING the links between improved sexual and reproductive health, provision of universal education, especially of girls, women empowerment and socio-economic development, poverty reduction, environmental protection and overall health and development;

URGE various stakeholders, including ministers, parliamentarians, health programme managers, service providers, donors, the media and others in all countries in our region, as a matter of urgency to: devote sufficient priority, commitment and resources to interventions, policies and strategies for reducing maternal mortality, including among others ensuring a continuum of care; access to quality family planning, counselling, information, services and commodities that promote informed choice; emergency contraception; prevention of unsafe abortion and provision of post-abortion care; access to ante-natal and post-natal care; provision of emergency obstetric and newborn care; ensuring availability of transport, access to skilled birth attendants, and safe blood and blood products; provide a separate annual incremental budget line for reproductive health within the health budget that adequately supports services, and strengthen national capacity in management and security of commodities, support forecasting, procurement and distribution of essential commodities including contraceptives on the basis of sound logistics, service and demographic data; ensure that sexual and reproductive health and rights, and research, which includes family planning, maternal health, prevention and control of sexually transmitted infections and HIV, and prevention of mother to child transmission, are integrated within national health strategies and action plans, to the fullest extent possible; establish policies and programmes that care for vulnerable groups, such as adolescents, underprivileged groups, the urban poor, ethnic minorities, marginalized communities, populations in conflict, post-conflict and disaster situations, and address their reproductive health needs; engage parliamentarians, sensitize the media, involve men and mobilize the extended family, community groups, religious and civil society leaders, the private sector, social marketing and relevant organizations to participate in the introduction and scaling up of interventions for improving sexual and reproductive health, and the elimination of gender-based violence; introduce programmes and policies that support HIV prevention and care, including comprehensive condom programming; and support HIV and reproductive health education in upper primary and secondary schools; train and retain health care providers for the delivery of an integrated and comprehensive range of reproductive health, including family planning services; and increase coverage for services, including through community-based initiatives; develop and implement national strategies for rapid production, deployment and retention of skilled health care providers and mid-wives and incorporate Emergency Obstetric and Newborn Care in pre-service training at all levels of health care delivery system; ensure that national essential medicines lists include reproductive health commodities; and support quality assurance in the production and supply chain; institutionalize monitoring and evaluation (M&E) and allocate adequate human and financial recourses, including the identification through M&E, and sharing of best practices.

In conclusion, we want to reiterate and commit to improving the health of women, men and young people in our countries. As parliamentarians, policy-makers and media professionals, we wish to advocate for greater awareness and a stronger commitment to achieving the MDGs, in particular MDG 5, which shows the least.

Signed by Afghanistan, Bangladesh, Bhutan, India, Maldives, Nepal, Pakistan and Sri Lanka on 30th day of July in the year 2009, Kathmandu, Federal Democratic Republic of Nepal.

In the subsequent chapters are described health care and health tourism aspects in India, neighbouring countries in ASEAN, Philippines and Korea. Below are described some aspects about the health care in Pakistan, Myanmar and Bangladesh.

MEDICAL CITY IN PAKISTAN

Sharif Medical City Hospital (SHCH), Lahore was established in 1997, a vision of founding father Mian Muhammad Sharif to build a multidiscipline hospital of international standards. This hospital is 360 bed tertiary care center. This is the first hospital established on the concept of a "Medial City" in Pakistan. This has the unique advantage of offering comprehensive medial facilities under "one roof". The main hospital along with allied campus buildings, including staff residences, and a planned medical college, are situated on 80 acre land on a canal bank, in green and pollution-free idyllic surroundings.

SMCH is a centre of excellence for Kidney Transplant and more than 700 successful kidney transplants, both adult and children have been performed so far. International guidelines and standards are observed for patient selection, pre and post-transplant management. End Stage Kidney Failure is now of epidemic proportion both in developed and developing countries. To sustain life, patients with this condition need dialysis or transplant. Unfortunately, both modalities of treatment are life long and expensive.

Kidney Transplant provides:

- Freedom from dialysis.
- Better quality of life.
- Fewer restrictions on diet and routine activities.

Sharif Medical City has one of the most advanced and renowned kidney transplant programs in this part of the world and is a centre of excellence for Kidney Transplant, both for adults and children. International guidelines and standards are strictly observed for patient selection, pre and post-transplant management.

Renal Transplant Package Includes the following :

Evaluation for transplant by consultants

- Nephrologist
- Internist
- Cardiologist
- Transplant Surgeon/Urologist
- Critical Care Medicine and Anesthesiologist
- Dentist
- Gynaecologist (for women)

Pre-transplant evaluation of chronic kidney failure patients

- **Biochemistry**: Renal Function, Bone, Liver Enzymes, Blood Sugar, Lipid Profile, TSH, PTH and Iron Profile
- Hematology
- Immunology
- Virology, HCV, HBsAg, HIV, CMV, EBV
- Microbiology
- Cardiological Evaluation—ECG, Doppler, ECHO, Angiography if needed.
- Radiological Diagnostic Evaluation
- Histopathology (if required)

Pre-op work up of patient

- Blood Group
- DNA Tissue Typing of recipient and donor
- Cross Matches with Potential donor upto three
- Radiology Evaluation for fitness of patient and donor
- Cardiology evaluation for fitness (ECG, ECHO, ETT, Thallium Stress Test and Angiography if required)

Transplant surgery

- Transplant Surgery Team Fee
- Transplant Anesthesia Fee
- Transplant Post-Operative Care Team Fee
- ICU/CCU Care Fee
- All laboratory investigations including Cyclosporine level, Serial ultrasound and Dopplers of Transplant Kidney.

Cost of Renal Transplant

The cost of a renal transplant at Sharif Medical City Hospital includes :

- Stay upto 3-4 weeks (upto 7 days post-transplant)
- Meal Charges (All three times meal + Tea + Soft drink + Mineral Water)
- Medication—Pre- and Post-Transplant (all Inclusive) before and 4 days after transplant. Simulect injection only if required has extra charges (patient will be informed accordingly)
- Maintenance dialysis.
- Investigations and surgery.
- Consultations of Nephrologists and Transplant Team

Patient will be required to pay

There will be extra charge for the following for which you will be duly informed and consented received for:

- Simulect Injection (if needed)
- Any specialized/invasive investigations like Coronary angiography, etc.
- Extra Cross Match with donor of US $ 100 each
- Any extra surgery, if needed
- Laundry Services
- Patient facilities
- Central Air-conditioning, ensuite private room
- Helpers and Valets (24 hours on duty)
- Antiseptic and Disinfection Protocol
- Airport Pick-up and Drop-off facility
- 24 hours house keeping and Kitchen Staff
- Fully functional Kitchen and freshly made all meals, beverages and mineral water provided.
- Exclusive Executive Lounge.
- Local Telephone, Fax and Internet services.
- 25 Channel Cable TV
- General and Provision Store
- Cafeteria
- 24 hours Hospital Security
- Uninterrupted Power supply

Events once the patient arrives

After patient's arrives, the following arrangements are made:

- Excellent services of Interpreters. Official language of the hospital is English.
- Introduction on the arrival at Sharif Medical City Hospital.

- Ensuite private rooms + all meals and mineral water provided.
- Complete medical examination.
- All pre-operative investigations arranged, medical treatment and maintenance of dialysis continued.
- Patient examined by all relevant consultants for initiation of Transplant work-up.
- The potential recipient and donor undergo extensive investigations of international standard of clinical care.
- Informed consents in writing obtained.
- Once Tissue Typing and Cross Match results available, the donor undergoes complete clinical, laboratory and radiological investigations before the suitability for kidney donation is established.
- Post-Transplant Care.
- Recipient and donor shifted to ICU for close monitoring and management.
- Recipient shifted to room after within few days.
- Recipient undergoes regular laboratory tests, radiological investigations and closely monitored by Nephrologists and Surgical team.
- Once discharged from the hospital, the patient is provided with detailed discharge summary, list of medications and photocopies of important investigations.
- Patient receives detailed advice for follow-up.

Myanmar: private hospitals

The Myanmar Health Ministry has re-granted business licenses to more private hospitals and clinics as well as other health service centers in the country to run in 2010 after such grant was suspended for a time, sources with the health department said. Health care-related facilities, medical equipment and qualified health care staff shall be in place by the time when it starts operation as prescribed, the sources said. Such measures shall be carried out nationwide by the central private health care department to be organized, it also said. There are altogether 50 private hospitals, over 300 special health care centers and over 1,800 clinics operating in the Yangon division, statistics show. Meanwhile, a private special treatment hospital in a new satellite town in Myanmar's new capital of Nay Pyi Taw is under construction to add to the developing health facilities there. The Okdarathiri Myothit Private Hospital of Singapore-standard is being built to become the first of its kind in the new capital.

Aimed at developing private health care services and utilizing effectively the resources of private sector in providing such services to the public in accordance with the national health policy, Myanmar permits systematic running of private health care services which include private clinic service, private hospital service, private maternity home service, nursing home service and private mobile health care service. For the development of the health sector, Myanmar has drawn up its health vision 2030 with the aim to provide comprehensive health care for the entire people.

BANGLADESH

City Hospital Ltd.

It started in 1999 as 20 bed Specialized Burn and Plastic Surgery Hospital at 69/I/1, Panthapath, Dhanmondi, Dhaka-1205, then shifted to Lalmatia, Dhaka in 2006 as 150 bed general hospital including 24 bed Burn and Plastic Surgery (8 High Dependency Unit beds and 16 general beds) and 8 bed General Intensive Care Unit (I.C.U). In terms of quality of services and treatment, it is now considered as a centre of excellence in medical and hospital care. It has world class treatment facilities as well as cost effective treatment solution in Bangladesh. Presently they have different specialties like Medicine, Diabetes and Endocrinology, Gynaecology and Obstetrics, Nephrology, Urology, ENT, Gastroenterology, General and Laparoscopic surgery, Burn, Plastic and Cosmetic Surgery, Oncology, Neuromedicine and Physiotherapy. A number of reputed and experienced physicians, surgeons and other health professionals are providing their best support round the clock. They have ICU facilities, 6 operation theaters with modern equipments and central gas supply and other supporting facilities. We also have a full-fledged diagnostic complex with sophisticated modern analyzers and imaging equipments. not only modern machines but men behind the machines are also very important factor. So, we have recruited highly qualified team of technicians, biochemists and other professionals having proper background and experience in respective fields under the supervision of specialists. Round the clock Emergency, Outdoor, Pharmacy, Cafeteria and Food services are also available.

OTHER HOSPITALS AND CLINICS IN BANGLADESH

Al-Raji Hospital Ltd.
Farmgate, Dhaka
Phone: 8119229, 9117775

Apollo Hospitals
Plot 81, Block E, Bashundhara R/A
Dhaka-1229

Aysha Memorial Specialized Hospital
74F/74F Peacock Square
Air Port Road, Mohakhai, Dhaka
Phone: 9122689-90, 9131742

Bangladesh Medical College
House# 33/35, Road# 14/A
(New) Dhanmondi R/A, Dhaka
Phone: 9118202, 8115843

BIRDEM
Shahbagh, Dhaka
Phone: 9661551-60, 8616641
Central Hospital
House# 2, Road# 5
Green Road, Dhanmondi, Dhaka-1205
Phone: 9660015-19, 8619321

China-Bangla (JV) Ltd.
House# 15, Shayesta Khan Avenue, Sector# 4,
Dhaka, Phone: 8913674, 8913606

City Dental College and Hospital
1085/1 Malibagh, Chowdhurypara
Dhaka-1219, Phone: 9341662-4, 9338470

CIty Hospital (Pvt) Ltd.
69/1, Public Colleger Goli
Panthapath, Dhaka
Phone: 8617852

Crescent Hospital and Diagnostic Complex Ltd.
Address: 22/2, Babar Road
(Opposite of Sohrarwardi Hospital),
Mirpur Road, Dhaka
Phone: 8119775, 9117524

Dhaka ENT (Ear Nose Throat) Hospital
Dhanmondi, Dhaka
Phone: 8613936, 8617593

Dhaka Eye Hosptial, BNSB
Mirpur-1, Dhaka
Phone: 8014476

Dhaka Shishu Hospital
Sher-E-Bangla Nagar
Dhaka-1207, Phone: 8116061-2, 8114571-2

Dushtha Shasthya Hospital (D.S.H)
21/1 Khilgi Road, Mohammadpur-1207
Dhaka, Phone: 8124952

Gana Shasthya Nagar Hospital
House# 14/E, Road# 6, Dhanmondi
Dhaka-1205, Phone: 8617208
Gene Cure Health Care Ltd.
37, Kemal Ataturk Avenue, Banani
Dhaka-1213, Phone: 8853707

Green Hospital
House# 31, Road# 6, Dhanmondi
Dhaka, Phone: 8612412

Holy Family Red Cresent Hospital
Eskaton, Dhaka.
Phone: 8311721-25

ICDDRB
Address: Mohakhali, Dhaka
Phone: 8811751-60

Islamia Eye Hospital
Farmgate, Dhaka.
Phone: 8112856, 9119315

Marks ENT Clinic and General Hospital
Mirpur, Dhaka.
Phone: 9872241, 9871527

Medinova Medical Services
Address: House# 71/A, Road# 5/A, Dhanmondi
Dhaka-1209. Phone: 8620353-7, 8618583

Modern Clinic of Surgery and Midwifery
Gulshan, Dhaka
Phone: 9883948

Monowara Hospital (Pvt) Ltd.
Siddheswari, Dhaka
Phone: 8318135, 8319802, 83

National Heart Foundation Hospital
Plot# 7/2, Section# 2, Mirpur, Dhaka
Phone: 8010491, 8014914

National Heart Institute
Shyamoli, Dhaka
Phone: 9122560-72, 8114089

National Institute of Cardiac Vascular Disease
Ser-E-Bangla Nagar, Dhaka
Phone: 9122560
Nibedita Shishu Hospital Ltd.
Wari, Dhaka
Phone: 7119473

P.G. Hospital (BSMMU)
Shahbag, Dhaka
Phone: 8614001-5, 8614545-9

S.P.R.C Hospital
New Eskaton Road, Dhaka
Phone: 9339089, 9342744

Samorita Hospital Ltd.
89/1, Panthapath, Dhaka-1215
Phone: 9131901, 9129971

Shahid Suhrawardy Hospital
Ser-E-Banglanagar, Dhaka
Phone: 9130800, 9122560-78

South Asia Hospital Ltd.
25, Green Road, Pantahpath
Dhaka-1205, Phone: 8616565, 9665852

Stone Crash Hospital
Dhanmondi, Dhaka
Phone: 503948, 8618388

Universal Medical Hospital
Nurer Chala, Besides Kolotan Public School
Notun Bazar, Dhaka
Phone: 8813375

Uttara Central Hospital
Sector : 1, Uttara, Dhaka
Phone: 8911551

Z.H. Sikder Women's Medical College and Hospital
Monica Estate (Western Side of Dhanmondi)
Dhaka-1209, Phone: 8115951, 8113313

Labaid Specialized Hospital
House# 1, Road# 4, Dhanmondi
+880-2-8610793-8, 9670210-3, 8631177, 01819-215890
http://www.labaidgroup.com/

Square Hospitals Ltd.
18/F, West Panthopath
Dhaka 1205, Bangladesh
Phone: +880 2 8129334, +880 2 9146248
Emergency: +880 2 8144466
Email: info@squarehospital.com
Labaid Cardiac Hospital
House# 1, Road # 4, Dhanmondi, Dhaka-1205
+880-2-8610793-8, 9670210-3,
8631177, 01819-215890
http://www.labaidgroup.com/lch.php

Ibn Sina Hospital at Sankar
House #68, Road #15/A
Dhanmondi R/A, Dhaka 1209
Phone: 8119513, 8113709, 01817144609,
01817144612 (ICU)

Ibn Sina Hospital Fouad Al Khatib Unit
2/2, Kallyanpur Bus Stand
Mirpur Road, Dhaka 1207
Phone: 9007188, 9004317

Ibn Sina Diagnostic and Imaging Center
House 48, Road-9/A
Dhanmondi R/A, Dhaka
Tel: 9126625-6, 9128835-7

Ibn Sina Medical Imaging Center
House 58, Road-2/A
Dhanmondi R/A, Dhaka
Tel: 9663289, 9666497, 8628118, 8618262, 8610420

Other Institutions
Anjuman-e-MofidulIslam 9336611, 248166, 239808
Bangladesh Diabetic Society 9661551-60
Al-Baraka Kidny Hospital 9350884, 9351164
Al-Biruni Hospital 8118905, 9115958
Al-Manar Hospital 9121387, 9121588
Al-Markajul Islamic Hospital 9129426, 9129217
Al-Maghraby Eye Hospital 9135451-2, 8114142
Al-Rajhi Hospital (PVT.) Ltd 8119229, 9117775
Bangkok Hospital 9139777, 9134982, 8111154
BARDEM (Shabagh Avenue) 8616641-50
BDF Hospital 8113431 8323730
Bangladesh Diabetic Society 9661551-60

Bangladesh Diagonostic and Medical Centre 9335838, 8322249
B.N.S. Eye Dhaka 8014476
Bangladesh Medical College Hospital 9118202
China-Bangla Hospital 8913674 8913606
Cholera Hospital 600171-8
CMH (Dhaka) 9871469
Chritian Medical Hospital 9886298 8813375
Dhaka Medical Collage 500121-6 505025-29, 502529
Fire Service for Ambulance 9555555 9556666
Green Hospital 8612412 8619068
Holy Family Red Cresent 8311721-5 8315007-8
Hospital For Infection Disease 602429
ICDDRB B 8811751-60
ICDDRB B (Ambulance) 8811751-59
ICDDRB B (Director) 8823031
ICDDRB B 8811751-59
IPGMR 8614545-9 8611737-41, 8614001-5
Islami Bank Hospital 8317090 8321495
Islamia Eye Hospital 9119315 8112156
Lion Eye Hospital 9129127
Lab Aid Cardiac Hospital 880-2-8610793-8, 8629782
Maternity Hospital (Azimpur) 503329
Mirpur General Hospital 9007873 8015444
Mitford Hospital 7319002-6
Monowara General Hospital 239446 244717
Monowara Hospital (Pvt) Ltd. 8318135 8319802
National medical Institute Hospital 237300 233469
Orthopedic Hospital 9112150
Railway Hospital 409341-9
Royal Hospital (Pvt) Ltd. 8313096
Salimullah Medical College Hospital 7319002-6
Samorita Hospital 9131901
Shahid Suhrawardi Hospital 9122560-78 9112086, 8114856, 9130800
Shahid Suhrawardi Emergency 9130050
Shishu Hospital 8116061-2 9119119
South Asian Hospital 8616565
Stone Crash Hospital 8618388
Heart Hospital 9801874 9803302
T.B. Hospital (Mohakhali) 608031-4
Women and Children`s Hospital and Research Centre 9115458 9121077
Yamagata Dhaka Friendship Hospital 9129354
Aroggaya Niketan 9333730
Compath Clinic 8617844 9660086, 508651
Comfort Diagnostic Centre 8616045 9660111
Cosmopolitan 601774

Dhaka Monorog Clinic 9005050
Dipham R & S Centre 8117772-3 9125811
Enayet Hospital 509313 509586
Gulshan Mother and Child Clinic 8822738 8812992
Ibn Sina Clinic 8119513
Judi Maternity 9113322
Medi Aid Clinic 9112076 8118456
Medistone Clinic 405092
Paltan Poly Clinic 9557385
Peeriess Diagnostic Treatment Centre 9550441
Retina Eye Centre (Clinic) 9884588 9884566
Rajdhani Clinic 413525
Rusmono Clinic 418268 418205
Sclavo Medical Centre 9351404 8311830, 418409
Shefa Nursing Home 9111758
Shumana Clinic 245534
The Eye Clinic 9333238
Trauma Centre 327257 8116969
Uttara Heart Centre Pvt. Ltd. 9118138 8911875
Bikalpa Dental Clinic 606634
Capital Dental Clinic 328888
Capital Dental and X-ray Clinic 501531 328888
Dental Clinic (Chittagong) 634837
Dental Clinic (Tajmahal Road) 326433
Endo Dental Clinic 413851
Fatema Dental Care 9342033
Flowrence Dental Care 9342033
Intimate Dental Clinic 8612136
Mukul Dental Clinic 500007
National Dental Care 328888
Oroni Dental Clinic (Mirpur) 8014760
Palashy Dental Clinic 501892
Popular X-Ray 506089
Ratan Dental Clinic 8614898 508000
Shajahanpur Dental Clinic 9332125
The Dental Surgeons Ltd. 415458 9342275
U.S Dental Clinic 8912891 8918090

Chittagong [+880-31]
C.M.H 681551-9 618851-4, 680359
CTG Medical College Hospital 616891-5
Diabetic Hospital 617495
Eye Hospital Ctg 616625 615710-2, 636061
Infection Diseases Hospital 751733
Lions Eye Hospital 616652
Memon Hospital and Maternity 617169

Panaroma Hospital 619921 630549
Pahartaly Hospital 615710
Police Hospital 616379
Port Hospital 505021-9
Railway Hospital 720121-39 722220
Red Cross Maternity Hospital 631419 634545, 636886, 682186
Shishu Hospital 711236 720063
T.B Hospital (Fauzdar Hat) 751444
University Hospital 659071

Khulna [+880-3]
Ali Clinic 724066
Al- Faruq Health Centre 732083
Arogya Niketan 731366
B.N.S.B. Eye Hospital 785889
City Nursing Home 724329
Community Eye Hospital 725355
C.S.S. Eye Hospital 731220 722355
Cure Home General Hospital (Pvt) Ltd. 723542
Diabetic Hospital 721966
Diarrhoea Hospital 722556
Doctors Clinic 723215
Doulatpur Poly Clinic 774887
Dr. Amanullah Clinic 721283
Eye Hospital (Rupsha) 722355
Fair Health Clinic 761617
Garib-e-Nawaj Clinic 720081-3 721784
Green Maternity Clinic 721016
I.D Hospital 774716
Khan-A-Sabur Cancer Hospital and Research Institute 760607
Khulna Children`s Nursing Home 723572
Khulna Clinic 730562
Khulna Disabled Hospital 761486
Khulna Maternity and Health Centre 731533
Khulna Medical College Emergency 761509
Khulna Medical College Hospital 761531-5 761509
Khulna Pain Centre 720415 720711
Khulna Pangu (Dis-Able) Hospital 721019
Khulna Police Hospital 723505
Khulna Sadar Hospital 723876 723433
Khulna Sergical Clinic 722568 724450
Khulna Surgical and Medical
Hospital (Pvt) Ltd. 723966 724450, 722568
Khulna Shishu Hospital 724275
Khulna Skin Care Centre 730166
Khulna T.B Clinic 731105 761105

Khulna T.B Hospital 762552 774552
Khalishpur Clinic 762109 761637
Kinder Clinic 732212 725552
Linda Clinic 724066
Marie Stopes 721902
Matri Mangol Clinic 721688 762109
Maternity Hospital (Headquarter) 722556 720444
Medicare Diogonastic Cintre 722678
Mery Stop Clinic 731190
Metropolitan Clinic 723075
Mishu Clinic 721270
Mohanagar Diogonastic Clinic 723852
Monisha Clinic 760977
Nabila Clinic 730950
Nahar Clinic 731478 720740
Nargis Memorial Clinic 723499 720379
Nazma Clinic 725042-146
Niramoy Clinic 730220
Popular Nursing Home 761456
Pyramid Clinic 783238
Quior Home 723542
Railway Hospital 723231
Raj Surgical Clinic 720782
Sadar Hospital 724525 720133
Samela Memorial Clinic 760956
Seba Clinic 724267 724269
Shatadal Clinic 724930
Shapla Clinic 724857
St. Martin Pathology 724065
Upasam Hospital 720778
Auro Diagnostic Complex 731744
Basundhara Diagnostic Centre 720075
Biswas Investigation Centre 763648-111
C.T Imaging Centre Khulna Ltd. 731150
Doctors Diagnostic Centre 723655
Doha Physiotherapy Centre 732355
Fatema Health Care Centre (Pathology) 730265
Jamuna Diagnostic Centre 760757 731771
Khulna Diagnostic Centre 732228
Lab-Tec Diagnostic Centre 724246
Medicare Diagnostic Centre 722678
Mohanagar Diagnostic Centre 723852
Padma Diagnostic Centre 724907
Rangdhanu Diagnostic Complex 731658
Sandhani Diagnostic Complex 724819
Sent Martins Pathological Laboratory 724065

Setu Diagnostic Centre 730310
Standard Pathology 725848
Sundarban Diagnostic Centre 722079
Tot Pathology 725141
Ultra Diagnostic Complex 720600 722369
Medical College Hospital
(Emergency) 761509 761531-3

Feni [+880-331]
Adhunic Sadar Hospital 74866
Baptist Mision 74176
Diabetic Hospital 74870
Feni Medical College Hospital 73085
Meri Stop Clinic 73380
T.B. Clinic 74137
Cox`s Bazar
Hospital Enquiry 584

Sylhet [+880-821]
I.D Hospital 716602
Maternity Hospital 716214
Medical College 717055 717051
Sadar Hospital 717061-5
Faridpur
Hospital Enquiry 3152
Red Crescent Enquiry 2539
Kushtia
Hospital Enquiry 3049
Mymensingh
Medical College - PABX 5702-5
Barisal
Red Cresent Hospital 2343
Sadar Hospital Enquiry 2101

Bogra [+880-51]
Hospital Enquiry 6333
Comilla
General Hospital 5022
Jessore
Ad-Deen Hospital 72803-6
Daratana Hospital 3812
Diabetic Hospital Jessore 6273
Dipa Clinic 5140
Fatima Hospital 5056
Garib Shah Private Hospital 72524
General Pathology and Diagnostic Centre 5615

Hasina Clinic and Nursing Home 5737
Janaseba Complex and Pathological Laboratory 3664
Jessor Eye Clinic 5990
Mother and Child Health Care 3138
Nova Medical Centre 72233
P.K.S. Clinic 5001
Police Hospital Jessor 76191
Prime Diagnostic Complex 6277
Sadar Hospital 5056
T.B. Clinic 76779
T.B. Hospital Jessore 6779
Uniqe Diagnostic 5030
Uttara Private Hospital 6347

Noakhali [+880-321]
Hospital 6027
T.B Hospital Enquiry 5560 5220

Rajshahi [+880-721]
Medical College Enquire 774354
Sadar Hospital 779155
TB Hospital 779133

Dinajpur [+880-531]
General Hospital 4023
Police Hospital 3283

Chandpur [+880-841]
Hospital Enquiry 3022

Pabna [+880-731]
General Hospital 5077
Mental Hospital 5581
Sadar Hospital Enquiry 6112
T.B Clinic 5588

Laxmipur [+880-381]
Adhunic Hospital 663
Sadar Hospital 211

Rangpur [+880-521]
Medical Emergency 3063
Sadar Hospital 3043

Tangail [+880-921]
Hospital Enquiry 3038

Rangamati [+880-351]
Hospital Enquiry 2220 3122

Natore [+880-771]
B.A.V.S Hospital 2373
Baptist Med Mission Hospital 2386
Diabetic Hospital 6714
Mahmood Clinic 2778
Police Hospitel 6968
Sadar Hospital 6912
T.B. Clinic 2326

Sources

Guljit, K. Arora. "Globalization and health effects in SAARC region, evolving a framework of analysis". *International Journal of Economic Development*. FindArticles.com. 08 May, 2010.

Arora, G.K. 1995. "Environment Extremism or Economic Development". *Mainstream*, Delhi, April, 22, 1995, pp. 23-30

Arora, G.K. 2002. Globalisaion, Federalism and Decentralisation—Implications for India, Delhi Bookwell.

Arora, G.K. 2002. Globalisaion, Employment Restructuring and Skill Formation: Emerging Challenges for India. Paper presented at Indian Labour Conference, Dec. 15-18 Dec. (Abstracted in *Indian Journal of Labour Economics*, Oct.-Dec. 2002, Vol 45, No. 4, 2002, pp. 1317-18.

Bagchi, Amiya Kumar. 1999. "Globalization, Liberalisation and Vulnerability", *Economic and Political Weekly*, Nov. 6, pp. 3219-30.

Bhat, Ramesh. 2000. "Issues in Health—Public Private Partnership." *Economic and Political Weekly*. 34(52 and 53): pp. 4706-16.

Buss, Paulo Marchiori. 2002. "Globalisation and disease: in an unequal world, unequal health!" Cadernos de Saude Publica. 18 (6): pp. 1783-89.

Chaturvedi Sachin and Gunjan Nagpal (2003): "WTO and Product-Related Environmental Standards—Emerging Issues and Policy Options", *Economic And Political Weekly*, January 4.

Cornea, Giovanni Andrea. 2001. "Globalisation and health." Bulletin of the World Health Organisation. 79(9): pp. 834-41.

Dollar, David. 2001. "Is Globalization good for your health." Bulletin of the World Health Organisation. 79(9): pp. 827-33.

Government of India, Planning Commission (2002) : Special Group on Targeting Ten Million Opportunities per year over The Tenth Plan Period. Planning Commission, New Delhi.

———. 2002. Tenth Five Year Plan. Planning Commission, New Delhi.

Government of India. 2003. Economic Survey, 2002-03. Ministry of Finance, New Delhi.

Gumber, Anil. 2000. "Structure of Indian Health Care Market: Implications for Health Insurance Sector". WHO Regional Health Forum. 4 (1and2): pp. 26-34.

Gumber, Anil. 2002. "Economic Reforms and the Health Sector: Towards Health Equity in India." In *Reform and Employment*. Eds. Institute of Applied Manpower Research. New Delhi: Concept Publishing House, pp. 235-284.

Harriss, J (1999): "Comparing Political Regimes across Indian States—A Preliminary Essay". *Economic and Political Weekly*. Nov. 25.

Heiskanen, Veijo (2001, ed.): "Introduction", The Legitimacy of International Organizations. New York, United Nations University Press.

Howse, Robert 2001): The Legitimacy of the World Trade Organization. In Jean-Marc Coicaud and Veijo Heiskanen (2001, ed.), *The Legitimacy of International Organizations*, New York, United Nations University Press.

Junne, G.C.A. (2001): International Organizations in a period of globalization: New (problems of) legitimacy. In Jean-Marc Coicaud and Veijo Heiskanen (2001, ed.), *The Legitimacy of International Organisations*, New York, United Nations University Press.

Makinda Samuel (2000): "Recasing globalization governance". In Ramesh Thakur and Edward Newman (2000, ed.) *New Millennium, New Perspectives—The United Nations Security and Governance*, New York, United Nations University Press.

Matowe, L. and David R Katerere. 2002. "Globalization and Pharmacy: A View from the Developing World". *The Annals of Pharmacy*. 36: pp. 936-38.

Petras, James and Henry Veltmeyer. 2001. Globalization Unmasked. Delhi: Madhyam Books.

Research and Information Systems for the Non-Aligned and Other Developing Countries (2003): *World Trade and Development Report*, 2003, Delhi.

Sampson, Gary P. (2001): "Overview", In Sampson G.P. (ed). *The Role of the World Trade Organization in Global Governance*. New York: United Nations University.

Satapathy, C (1999): "Trade Sanctions and other Barriers to Free Trade". *Economic and Political Weekly*. Dec 18.

Sen, Gita, Aditi Iyer and Asha George. 2002. "Structural Reforms and Health Equity". *Economic and Political Weekly*. 37(14): pp. 1342-52.

Sundaram, K (2001): Employment-Unemployment Situation in the Nineties. *Economic and Political Weekly*, 21 March (XXXVI, 11), pp. 931-40.

Sutherland, Peter *et al.* (2001): "Challenges Facing The WTO And Policies To Address Global Governance". In Gary P. Sampson (ed.) *The Role of the World Trade Organization in Global Governance*, New York, United Nations University.

U.N.D.P. 2004. Human Development Report, 2004. Geneva.

United Nations, UNCTAD (1999): Trade and Develoment Report, Geneva.

World Bank (2003): World Development Report, 2003. Washington D.C.

World Health Organisation (1997). Think and Act Globally and Intersectorally to Protect National Health. Geneva: WHO.

APPENDIX

ASIAN MEDICAL CITIES IN HEALTH TOURISM

The birth of new technologies has transformed the globe's vast population into a boundary-less "Global Village Community." From a 'consumer' point of view, it is now possible to take advantage of both cheap airfares and often higher standards or more affordable medical treatment in foreign countries, than those available in their own countries. From a patient perspective, the benefits of global health care are numerous. Though cost is the over-riding factor, the wait for surgeries in some developed nations can also be annoying. USA, Canada and Great Britain have reported a surge in the number of people traveling outside the country to avoid long queues in the National Health Service, which can often be for a year or more for some surgical procedures. The South East Asian countries such as Thailand, Malaysia, Singapore, Korea and Philippines are the popular destinations for medical treatment. India is positioning itself as the primary destination for advanced medical procedures in the world. Some of Indian hospitals are also competing with their Asian peers to get a slice of the cake in the booming health tourism market for international patients.

Asia leading

Health tourism is a promising new industry in Asia, offering prospects for private hospitals facing saturation in patient growth. It is with a clearer view of the addressable market potential, internal strengths and limitations, as well as the level of external competition, that health care providers may best move forward to realize this potential. Health Care providers may now consider the medical quality of their services, how non-medical services are key to encouraging patient access, and the various marketing options available to them. Thailand's Bumrungrad Hospital was among the first in the region to focus on attracting foreign patients. Thailand's Bangkok Medical Centre is also excelling in health tourism (see appendices at the end). The Malaysian Government has successfully exerted its leadership to facilitate and encourage hospital industry development, with the formation of National Committee for the Promotion of Health Tourism. The Hong Kong Government is starting to consider to possibility of marketing its Traditional Chinese Medicine (TCM) capabilities to the region, while concerted efforts have similarly been launched by government agencies in Singapore to market its world-class medical capabilities. In countries such as Thailand, the onus remains on the private sector to analyze available opportunities, spearhead sectoral development, and formulate strategies to improve their competitiveness.

With the tightening of immigration rules and security checks, the US has seen a decline in the number of foreign patient visits. More patients, especially those in the Middle-East, are moving towards alternatives like

Thailand. Over 100,000 foreign medical tourists visit Malaysia annually, while Singapore and India are also starting to experience positive growth in patient visits as a result of their aggressive marketing initiatives to source countries like Indonesia. However, Thailand leads the Asia-Pacific region. Thailand is able to attract a large volume of patients as it has a variety of existing tourist attractions for recuperating patients, a relatively low cost of living, expat-friendly locals, and a respectable quality of health care in cosmetic surgery.

Industry's best practices for International patients

Medical tourists expect the highest possible quality of care, having traveled great distances to seek world-class doctors and hospitals. Many leading hospitals have expounded on this by branching their medical expertise into super-specialization. For instance, some Australian hospitals focus not only on cancer, but perhaps on specific variations of skin cancer. This also builds credibility and buy-in, when the referring doctors are trained in the post-procedural stage to provide a continuum of patient care. Even nursing teams are trained to specialize as oncology nurses, while the cross-fertilization of medical teams such as with dermatologists, radiologists and oncologists ensures that all complications are completely accounted for. Medical quality is also supported by hardware and software investments. Hardware investments include the purchase of cutting-edge technology such as MRI or Gamma Knife machines. Software refers to the intellectual output of the hospitals as demonstrated by the latest medical research.

Non-medical services

Many hospitals offer airport pick-up services for patient convenience. Hospital reception areas are fitted as luxuriously as five-star hotels; Bumrungrad Hospital in Thailand for instance even features a Starbucks café and McDonald's outlet. Bangkok's Piyavate Hospital may even feature spa facilities that offer a holistic wellness experience. Western-style hospitals such as in the US, UK or Australia feature their own on-site accommodation, both for patients in the aftercare stage, as well as for their relatives. Similarly, many Asian hospitals that do not manage their own accommodations also offer link-ups with different hotels, hostels, etc. Apart from bedside manners, hospital staff members are also being recruited to accommodate to their religious, dietary and cultural needs.

Hospitals that are successfully attracting foreign patients enlarge their geographical footprints with representative offices or agencies in other countries. For example, Cromwell Hospital in the UK has representatives in India and Pakistan, while hospitals in Singapore are also setting up offices such as in Indonesia or the Middle-East. These agents help establish and maintain relationships such as with local hospitals, doctors, embassies, sponsor corporations, or insurers. Participating in different events also facilitates such relationships. For instance, trade shows, exhibitions or training seminars allow health care providers to share their medical expertise.

With budget air travel and the Internet providing access to information about cheap or specialist treatment overseas, medical centers across Asia are vying with each other to become regional or even global hubs for health care. Singapore is aiming to attract one million foreign patients per year by 2010 while India is gunning to be a top medical tourist destination, benefiting from its huge base of medical professionals and low costs. Pioneering stem or embryonic cell work is attracting patients to South Korea and China to undergo treatment that is not available, or legally permissible, in many other countries. The work may be controversial but it is providing new hope to paralyzed patients.

Medical tourism as an engine of economic growth

In the past 30 years or so, the costs of health care have soared in developed countries, especially the United States. Americans and, to some extent, the British, Canadians, Australians began to look for ways to reduce these expenses. Certain services and procedures in American hospitals are now being contracted out to Third World countries, from transcriptions of medical records to the reading of X-rays. Medical tourism presents an opportunity for hospitals to fuel economic growth by tapping the potential of the international patient market. To attract foreign patients, health care providers may consider leveraging on both business and clinical considerations. The advancement in medical technologies, increased patient mobility and demand for immediate quality health care is arousing interest among health care providers globally. To set-up world class medical tourism centers, massive investment in health sector is called for. This will not only improve health care for the countrymen, but also attract patients from all over the world on the strength of quality, promptness and economy.

However, needs can vary widely between the 'essential' health care seekers—traveling by necessity, because treatment is not available or unaffordable locally—and the 'premium' medical tourists, who are typically looking for wellness or cosmetic procedures and may want first-class flights and exclusive add-ons. Pacific Health Care Holdings Patient Relations Manager Alison Lim says, our International Patient Liaison Centre has seen an increase in these "premium" medical tourists seeking high end elective treatments like titanium dental implants, complex cosmetic procedures as well as deluxe health screening. An emerging trend is the bundling of five-star health care services with unconventional post-operation treatment. India is providing traditional recuperation forms such as yoga and naturopathy, while Thailand is promoting its ancient Thai herbal remedies to the West, Middle East and Far East. To create awareness and market their medical services, Singapore's Raffles Hospital works with 50 agents in 12 countries. Parkway Group Health Care has marketing offices in 15 countries including China, India, Bangladesh, Sri Lanka, Vietnam, Brunei,

UAE, Brittan, Russia, Canada, Indonesia and Malaysia, which last year helped attract over 17,000 indoor patients and 140,000 outpatients.

Top 10 in medical tourism

- Bumrungrad International Hospital in Bangkok
- Buchinger Clinic in Germany
- All India Institute of Medical Sciences in Delhi
- The Fyodorov Clinics in Russia
- A Technology Prescription: Denver Health
- Brigham and Women's Hospital
- Sourasky Medical Center in Tel Aviv
- Hôpital Edouard Herriot in Lyons
- Hospital for Tropical Diseases in London
- Mount Sinai Medical Center

The medical tourism policy can draw strength from recommendations that the corporate sector has been making in India, and specifically from the "Policy Framework for Reforms in Health Care", drafted by the Indian prime minister's Advisory Council on Trade and Industry, headed by Mukesh Ambani and Kumaramangalam Birla. Certain other Asian countries have taken Giant strides in promoting medical tourism in their respective countries. However, the current market for medical tourism in India is mainly limited to patients from the Middle East and South Asian economies, besides the NRIs from all over the globe. Analysts say that as many as 1,50,000 medical tourists came to India in the year 2005 and over 2,00,000 in the year 2006. Afro-Asian people spend as much as $20 billion a year on health care outside their countries—Nigerians alone spend an estimated $1 billion a year. Most of this money is spent in Europe and America, but it is hoped that this would now be increasingly directed to developing countries like India.

The foreign patients come from SAARC region, Afghanistan, Ethiopia, Nigeria, Tanzania, other parts of Africa, CIS countries and the Middle East, especially Oman and Yemen. As per New trends from 2003, patients from the US, UK and Canada, escaping high costs and waiting lists are coming to India. Also from Europe, Australia and New Zealand for procedures not covered by insurance such as cosmetic surgery, obesity treatment, and new techniques like hip resurfacing Around 30 private tertiary hospitals, mainly in Delhi, Mumbai and Bangalore; but also Chennai, Calcutta Thiruvananthapuram, Coimbatore and Hyderabad. It Includes hospital groups like Apollo, Wockhardt, Fortis, Max, Escorts. At an Indian medical tourism expo in the UK last year, 25 per cent of visitors were seeking medical treatment in India. India's Apollo is setting up hospitals in joint ventures in Dhaka and Colombo; and clinics in Yemen and Saudi Arabia Parkway Holdings of Singapore in tie-up with Apollo in Calcutta; with Asian Heart Institute and Research Centre in Mumbai; International chain Columbia Asia has a 75-bed multi-speciality hospital in Bangalore.

Indian corporate hospitals have a large pool of doctors, nurses, and paramedics ensuring individual, personalized care for all. The highly skilled personnel, with wide experience and international exposure excel in cardiology and cardio thoracic surgery, joint replacement, orthopedic surgery, gastroenterology, ophthalmology, transplants and urology to name a few. The various specialties covered are Neurology, Neurosurgery, Oncology, Ophthalmology, Rheumatology, Endocrinology, ENT, Pediatrics, Pediatric Surgery, Pediatric Neurology, Urology, Nephrology, Dermatology, Dentistry, Plastic Surgery, Gynecology, Pulmonology, Psychiatry, General Medicine and General Surgery.

Bangkok; the hub of medical tourism

Catch some sun, take in a few golden temples, and get a new hip— a new slogan coined by the Thailand Tourism, to promote medical tourism. It's an increasingly popular itinerary for foreign visitors who are flying into Thailand in ever greater numbers to get quality hospital care at bargain prices, part of a 'medical tourism' boom that is turning into a multi-billion dollar industry in Asia. The kingdom is one of several countries in the region cashing in on its ability to use cheap but highly skilled labour, affordable hospital accommodation and offer specialist treatments. Of a total of one million patients each year at Bumrungrad, nearly 50 percent are foreigners with Americans making up the biggest group, followed by patients from the United Arab Emirates, Bangladesh, Oman, Britain, Japan, Australia, Cambodia and Myanmar. Among Americans, back surgery and hip and knee replacements are the most popular procedures at Bumrungrad, while many Australians seek plastic surgery. Bumrungrad International Hospital offers a full spectrum of services from executive health tests to cardiac packages, cancer therapy, eye surgery, liposuction and other cosmetic options. Bumrungrad has more than 700 internationally-trained and board-certified doctors, and a complete range of health care services and facilities.

Which Thai Hospital is Best: Bumrungrad *vs.* Bangkok Hospital

Charles Runckel writes about two leading hospitals in Bangkok, Thailand. Thailand is the world leader for medical tourism, but which hospital within Thailand is best for you? This article, part three of a series on Medical Tourism, explores the top two choices. While there are many hospitals in Thailand that cater to medical tourists, these are two full-service facilities that have strong reputations for quality and experience with foreigners. The aspiring medical tourist should consider these two before any other Thai hospitals, even ones with a slightly lower cost, as they are the gold standard for medical tourism not only in Thailand but worldwide.

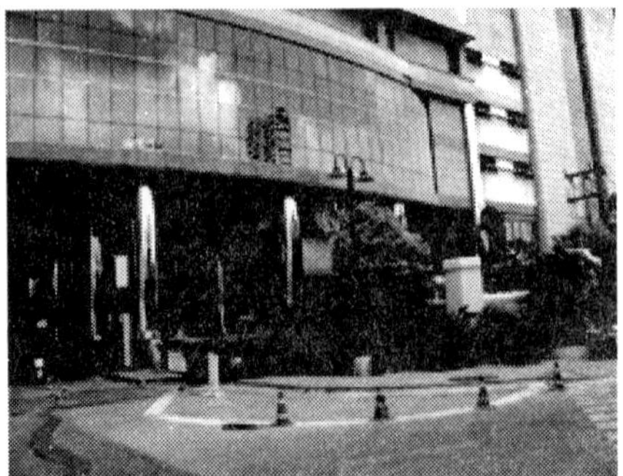

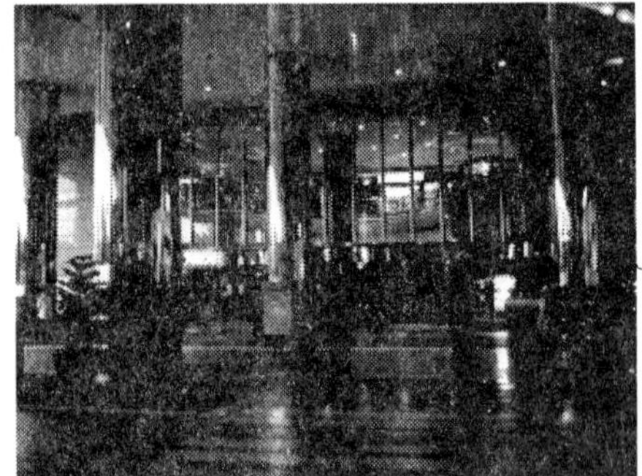

Pictures (top) Bumrungrad Hospital's main building and entrance

Pictures (below) Bangkok Hospital's Buildings and one of their entrance

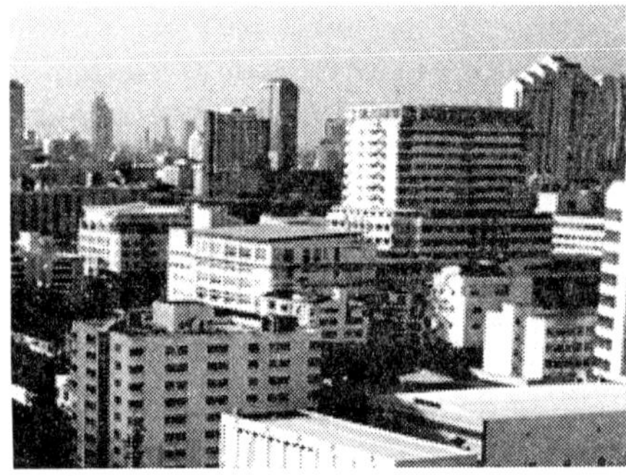

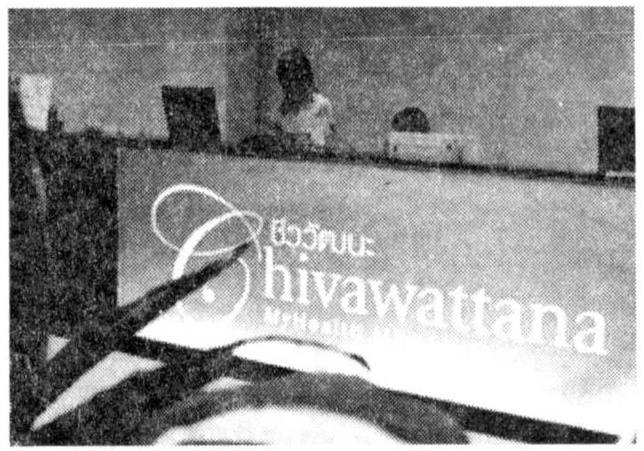

Background and Location

Bumrungrad Hospital treats over 400,000 foreign patients every year and has made medical tourism its major focus. The monolithic hospital consists of a large tower and several associated buildings adjoining, all conveniently located in downtown Bangkok. The hospital is within walking distance of Bangkok's Skytrain (light rail system) but only barely, and given the heat usual in Thailand most patients are strongly advised to take a taxi. International patients are so much a part of Bumrungrad's focus that they recently broke from their single tower architecture and built a separate International Tower that caters specially to foreigners with a brand new Physical Exam wing and upgraded VIP rooms.

Bangkok Hospital Group is a network of Thai hospitals focused on Bangkok and sprawling into the provinces and even Cambodia, though the portion of this that is most important to foreigners is their Bangkok Hospital Medical Center (BMC) complex. This campus consists of their International Hospital as well as their main General Hospital and a collection of specialty hospitals, including their Heart Hospital, Rehabilitation Center and Dental Clinic. The BMC is a series of adjacent buildings connected by skywalks and, apart from the main General Hospital building, are new having been built in the past five years. The

BMC is located near, but not walking distance from, several Sky-train and subways stations, so a taxi is in order in this case as well. While BMC and Bumrungrad treat about the same number of total patients each, a lower proportion of BMC's patients are from overseas and total only 150,000 annually, though these are often for more serious treatments.

Layout and Impressions

Bumrungrad Hospital is, as previously mentioned, monolithic. Visitors enter into the lobby of the main tower at the ground floor, but this and the next floor contain mostly restaurants, coffee shops and the cafeteria. The Hospital portion does not begin until the third floor, where the patient is greeted with a larger lobby and registration area. Elegantly uniformed staff register new patients with digital cameras—both Bumrungrad and BMC are very tech savvy hospitals with test results updated and delivered electronically and pictures of each patient checked at every stage to avoid foul-ups. This registration area is both the point of entry and exit, and next to registration are desks for checkout and a pharmacy.

On every floor of Bumrungrad runs a long, wide hallway with specialty clinics and divisions branching-off, generally four to six per floor. Each has its own lobby, which looks out onto the hall. The older main tower and new international tower are quite different, with the older tower very much feeling like a mature hospital, with traditional waiting areas and layout, while the new wing is decidedly more modern and up-to-date, from the lobbies and hallways to furnishings in patient rooms.

Upon walking into BMC's main building, one is immediately greeted with the registration staff. They are far more eager to register you than those at Bumrungrad, though this has a strong basis in necessity. Upon registration, a patient's schedule will likely initially take them to another building, or several buildings if they have multiple appointments. The BMC staff then ensure that you are taken to the right building or floor of the main structure. There are enclosed walkways between the buildings, however most patients are initially led to the shuttles, which are over-sized gold carts or minivans that scoot patients around the campus.

Each division, clinic or specialty hospital at BMC has its own modular area with it's own independent registration and cashier services (so you don't have to go through the main lobby at all, if you know where you're going). These lobbies, especially in the newer buildings, are considerably more aesthetically appealing and pleasant to wait in than many of Bumrungrad's specialty clinic lobbies, mostly due to their smaller size, more updated furnishings and clever architectural design. Like Bumrungrad, there is a clear difference in ambiance between their older General Hospital building and the new, adjoining specialty centers.

The famed, or infamous, Bangkok Hospital Phuket is renowned as a world leader in sex-change operations, but is also a state-of-the-art hospital for more mundane purposes and nothing beats Phuket's beaches for physical therapy and recuperation after a surgery in Bangkok, which the Phuket Hospital supervises and coordinates.

One of many MRI scanners at the Bangkok Hospital

Unlike many other aspects of a hospital experience, the sheer technical capabilities of a hospital are somewhat easily quantified, and it is in this aspect that Bangkok Hospital most outshines its competitor. BMC has focused a tremendous amount of resources to being on the cutting edge of medical technology, and while Bumrungrad is certainly not unsophisticated, there is general agreement that Bumrungrad is a solid step behind BMC technologically. BMC's hi-tech drive falls into two general areas: advanced imaging and non-invasive surgery. Their advanced imaging options include at least seven MRI scanners in their main campus alone. Each department receives its own specialized diagnostic equipment, unlike many hospitals which must pool resources, including Digital Mammography and a brand new 128-slice CT scanner currently being installed. It is peerless in South-East Asia, and BMC boasts one of Thailand's only two clinical PET-CT scanners. The non-invasive offerings include state-of-the-art radiation systems such as the Novalis device for brain tumors and robotic laparoscopic surgery for both heart and joint operations (with different robots, of course). Bumrungrad simply does not compete in this field, which gives BMC a decisive advantage in the specific operations these advanced machines enable; reducing risk, discomfort and hospital stay time.

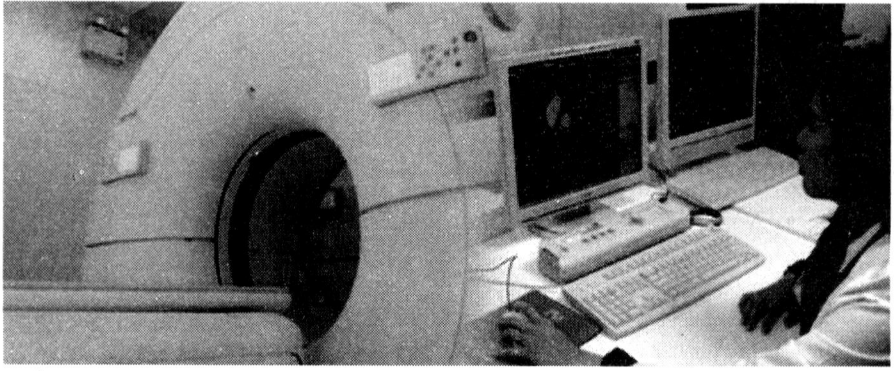

Reputation and Marketing

Bumrungrad is probably the best-marketed hospital in the world. Their fame is well deserved, but their marketing staff and management have put a tremendous effort in being "The" medical tourist hospital that potential patients in the Western world have heard of, specifically through news reports on ABC and CBS as well as multiple appearances in Newsweek. BMC, in contrast, is more famous within Thailand and elsewhere in Asia and the Middle East. Both hospitals treat approximately the same total number of patients—about 1 million a year—however Bumrungrad began courting foreign patients much earlier than BMC and now draws 400,000 foreign patients a year to BMC's 150,000-250,000. It is worth noting that different hospitals use different metrics to calculate these numbers (visits vs. patients) so these comparisons must be taken with a grain of salt, however it is commonly accepted that Bumrungrad's proportion is higher than BMC's, though not by as much as the disclosed numbers suggest. While BMC's focus for the future includes increasing the proportion of foreign patients, the target countries of both hospitals will likely remain the same with Bumrungrad focusing on the US and BMC focusing on the Middle-East and Asia, affecting the level of marketing in each area.

Part of Bumrungrad's early marketing included aggressive pursuit of international certification, and as a result Bumrungrad correctly claims a number of regional "Firsts" with various international credentialing organizations. In many ways, Bumrungrad was a trendsetter and these certifications were necessary when no one had even heard the term "medical tourism" and there were serious doubts about the quality of a Thai hospital. Today, the first and second tier of Thai hospitals are firmly within international standards and rising acceptance of medical tourism make this less necessary. BMC has, itself, a slew of acronyms attesting to its quality, many of which overlap Bumrungrad's, and comparing certifications should be less important to the potential medical tourist than other aspects of reputation, but for a nervous first time medical tourist Bumrungrad's list of "firsts" can be welcome reassurance.

The savings on one 'major tooth repair' can pay for an economy level 2 week vacation including air.

- Root canal and cap front tooth 14,000 thb US$354. AUD$481. EU284.
- Significant dental work (2 teeth) would result saved money in your bank account + the vacation!
- Very simple but necessary dental procedures from cleaning to cosmetic.. available at significant savings.
  - Diagnostics, imaging, lab analysis, physical rehabilitation, cosmetic surgery, dental.. all 80% off US pricing.

Anonymous violent crime/robbery, common in the West, is all but unknown in Thailand.

- Most "Thailand Citizen US Educated Doctors" return to Thailand after graduation from their US Medical School.
- Plus, access to top Thai specialists within 24 hours is pretty reassuring
- .. no waiting, ever, for anything! + a free tasty lunch!
- The Dell computer system at Bumrungrad is equal to any in the world.
- Orthopedic images, blood work, diagnostics, specialist notes.. all are available across the network.
- No carrying film/records to a specialist.. it's in the system and instantly available.

- Doc suggests additional imaging:.. OK, he orders it, the test is completed and you are back in his office getting his interpretation within 24-48 hours.
- Doc orders a CAT scan and it's completed the next morning and immediately it's in the computer system!.. !!
- Appointments are coordinated system wide.. smooth patient flow.. no bottle necks.. no waits, respect.. professional! + smiling happy Health care team and bilingual clerical staffing.

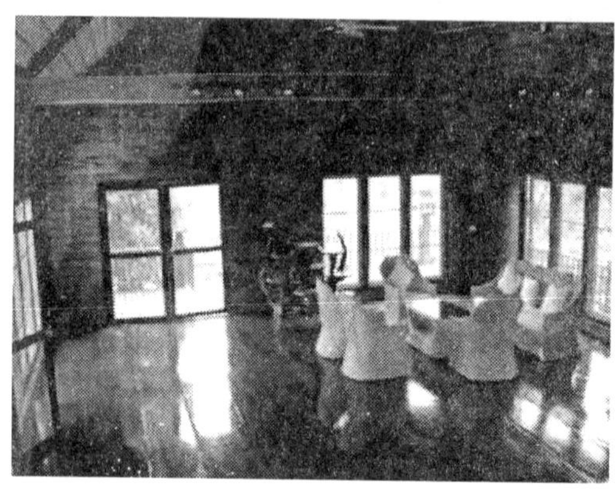

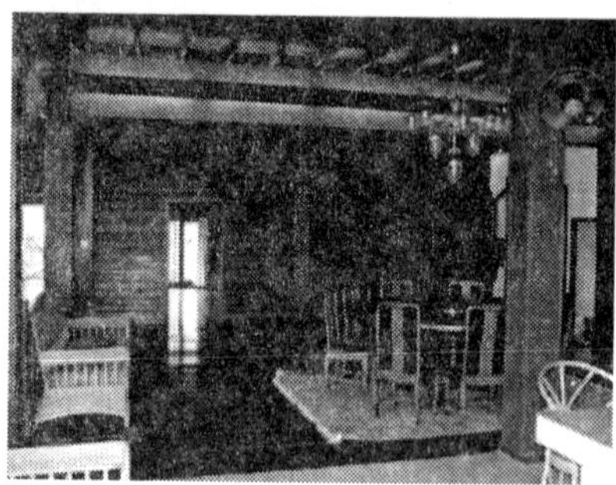

In the Chiang Mai/Chiang Rai area some incredible Lanni Thai style house are available for short-term rental.. quite marvelous houses built from 100% teak. The house above rents for 17, 000 Thb (US$400, Euro 325 per month)

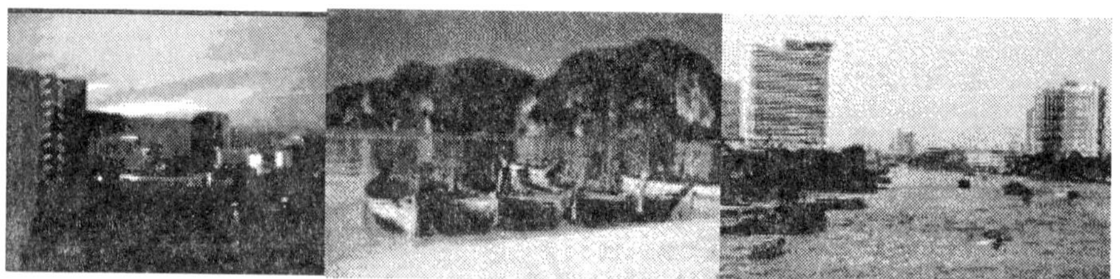

Golden Triangle **Beaches** **Bangkok**

Bangkok is a wonderful mix of Ancient Far East and Ultra Modern West

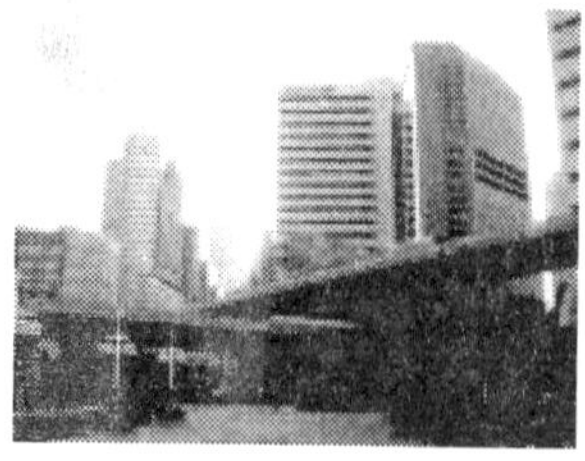

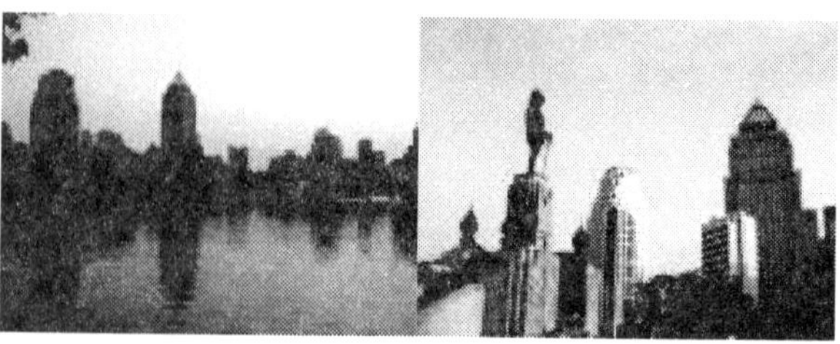

Thailand can provide an "extremely cost effective" Health Vacation.

- Grand Imperial Travel of Bangkok offers Executive Medical Tourism Packages!
    - They assist with appointments and suggest hotels/apartments near your medical provider.
    - They pick you up at the airport, provide a cell phone for your stay, provide a personal guide for both tourist outings and medical appointments.. all for a flat fee.
- Bumrungrad and Bangkok Hospital compare well to US Med Center Hospitals.. and far better than rural US hospitals.

Bumrungrad Hospital, is very foreigner friendly. Said to be #1 in Asia! Bangkok Hospital, off New Petchaburi Road, is foreigner friendly and comparable to most western hospitals. Private hospital room is $60. per day. A few extra days in the hospital, no problem. Many Japanese companies send their employees to Thailand for annual physicals as well as long-term medial care modalities. The savings on medical fees and the high quality medical care makes the air fare inconsequential. See attached appendix to this chapter for more details on Bumrungrad.

Dental experiences vary greatly. These clinics offer modern equipment and a full range of 'pain reduction techniques'.

- Asavanant Clinic
- Bangkok Dental Hospital
- Siam Family Dental
- The Dental Hospitals on Suk Soi 55, Suk Soi 49 and Suk Soi 39 as well as the Dental clinics at Chula Hospital and Bumagard Hospital are professionally staffed and equipped well.

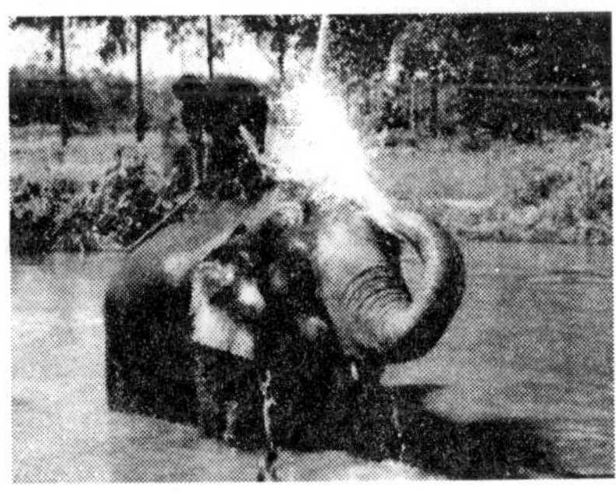

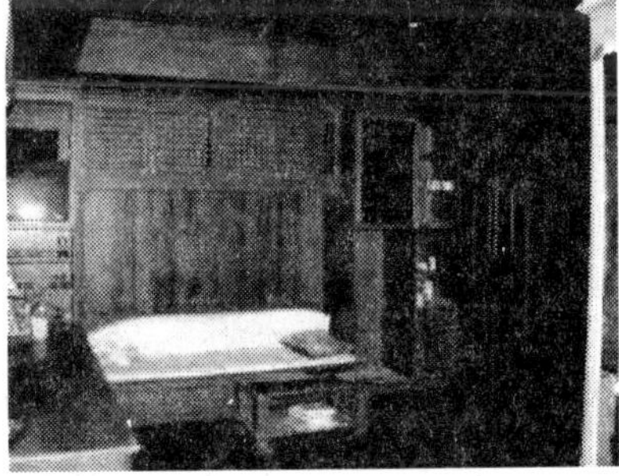

- Bumagard Hospital has serviced apartments adjacent to the hospital.. hospital staffed rehabilitation apartment suites for less than $100 per day.
- Affordable 24/7 out patient nursing. $100. per day can provide luxury hotel accommodations, gourmet meals and 24 hour 'private duty assisting provider'.

More than 150,000 North Americans and Europeans currently seek medical treatment overseas each year, estimates Josef Woodman, author of the forthcoming "Patients without Borders." For invasive surgeries, preferred destinations include India, Thailand, Singapore and Malaysia. Large hospitals, such as Bumrungrad and the Apollo chain in India, actively court American, European and Middle Eastern patients. Bumrungrad arranges limousines to pick up patients at the airport, and sheiks and princes congregate in the Platinum Lounge of Apollo's Delhi hospital. Abacas International, a leading travel facilitator, reports that medical tourism to Asia could generate billions of dollars.

Businesses are taking notice. At least 40 corporations have signed on to the overseas plan that United Group Programs, a health insurer in Boca Raton, Florida, began offering six months ago. Sending an employee abroad can save 80 percent of the costs of a procedure; a $50,000 angioplasty in the United States costs less than $6,000 in Mohali, Chandigarh India, according to Global Choice Health Care, a firm that arranges foreign medical procedures. Walk-in patients see a specialist in 17 minutes on average. Since 75 percent of hospital revenues are paid by patients directly, health and insurance companies have no say in treatment. Low labour costs allow Thai hospitals to employ more staff.

In Australia, Europe and North America, "complementary and alternative medicine" (CAM) is increasingly being used in parallel to modern medicine, particularly for treating and managing chronic disease. Concern about the adverse effects of chemical medicines, a desire for more personalized health care and greater public access to health information, fuel this increased use. For the past six years, persons from over two hundred countries with difficult and chronic conditions, i.e. diverticulitis, cancer, and incurable autoimmune diseases such as Systemic Lupus Erythematosis (SLE), Multiple Sclerosis (MS), Lou Gherig¡¯s Disease (ALS), have been motivated to explore the options Traditional Chinese Medicine (TCM) offers them at Huai Hua Red Cross Hospital. Since these conditions are chronic and often times incurable, they have led many patients and/or their family members to seek and decipher complex, baffling, and, obscure medical information and to explore options encountered beyond the diagnostic and treatment scope generally available to them. Despite their diverse cultural backgrounds, many persons reach this intersecting destination at the time-honored tradition of TCM and the Huai Hua Red Cross Hospital for Difficult and Chronic conditions.

Five million tourists for health treatment

According to the Tourism Authority of Thailand (TAT), at least five million tourists come to the country annually for medical treatment. Various plastic surgery clinics could attest that the number of both Thais and foreigners undergoing dental and plastic surgeries, lasik, and other physical enhancement procedures is increasing. Aside from these, Thailand has earned its reputation as an excellent location for spa services. "The growth of spa business is a good sign that tells us that we can respond to customers' needs," Mr. Apichai added pointing to Proud Asia 2008 as an excellent venue where the international community can actually see the advancements that Thailand has taken the field of medical tourism.

"Beauty business will continuously grow as both men and women care about their looks," President of Thai Society of Cosmetic Dermatology and Surgery, Dr. Thada Piamphongsan, said, adding that Thailand has more advantages than other countries in Asia when it comes to offering the best quality medical and beauty services but at cheaper rates.

"Proud Asia 2008 is definitely not just the usual exhibition event on beauty and health care products and services we see here and in other countries. What makes this event extraordinary is the fact that we are going to have a grand showcase of the latest innovations of products and services in the field of medical tourism, spa and wellness. Everybody will be here-the expert in medical tourism, the best spa and wellness providers, and the most highly interested buyers. "The event promises to be a big one for both suppliers and buyers and the most important thing is that it will be held right here in Bangkok. This means that the Kingdom will again have the chance to prove to the international community that Thailand has sufficient MICE infrastructure to be the best venue for this kind of trade exhibition and conference. Proud Asia 2007 is a huge event that will help the country achieve its goal of becoming a regional hub for exhibitions and conventions business and Mice market," said Mr. Vithaya.

Health tourism boom takes Singapore by storm

Singapore on the other hand makes world headlines for performing complex neurosurgical procedures and delivering cutting-edge medical treatment by the region's leading health specialists. The Republic's reputation for high quality medical facilities and well-trained doctors pulled in more than 370,000 visitors in 2004. The cost of treatments in Singapore, such as a hip replacement, can be less than a third of the price in the United States. In some cases, the cost is less than a tenth of what people would pay in America or Europe.

Raffles Hospital, has gained fame in recent years for highly publicized operations to separate conjoined twins, exemplifying the highly skilled expertise available.

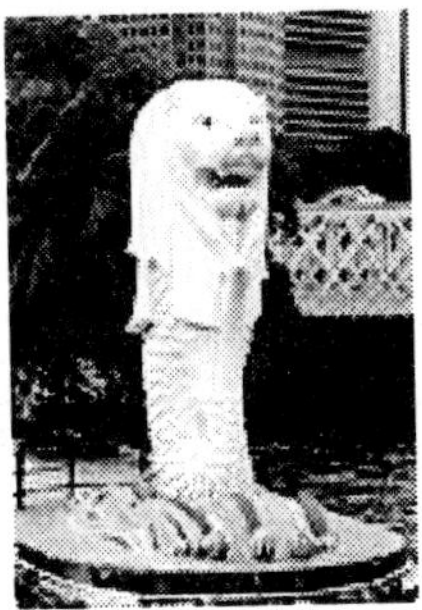

The tiny island of Singapore, having a populace of 4.4 million, is fast positioning itself as a medical tourism hub. The authorities are ambitious of serving one million foreign patients annually by 2012 and generate USD 3 billion in revenue.

Parkway hospitals group is Singapore's largest private health care group in Asia, owning three tertiary care private hospitals: East Shore, Gleneagles and Mount Elizabeth. The magnificent façade of these hospitals are complemented by equally competent doctors and excellent services with world class equipment. Incidentally, quite a few patients come from India for liver transplant. Nitin Saxena, who brought his father all the way from Delhi to Gleneagles for a liver transplant, opines unlike Indian hospitals, the services and facilities value for money.

Stem cell transplant is yet another field developing rapidly on the health map of Singapore. The haematology and stem cell transplant centre of Mount Elizabeth Hospital has pioneered stem cell treatment for patients with advanced cancer tumours. Headed by director Dr. Patrick Tan, a world renowned specialist in the field of oncology, cost of treatment here ranges from USD 72,000 to USD 90,000 per person, compared to USD 235,000 for similar treatment in the US. Recently, a 12-year-old girl from Delhi underwent cord blood transplant at the centre. As a mark of hospitality, hospital staff goes to receive patients and their relatives from the airport, make arrangements for their stay and even provide with language whenever required.

The medical tourism boom is just not restricted to Singapore alone. Current trend of economic developments in the Asian region, higher life expectancies, an ageing population and an ever-increasing awareness of the benefits of the quality health care have given a shot in the arm to the Asian health care industry, taking it to witness an unprecedented growth. Presently, there are only 140,000 hospitals serving an Asian population of 3.5 billion. With Asian population expected to grow to 5.6 billion by 2050, the consumer expenditure on health care services and goods will increase from US$90 billion in 1999 to US$188 billion in 2013. Malaysia is targeting the Middle East and China to generate whopping revenue of 2.2 billion by 2010. These emerging markets prove that there's immense potential in the Asian health care business, remarked Ms Tan-Hoong Chu Eng, MD, Parkway Promotions Pte Ltd., a subsidiary company of Parkway-Holdings Ltd. the largest private health care group in Asia.

Demand for health care is rising in the Middle East with millions of dollars spent in establishing specialised hospitals and clinics, expanding existing facilities and adopting world class technology in Bahrain, Kuwait, Yemen, Oman and Qatar. In the UAE, for instance, the government plans to double the bed capacity of public hospitals to achieve a target of one for every 300 people by the end of the decade.

The Philippines Faith Healers

The Philippines probably beat other countries to this idea of medical tourism bit many years ago. I recall how in the 1970s, faith healers like Tony Agpaoa were already offering tour packages for people coming in from Europe and Japan who wanted the faith healers' services. Agpaoa even had his own little hotel in Baguio City so patients didn't have to look for their own accommodations. The faith healing packages eventually went into decline, and last I heard, it was our faith healers who were going to Eastern European countries to do their road-show healing.

Earlier this year, then-secretary of tourism Roberto Pagdanganan announced that the Department of Tourism was teaming up with the Department of Health, specifically the Philippine Institute of Traditional and Alternative Health Care, to promote medical tourism. At that time, he said only the St. Luke's hospital had been accredited for their program but Asian Hospital, Capitol Medical Center, and Medical City had also applied. Our medical and nursing curricula are certainly tougher than many of our neighbours' in Southeast Asia. Who knows, maybe medical tourism can convince a few more Filipino health professionals to stay rather than migrate.

Malaysia

Malaysia raked in RM 203.6 million in hospital receipts last year from nearly 300,000 foreign medical patients. Health Ministry parliamentary secretary Datuk Lee Kah Choon said Penang's portion of the takings amounted to RM 129.9 million or 63.83 per cent of the total. The other cities involved were Kuala Lumpur, Malacca and Johor Baru. "We are expecting double-digit growth for hospital receipt figures this year," he said after witnessing the signing of a clinical research collaboration between YSP Industries Sdn Bhd and Penang-based Infor Kinetics Sdn Bhd here. Among the types of treatment sought are for heart ailments, cosmetic surgery, and wellness treatment at spas. "Patients include those from Indonesia and Singapore. The government is studying ways to make medical tourism more attractive to invest in." Health Care tourism in Malaysia took-off in an aggressive manner in 2002 when Tourism Malaysia began promoting it overseas. "This includes tax-relief on the purchase of medical equipment or capital allowance on costs for new buildings," he said, adding that the proposed breaks were to reduce the "burden" on these institutions to enable them to continuously invest in upgrading their services. The Health Ministry is pursuing international accreditation for two Kuala Lumpur hospitals to boost medical tourism.

Several other countries in Asia and other continents are also working for medical tourism.

Common surgical interventions sought by foreign medical tourists

Globalisation has promoted a consumerist culture, thereby promoting goods and services that can feed the aspirations arising from this culture. This has had its effect in the health sector too, with the emergence of a private sector that thrives by servicing a small percentage of the population that has the ability to "buy" medical care at the rates at which the "high end" of the private medical sector provides such care. However, for patients and profits to increase, India must remedy negative first impressions and persuade doubters that millions of the country's poor and ailing won't be left behind.

The following services are visibly noticed.

Bone Marrow Transplant

Major hospitals in India have oncology units comprising surgical oncology, medical and radiation therapy as well as the crucial Bone Marrow Transplantation (BMT). The BMT unit with high-pressure Hipa filters has helped achieve a very high success rate in the various types of transplantation. Cord Blood Transplant and Mismatched Allogeneic Stem Cell Transplant have been performed successfully, a feat that is remarkable and significant, considering the fact that the treatment costs one-tenth of what it does in the west. Special surgeons are available for individual organs. Plastic surgeons of repute provide treatment for head and neck cancer, breast cancer and other malignancies. Facilities offered include tele-therapy, which includes simulation work stations to ensure high precision and safety during treatment at the 18 MV linear accelerator or tele-cobalt machines, brachy therapy and 3-D planning systems. In orthopedics, the Ilizarov technique is practiced for the treatment of limb deformities, limb shortening and disfiguration.

Cardiac Care

Cardiac care has become a specialty in India with institutions like the Escorts Heart Institute and Research Centre, All India Institute of Medical Sciences and Apollo Hospital becoming names to reckon with. These centres have the distinction of providing comprehensive cardiac care spanning from basic facilities in preventive cardiology to the most sophisticated curative technology. The technology is contemporary and world class and the volumes handled match global benchmarks. They also specialise in offering surgery to high-risk patients with the introduction of innovative techniques like minimally invasive and robotic surgery.

Having accomplished what he set out to do with Escorts, Trehan is planning a multispecialty hospital in Gurgaon, on the outskirts of New Delhi, that's patterned on the Cleveland Clinic in Ohio and the Mayo Clinic in Rochester, Minnesota.

Interventional Cardiology

Interventional Cardiology is a specialty which uses imaging techniques and strategies for the diagnosis of the diseases of the heart and blood vessel. These novel, minimally invasive, non-surgical procedures make use of mechanical treatments for the diseases of the heart and blood vessels. These procedures are mostly performed under local anesthesia, have a considerably short hospitalization and recovery period with minimal post-operative pain and discomfort. Interventional Cardiology includes a number of procedures that can be performed to the heart by means of inserting a 'catheter' either in your heart or in one of your blood vessels of the groin, neck or forearm. Established in 2000, the Krishna Heart Institute and Specialty Clinic is known for its innovative diagnostics and treatment procedures, and its extensive work in areas such as cardiology and joint replacement. Located in Ahmedabad, Gujarat, this institute is one of Gujarat's leading medical facilities. Initially specializing in cardiac care, the institute has grown into specialized areas such as hip and knee replacement surgeries, plastic and reconstructive surgeries, Onco-surgery, and other invasive and minimally invasive procedures. The institute has an excellent record for providing quality medical care for its international visitors at affordable prices. An air conditioned lounge is on each floor and there is a cafeteria with an expert chef serving a selection of cuisines. The institute provides continuous central monitoring and International standard water filtration and distribution systems for pure water, hot and cold. This institute is only one of the several cenres of excellence in the field of interventional cardiology.

Peripheral Angioplasty or Percutaneous Transluminal Angioplasty (PTA)

Peripheral Angioplasty is a minimally invasive procedure which is used to open narrowed arteries of the legs (most commonly iliac arteries causing cramps when walking, known as claudication), those to the brain known as the carotid arteries (causing stroke) and the arteries to the kidneys (causing high blood pressure). These conditions belong to the group of Peripheral Vascular Disease. Another condition may be ballooning of the artery called aneurysm. Aneurysms commonly occur in abdominal aorta where it manifests itself with abdominal pain or tenderness and a throbbing mass in the abdomen. Peripheral Vascular Disease is diagnosed by a procedure called angiogram which is similar to Coronary Angiogram. Peripheral Angioplasty is very similar to Coronary Angioplasty where arteries of the heart are narrowed due to atherosclerosis (Coronary Artery Disease). The blockage in the arteries is caused by deposition of fat in the form of plaques which accumulate along the arterial wall. Cost of procedure performed in the US: $18,171.

What does the procedure for Peripheral Angioplasty involve?

The procedure for Peripheral Angioplasty usually comprises of three steps: Step one of Peripheral Angioplasty, also known as artherectomy involves removal of blockage (plaque) from your peripheral artery either by laser or with specialized instruments to cut the plaque away and clear the arterial channel. The second step of Peripheral Angioplasty makes use of a balloon. An un-inflated balloon is inserted with the help of a guide wire to the site of blockage. The balloon is then inflated, which as a result enlarges the blood channel and increases blood flow through the artery. It is interesting to note that Peripheral Angioplasty can reduce a 70-90%

blockage to about 20-30%. Step three of Peripheral Angioplasty consists of implanting a mesh stent which is tightly mounted on the Peripheral Angioplasty balloon into the walls of blocked artery.

If you have been diagnosed with intermittent claudication, i.e. aches, pain, cramps, or tightness in the calves, thighs, hips or buttocks when walking, which is relieved with a few moments rest, if you have leg ulcers or gangrene, if you have an aneurysm (abdominal aorta or cerebral artery), if you are a smoker who experiences numbness, tingling or coldness of legs and feet, if you suffer from high blood pressure, diabetes, high cholesterol, a family history of heart or vascular disease, and are overweight with symptoms of peripheral vascular disease, then you are an ideal candidate for Peripheral Angioplasty.

Peripheral Angioplasty has a success rate of almost 95% with the chances of re-stenosis occurring in 5% of the patients. This procedure is less painful and allows you to go back to your daily activities quickly. This means that you will not have the symptoms of Peripheral Vascular Disease any more. Insertion of Drug Eluting Stents have potentially improved the clinical outcome of the procedure of Peripheral Angioplasty. Peripheral Angioplasty has revolutionized the treatment of Peripheral Vascular Disease. Implantation of stents during angioplasty procedure reduces the chances of re-stenosis of the artery tremendously. The procedure of Peripheral Angioplasty is certainly not a treatment for Peripheral Vascular Disease, however, accompanying lifestyle changes can definitely reduce your chances of further problems and complications. Cost of procedure performed in the US: $18,171.

What is Coronary Angiography?

Coronary Angiography is a procedure in which a non-ionic contrast dye is injected into the coronary arteries. This allows your cardiologist to visualize the coronary arteries on an X-ray and view the flow of blood through them.Cost of procedure performed in the US: $3,000 to $6,000. During the procedure of Coronary Angiography, you might experience some flushing and/or palpitation which will subside quickly. If you have chest pain which may or may not be increasing in intensity and duration, if you have unexplained pain in your jaw, neck or arm, if you have congenital heart disease or congestive heart failure, if you are planning to have heart valve surgery, if you have problems with your blood vessels like aortic aneurysm, if you have suffered a traumatic injury to your chest, then you are an ideal candidate for Coronary Angiography. Coronary Angiography is a relatively harmless procedure that can unfold tremendous amount of information and detail about the structure and function of your coronary arteries. Coronary Angiography is a diagnostic procedure that is used to confirm the diagnosis of the diseases affecting your heart and blood vessels. This procedure is also used to determine the extent and severity of your disease, and to help plan your treatment.

Risks of Coronary Angiography

- Allergic reaction to the contrast dye
- Irregular heart beat (arrhythmias)
- Heart attack and death during the Coronary Angiography procedure
- Stroke
- Injury to the internal wall of the artery where the catheter was threaded in
- Perforation of coronary artery
- Kidney damage
- Excessive bleeding (hemorrhage)
- Infection
- Blood clots

Alternatives to Coronary Angiography

- Magnetic Resonance Angiography (MRA)—In this procedure detailed images of your heart are captured using radio waves in a strong magnetic field without the use of catheters or X-rays.
- CT Angiography—This method does not require catheterization within the heart reducing some of the risks associated with Coronary Angiography.
- Digital Subtraction Angiography (DSA)—This method combines the X-ray techniques of Coronary Angiography with a high-speed computer to improve the resolution of images obtained.
- Cardiac Catheterization—This procedure is very similar to Coronary Angiography and consists of passage of a catheter in the coronary artery.

What is Coronary Angioplasty?

Coronary Angioplasty or Balloon Angioplasty is a minimally invasive procedure in which the blocked or narrowed coronary arteries are opened (widened) to facilitate perfusion of the heart muscle. Coronary Angioplasty reduces the need for medication and to some extent eliminates chest pain due to Ischemic Heart Disease. Cost of procedure performed in the US $35,000. The procedure for Coronary Angioplasty usually comprises of three steps: Step one of Coronary Angioplasty, also known as artherectomy involves removal of blockage (plaque) from your coronary artery either by laser or with specialized instruments to cut the plaque away and clear the arterial channel. The second step of Coronary Angioplasty makes use of a balloon (thus the alternative term Balloon Angioplasty). In this step, an un-inflated balloon is inserted with the help of a guide wire to the site of blockage. The balloon is then inflated, which enlarges the blood channel and increases blood flow through the artery. It is interesting to note that Coronary Angioplasty can reduce a 70-90% blockage to about 20-30%. Step three of Coronary Angioplasty consists of implanting a mesh stent which is tightly mounted on the Coronary Angioplasty balloon into the walls of blocked artery. The balloon is then deflated and removed leaving the stent in place permanently to hold the artery open. In this procedure of Coronary Angioplasty, the coronary arteries are accessed through a puncture made in the groin (femoral artery) or arm (brachial artery). Usually the femoral artery is used. Depending upon the extent of coronary artery narrowing, all three steps may or may not be carried out. The procedure of Coronary Angioplasty can take 30 minutes to several hours depending on the number of blockages being treated.

Benefits of Coronary Angioplasty

- Quicker and less painful recovery
- Short hospital stay, does not require general anesthesia
- Small incision
- Coronary Angioplasty can be done under local anesthesia
- The chest cage does not need to be opened
- Chances of major post-operative complications like stroke are minimized as heart-lung machine is not used during the procedure of Coronary Angioplasty.

Risks of Coronary Angioplasty

- Allergic reaction to the dye
- Ruptured coronary artery
- Bleeding and infection at the site of insertion
- Arrhythmia
- Stroke
- Heart attack
- Kidney failure
- Rupture or dissection of the coronary artery
- Re-stenosis of the coronary artery requiring Heart Bypass Surgery

Why is Coronary Stenting performed?

Coronary Stenting is performed to hold your coronary artery open to facilitate flow of blood to the heart muscle and reduce your chest pain due to angina. The coronary stents physically hold your artery open and create a channel for your blood to flow through it easily. Coronary Stenting is usually performed as part of the Coronary Angioplasty procedure. So if you are an ideal candidate for Coronary Angioplasty, i.e. if one or more of your coronary arteries are blocked, if your chest pain due to angina is not well controlled with medications or if it is severe enough to disrupt your daily activities and also occurs at rest, then you are an ideal candidate for Coronary Stenting. Coronary Stenting has a success rate of almost 95% with the chances of re-stenosis occurring in 5% of the patients. This procedure is less painful and allows you to go back to your daily activities quickly. This means that you will not have chest pain any more and that your tolerance to exercise will increase. Drug Eluting Coronary Stents have potentially improved the clinical outcome of Coronary Stenting.

Benefits of Coronary Stenting

- Quicker and less painful recovery
- Short hospital stay, does not require general anesthesia
- Small incision
- Coronary Stenting can be done under local anesthesia
- The chest cage does not need to be opened
- Chances of major post-operative complications like stroke are minimized as heart-lung machine is not used during Coronary Stenting procedure
- Implantation of drug eluting coronary stents dramatically decreases the chances of re-stenosis and the need for a repeat procedure.

In the procedure for Drug Eluting Coronary Stenting, the implanted stent is coated with a medication that prevents re-stenosis. This type of stent consistently releases a chemical substance that prevents clot formation and narrowing of coronary artery. Drug Eluting Coronary Stenting has been 20-30% more successful than bare metal stenting. Cost of procedure performed in the US $37,000.

Benefits of Drug Eluting Coronary Stenting

- Quicker and less painful recovery
- Short hospital stay, does not require general anesthesia
- Small incision (Minimally Invasive procedure)
- Drug Eluting Coronary Stenting can be done under local anesthesia
- The chest cage does not need to be opened
- Chances of major post-operative complications like stroke are minimized as heart-lung machine is not used during the procedure of Drug Eluting Coronary Stenting
- Implantation of Drug Eluting Coronary Stenting has dramatically decreased the chances of re-stenosis and the need for a repeat procedure.

Dialysis and Kidney Transplant

Common diseases like diabetes, hypertension and chronic glomerulonephritis can lead to permanent loss of renal functions—with dialysis and renal transplantation being the frequent outcome. The emergence of new therapeutic interventions has created opportunities in India to manage the progression of renal diseases. Major hospitals in India like Holy Family Hospital, Jaslok Hospital, Apollo Hospital, Sir Ganga Ram Hospital, Batra Hospital, Bombay Hospital and Hinduja Hospital have departments of Nephrology and Organ Transplant equipped with the latest computerised dialysis machines, reverse osmosis water plant to provide pure and trace element-free water supply, as well as state-of-the-art facilities in the operating rooms and Transplant Intensive Care Units.

For those who need renal replacement therapy, the following services are also available.

Patients can also avail of the bicarbonate dialysis facility at these centres. Round the clock service is available at these hospitals for the critically ill patients in the intensive care units who may need fluid, electrolyte management and renal supportive therapy.

The cost of getting a dialysis is around Rs. 1700 to Rs. 1800 per dialysis whereas the same costs about $ 300 in the U.S.A. Similarly, a kidney transplant package in India is available for around Rs. 3 Lakhs, which is comparatively much cheaper than what it would cost abroad. Hemodialysis Chronic Ambulatory Peritoneal Dialysis (CAPD) Transplantation In addition to the basic haemodialysis facilities, the patients' requirements for other modalities of treatment such as— Continuous Arterio-Venous Haemofilteration (CAVH) Continuous Veno-Venous Haemofilteration (CVVH) Continuous Cycler-Assisted Peritioneal Dialysis (CCPD)

Gynecology and Obstetrics

Leading Indian hospitals with gynecology departments and women's hospitals have facilities for the prevention and early detection of gynecological disorders. Many hospitals have women check-up programmes designed to detect the earliest signs of disorders of the breast and the organs of reproduction as well as catering to the contraceptive needs of women. A mammogram, an ultrasound of the pelvis and a pap smear of the cervix are an integral part of any good medical check-up for women. Specialist medical as well as surgical care is available for all types of gynecological problems like menstrual abnormalities, prolapse, fibroids and other tumors of the uterus and ovaries, tubal re-canalization by microsurgery and care of the infertile couple. State-of-the-art gynecological surgery is available with world-class equipment and expertise using minimally invasive techniques.

Ectopic pregnancies, ovarian cysts and tumors, fibroids endometriosis, tubal blocks and even hysterectomies can be performed laparoscopically. Hospitals like Apollo have state-of-the-art IVF labs backed by highly experienced doctors who have been involved in the field of infertility and assisted Reproductive Technologies (ART).

Joint Replacement Surgery

Shoulder/hip replacement and bilateral knee replacement surgery using the most advanced keyhole or endoscopic surgery and arthroscopy is done at several hospitals in India including the Apollo Hospital, Sir Ganga Ram Hospital and Holy Family Hospital in Delhi, Bombay Hospital, Leelavati and Hinduja Hospital in Mumbai and the Madras Institute of Orthopaedics and Trauma Sciences. Some hospitals like Apollo in Delhi have Operation Theatres with Laminar Air Flow System, which compares with the best in the USA and the UK. A knee joint replacement costs only a quarter of what it costs in the UK. In the last 5 years arthroplasty has got established and has changed the face of osteoarthritis patients. More than 10 million people are supposed to suffer from this ailment in India alone. Dr. Dholakia was the first to introduce the technique in 1986. Ranawat performed surgery on the knees of the then prime minister of India in 2000. Now further advancement has occurred and new techniques have come in giving better results.

Neurosurgery and Trauma Surgery

Other routine procedures performed with excellent results are replacement arthroplasty, diagnostic and operative arthroscopy, spinal surgeries including. Harrington Rod Instrumentation for scoliosis, corrective and reconstructive procedure for poliomyelitis and cerebral palsy, micro-cascular surgical procedures and automated percutaneous lumbar distectomy. In addition, the advanced Luque technique is employed for the correction of complex scoliosis, and decompression and stabilisation of fractures of dorsal and lumbar spine with paraplegia, by neurosurgeons with excellent training and background. Many super-speciality hospitals in India like AIIMS, Ram Manohar Lohia Hospital, Vidya Sagar Institute of Mental Health and Neuro Sciences, Bombay Hospital, Jaslok Hospital, Nizam Institute of Mental Health and Neuro Sciences and Apollo Hospitals have advanced facilities devoted to the treatment of the entire range of brain and spinal disorders with highly experienced neurosurgeons, neurologists, neuroanaesthetists and neuroradiologists. Treatment of intra- and juxta-cranial, spinal tumours and vascular malformations, aneurysms and thrombolysis for brain attacks are done at these centres. Hospitals like Apollo employ state-of-the-art LINAC-based stereotactic radio surgery system outside the USA. The Clinic 6000 SR Linear Accelerator with XKNIFE system is a highly sophisticated computer-driven technology used for removal of appropriately selected brain tumours, arteriovenous malformations and other abnormalities.

Osteoporosis

Several drug therapies now easily available in the market have been shown to be clinically effective in slowing down or reversing the bone-loss process. Leading hospitals in India are well equipped to detect and treat bone loss in its earliest states, so as to prevent the disease or lessen its impact. Doctors in leading hospitals have the expertise for the diagnosis and treatment of osteoporosis that involves an objective, quantifiable measurement of the patient's bone mass or bone density. Advanced technology called the DXA for bone densitometry is available. During a comprehensive bone valuation with DXA, the patient lies comfortably still on a padded table while the DXA unit scans one or more areas, usually the fractured spine or the hip. The entire process takes only minutes to scan depending on the number of sites scanned. It involved no injections or invasive procedures and the patient remains fully clothed.

Refractive Surgery

Refractive surgery is gaining popularity in India both among the public as well as among ophthalmologists. Till a few years ago only a few centres performed high volume radial keratotomy. Today, the highest international quality of eye care for cornea, cataract, squint and glaucoma is available in over 40 centres all over India. When it comes to reliability, India has the best ophthalmic surgeons with clinico-academic expertise honed to perfection in the best possible institutions. Apollo Hospital, Gurunanak Eye Centre, Dr. Rajendra Prasad Centre For Ophthalmic Sciences and Mohan Eye Centre in Delhi, Shankar Naytralaya in Chennai, L.V. Prasad hospital in Hyderabad are just some of the more popular eye care hospitals. The No Stitch Cataract Surgery with the most modern way of removing cataract through the use of Phacoemulsification procedure can be performed in India for as little as Rs. 20,000, for both the eyes, whereas the same surgery costs $ 45,000 in the USA. Facilities for PRK, myopia and astigmatism are now available in almost all parts of the country. Hyperopic and LASIK are available and even supra hard cataracts are treated using just 1 mm incision instead of the 3 mm incision size. Photo-refractive keratectomy or PRK treats the surface of the cornea with the Excimer laser while LASIK treats the inner tissue of the cornea. For this reason, with LASIK there is less area to heal, less risk of scarring, less risk of corneal haze, less post-operative pain and vision often returns very rapidly.

Urology

Several super specialty hospitals in India offer comprehensive Urologic services to diagnose and treat stone disease, Urologic cancer, incontinence, infertility, impotency and other urinary difficulties. Advanced methods such as lithotripsy for treating kidney and ureteric stones without surgery are available with complementary methods of treating stones endoscopically. Advanced machines like the Lithostar obvert the need for anaesthesia in the treatment of kidney and ureteric stones. High tech facilities for the treatment of prostate, bladder cancers, urethral strictures are also available. Investigation and treatment facilities for impotence and male/female infertility exist with specialized facilities for pharmacotherapy, cavernosometry and cavernosography, in addition to doppler studies for the assessment of blood flow.

Other surgeries

Removal of the gall bladder, the spleen, the bowel and other organs like the adrenals, an operation for prolapse rectum and hiatus hernia repair have become fairly commonplace in almost all the major speciality hospitals in India. Experts are easily available and accessible and the workload at most of these hospitals ensures that the doctors have enormous experience. High intensive care treatment at much cheaper rates than in the west is available at most of these centers.

Preventive Health Care

Preventive health care has been introduced for the first time in the country by Apollo Hospitals with hospitals in the metros of Hyderabad, Chennai and Delhi, within easy international air access. The professional chain also pioneered the concept of lifestyle clinics, established the first organ registry in the country and introduced non-invasive technique for treatment of lesions and tumours of the brain—Stereotactic Radio Surgery and Radiotherapy in the country. It recently installed a state of the art Cobalt Unit. Apollo Heart Hospital provides a complete network for cardiac patients. It has a total bed capacity of 500 beds distributed between Apollo Chennai, Hyderabad and Delhi. Apollo is linked to the Mayo Clinic and the Minneapolis Heart Institute, a premier heart institute led by the team of doctors who pioneered the Jarvik artificial heart.

Imaging with MRI, a hypertension research centre and facilities for hemodialysis and kidney transplantation are available at Akila Hospitals at Trichy. The hospital boasts a transplant team with 8 specialists, bone marrow transplant team along with five specialists on call to Sri Lanka, Sharjah, Kuwait and major Indian cities.

In Chennai, the Vijaya Heart Foundation's 79 beds have a state of the art cardiology and cardio-thoracic surgical unit manned by competent and experienced staff. The Vijaya Health Centre with 270 beds offers diagnostic facilities in laboratory, X-ray, ultrasound, treadmill, Endoscopy, C.T. Scan, M.R.I. and nuclear medicine.

Fasting

Naturopath doctors at such centres mean a minimalist diet of 300 calories per day—veggie broths and juices—for two weeks to several months, accompanied by blood tests, purges and other treatments. They say many hard-to-treat conditions, from arthritis to allergies and various skin disorders, benefit from the metabolic switch that takes place when the body starts living off its own reserves. Of the thousands guests who come to fast each year (half from southern Europe, America and the Middle East), about one-third arrive with serious ailments—the rest come to lose weight or cut stress.Fasting has lately gotten a boost from medical research. Clinical studies in Scandinavia have shown that fasting is an effective treatment for rheumatism—especially if followed by a vegetarian diet. In one study, pain and swelling came down by a third in a week and stayed that way for a year. Other studies have shown success in lowering blood pressure and treating chronic pain like migraine or arthritis. They have shown that when patients fast, stress hormones levels go down and serotonin levels rise (which may explain the "fasting high" many patients report). "The more we look into it, fasting seems to work like a reset button for the body's own self-regulating mechanisms," say Naturopaths.

$800 vs. $18

In the U.S., organizations such as the Joint Commission International (JCI) on Accreditation of Health Care Organizations, based in Oakbrook Terrace, Illinois, assess infection rates, the width of hospital corridors and the capacity of elevators. Dr. Trehan, Escorts' founder, says the hospital had a mortality rate of 0.8 percent and an infection rate of 0.3 percent in 2003. That compares with an observed mortality rate, or the rate of actual deaths, of 4.77 percent for heart valve surgery or coronary artery bypass surgery that included heart valves at New York-Presbyterian Hospital. Charging foreigners more than Indians is one way hospitals can make money to treat the poor, says Gautam Kumra, a McKinsey and Co. partner in New Delhi. An echocardiogram machine, used to picture the heart, costs about $200,000 anywhere in the world. Doctors can charge $800 per scan in the U.S.; in India, they charge 800 rupees, or $18, Trehan says. Fortis Health Care plans is setting up two hospitals on the outskirts of New Delhi. One will cater to overseas patients and charge them higher prices, says Harpal Singh, who adds the hospitals haven't set fees yet. Fortis is owned by brothers Malvinder and Shivinder Singh, who control India's largest drug company, Ranbaxy Laboratories Ltd. Harpal Singh is Malvinder Singh's father-in-law. One imbalance that works in India's favour is its lower salaries. A top cardiac surgeon in India makes about $330,000 a year compared with $5 million in the U.S., says Anupam Sibal, director at Apollo Hospital, New Delhi.

Cosmetic and Plastic Surgery

This is a surgical specialty that corrects disfigurement caused by burns, tumor, congenital defects, developmental abnormalities, trauma, infection, disease or injuries, improves appearance and self-esteem and restores function. Cosmetic and Plastic Surgery is mainly concerned with correcting problems and enhancing appearance of exposed areas of the body and the face. Reconstructive Plastic Surgery is another term that is used in this context mainly referring to surgical procedures that correct severe functional impairments, fix physical abnormalities, and compensate for tissue lost to trauma or surgery.

Some disfigurations corrected include hair restoration (hair implants, hair flaps, and scalp reductions), rhinoplasty (reshaping or re-contouring of the nose), stalling of the aging process (face lift, cosmetic eyelid surgery, brow lift, sub-metal lipectomy for double chin), dermabrasions (sanding of the face), otoplasty for protruding ears, chin and cheek enlargement, lip reductions, various types of breast surgery and reconstruction and liposuction.

The problem of loose upper arm skin usually occurs after weight loss. This problem is more common in people who have lost a lot of weight. If you were over weight, the skin of your arm has to stretch to accommodate the increased volume of your upper arm. After weight loss, the skin usually fails to tighten and sags. Brachioplasty is performed to correct this problem of loose hanging skin of your arms. Brachioplasty is performed as an outpatient procedure in the plastic surgeon's office under local anesthesia with sedation. The entire procedure of Brachioplasty takes about an hour per arm. The surgeon makes zigzag, elliptical or triangular incisions along the inner surface of upper arm. The space contained between the incisions is exactly the area of skin that would be removed. Removal of loose skin tightens the surface of the arm however, it does not remove the fat. That is why it is usually recommended that Brachioplasty be accompanied with liposuction as well to remove extra fat from your arms. Make sure that you make arrangements for some one to accompany you as you will be allowed to go home after a couple of hours following Brachioplasty procedure.

Benefits of Brachioplasty

- Brachioplasty will help you get rid of the extra fat and skin after losing weight. Although this requires you to undergo a Brachioplasty procedure, the results are well worth it. To be able to get the lean and shapely arms that you have always longed for, Brachioplasty is the best option available.
- Brachioplasty is performed under local anesthesia, does not require hospitalization and you can return to work and resume your daily activities within 2 weeks.

What is Body Lift?

Body Lift or Total Body Lift is a Cosmetic and Plastic Surgery procedure performed to reshape your body to it's natural curves and contours. Body Lift is a surgical procedure where the loose and hanging skin of the entire body is tightened and implants are inserted, all in one procedure. Body Lift basically reshapes the breasts, chest, arms, thighs, hips, back, waist, abdomen and knees after losing weight (for example those people who lose lot of weight after undergoing weight loss surgeries like Gastric Bypass, Laparoscopic Gastric Bypass, Gastric Banding), aging and multiple pregnancies. Body Lift can be:

- *Central Body Lift*—This procedure is also called Belt Lipectomy. In Central Body Lift, excess skin and fatty tissue is removed circumferentially from the belly, hips, back, buttocks, and outer thighs.
- *Lower Body Lift*—Lower Body Lift is performed to shape buttocks and thighs by removing excess skin and fat from these areas.

Body Lift can be combined with other Cosmetic and Plastic Surgery procedures like Liposuction, Power Assisted Liposculpture (PAL), Tummy Tuck, Thigh Lift, Arm Lift, Breast Reduction, Breast Augmentation, and Breast Lift. Skin Grafting may also be performed in places of the body where needed. These procedures not only remove excess skin and fat, they also improve the unsightly stretch marks and create an uplifted, shapely, youthful and fuller appearance.

If you have lost large amounts of weight (50-300 lbs.) and have loose, hanging skin on your face, breasts, back, belly and thighs, or if you want to lose weight (especially if you suffer from central obesity) that is resistant to diet and exercise, if you have folds of loose, hanging skin due to aging or multiple pregnancies that might pose a danger of cellulitis or abscess, then you are an ideal candidate for Body Lift. This procedure can either be performed in isolation or in combination with other body contouring and weight loss procedures like Liposuction, Tummy Tuck, etc. If you are severely obese, are a smoker or an alcoholic or do not have a stable mental state to undergo a major surgical procedure and follow post-operative instructions to obtain optimum benefit or if you are allergic to the medication used for general anesthesia, then you are not an ideal candidate for Body Lift.

Body Lift is performed in a hospital setting under general anesthesia and can take about 5-7 or may be 10 hours depending on what other cosmetic surgery procedures are performed along with it. The Body Lift surgery is usually performed to remove excess skin from the belly first, i.e. from the area between the belly button and pubic hair and tightening of abdominal muscles is also performed. Excessive skin is removed, belly button is repositioned, remainder of the skin is approximated and the incision is sutured. The surgeon will then turn you on your side, make incisions in your buttock and back area, remove fat and excess skin to try and normalize the curves and contours of your sides and back. Body Lift also involves Liposuction of the buttocks, thighs and abdomen areas. Lastly, your surgeon will work on the flabby arms (commonly called bat wings) and make them shapely. As mentioned above, Liposuction, Power Assisted Liposculpture (PAL), Tummy Tuck, Thigh Lift, Arm Lift, Breast Reduction, Breast Augmentation, Breast Lift and Skin Grafting can all be performed at the same time, whatever your need may be.

Body Lift is a comprehensive procedure that can take care of flabby, bulges in different parts of your body. The best results are obtained when Body Lift is performed by skillful and experienced cosmetic surgeons. This procedure is as safe as multiple shorter cosmetic surgeries. The contours of your body will be better defined and if you commit yourself to exercising regularly and eating sensibly, chances are that the results of Body Lift will be good for the rest of your life. Body Lift is a revolutionary surgical procedure that quickly, safely and effectively re-shapes the normal contours of your body. Most people who undergo Body Lift are quite satisfied with the results. The procedure of Body Lift is unified approach to treat and skin laxity as a result of aging, pregnancy and dramatic weight loss. Body Lift is a remarkable procedure which can help you get started on the way to a new, more fulfilling life of normalcy and a level of self-esteem that you may have never imagined.

Alternatives to Body Lift

- Liposuction is commonly used in both men and women to remove localized excess fat deposits that are resistant to dieting and exercise.
- Power Assisted Liposculpture (PAL)—Power Assisted Liposculpture uses a powerized cannula which moves back and forth through the fat tissue in a rapid motion.
- Tummy tuck, also known as Abdominoplasty or Panniculectomy is a procedure where large amount of skin and fat are removed from the middle and lower part of the abdomen.
- Thigh Lift is a procedure which is performed to remove loose and excessive (hanging) skin around your thighs and buttocks, thus to tighten them and improve it's appearance and texture.
- Arm Lift—Brachioplasty or Arm Lift is a procedure where loose and excess skin are removed from your arm.
- Breast Reduction is a surgical procedure designed to remove excessive fat, glandular tissue, and skin from large and pendulous breasts, making them smaller, lighter, and firmer.
- Breast Augmentation or Breast Implant Surgery is a surgical procedure in which the size and shape of a woman's breast is enhanced by inserting an artificial breast implant behind each breast.
- Breast Lift or Mastopexy is a surgical procedure which is commonly performed in men and in women to reshape sagging or drooping breasts and to give them a firm, youthful contour.
- Skin grafting is a surgical procedure by which skin or a skin substitute is used to replace the damaged skin or provide a temporary wound covering.

Body Lift is fondly called the Face Lift of your body. The resulting body contour shows a remarkable and significant improvement in the areas of the belly, pubic region, hips, back, and buttocks and will bring you to the range of normal body contour.

What is a Breast Implant?

A breast implant is a soft shell or a rubber sac that is filled with silicone gel or saline (salt-water). The feel of the implant is very natural and close to the feel of the normal breast tissue. They are available in several different sizes to accommodate different patient's needs and surgeon's preference. The surface texture of the implant can be smooth or contoured.

There are different approaches used for Breast Augmentation surgery: (1) Infra-mammary Breast Augmentation—This is the most commonly used approach for Breast Augmentation operation. In this approach an incision is made in the crease just below the breast where the breast tissue meets the chest wall. (2) Peri-areolar Breast Augmentation—In this approach a semi-circular incision is made around the lower part of the areola (areola is the dark area of skin surrounding the nipple). (3) Trans-axillary or Axillary Breast Augmentation—In this approach an incision is made in the armpit to insert the breast implant. (4) Trans-umblical or Umblical Breast Augmentation—In this approach, a breast implant is inserted through the umbilicus or belly button with the help of an endoscope.

Breast Augmentation surgery takes about 2-3 hours. Most commonly you can go home the same day or the following day. The sutures are covered with a gauze dressing to promote speedy healing. The outcome of Breast Augmentation is very satisfactory and successful. Your breasts will be enlarged for life. Clothes fit better and it certainly boosts your self-confidence and self-esteem. Some cases of leakage or breaking of the breast implant have been reported. In this case, a second Breast Augmentation surgery may be needed. The breast tissue is actually pushed to the surface as the breast implant is inserted behind the breast tissue. Following Breast Augmentation surgery it might become easier to perform breast self-examination to gain familiarity with your breast tissue. Of course, the obvious benefit Breast Augmentation is improved look of your breasts and your overall body image remains undisputed without any doubt. Breast Lift is designed to regain you youthful look and vigor. This procedure of Cosmetic and Plastic Surgery is used world wide by women as well as men to improve the appearance of drooping, sagging breasts. Breast Lift is performed in conjunction with Breast Augmentation to increase their size and give firmness. Breast Lift is a very popular surgery and the number of men and women undergoing Breast Lift has increased tremendously (214%) in the past five years. The beauty of Breast Lift is that it enhances your body image and maintains the normal shape of your breast as closely as possible. The operation for Breast Lift is an excellent option that reverses the changes that occur in your breast due to weight loss, pregnancy, breast feeding and aging. The goal of your plastic surgeon will be to restore the normal contour and firmness of your breasts as closely as possible. You will be extremely pleased with the results of Breast Lift surgery if you completely understand the procedure and make an informed decision but at the same time have realistic expectations.

What is Breast Reduction?

Breast Reduction is a surgical procedure designed to remove excessive fat, glandular tissue, and skin from large and pendulous breasts, making them smaller, lighter, and firmer. During Breast Reduction, the size of the areola is also reduced in proportion to the breast size. Breast Reduction is also performed in men for the correction of Gynecomastia.

Breast Reduction surgery is performed to alleviate both your physical and psychological problems due to large breasts. Physical problems include upper back and neck pain and discomfort, deep and sore indentations on the shoulder from bra straps, rashes on the under surface of the breast due to sweat and moisture and difficulty finding clothes or bra that fit you well. Psychological problems include feeling self-conscious due to large breasts. All the above reasons are definite indications for Breast Reduction surgery. Breast Reduction is also performed in men who have large breasts. Although certain health conditions and medications are known to cause male breast enlargements (Gynecomastia), there is no other known cause for this problem in men. If you are a woman who has large, pendulous breasts and are not planning on having any more children, if you have chronic headache, upper back or neck pain, then you are an ideal candidate for Breast Reduction surgery.

Benefits of Breast Reduction

- Breast Reduction surgery not only alleviates your anxiety of being self conscious about large, sagging breasts but it also relieves physical discomfort like chronic neck and back pain and skin rashes. Of course to say the least, Breast Reduction adds tremendously to your self-confidence and self-esteem as it enhances your body image and allows you to enjoy wearing clothes that you might have avoided to wear in the past. Breast Reduction also allows you freedom to enjoy sports and physical activities that might have been painful or uncomfortable due to bouncing of large and heavy breasts.
- You can feel the breast tissue better during Breast Self-Examination as the surrounding excessive fat surrounding the glands and ducts has been diminished.

2

India's Health Care Sector

The Indian health care sector can be viewed as a glass half empty or a glass half full. The challenges the sector faces are substantial, from the need to improve physical infrastructure to the necessity of providing health insurance and ensuring the availability of trained medical personnel. But the opportunities are equally compelling, from developing new infrastructure and providing medical equipment to delivering tele-medicine solutions and conducting cost-effective clinical trials. The scenario is improving, though haphazardly, that is giving the nation many tertiary care hospitals and opportunities of health tourism from the east as well as west.

It goes without saying that good health care is the basic need of any welfare state and also is the core of Human Development Index (HDI). Unfortunately even developed countries have not been able to provide good health care to all its citizens and the quality, accessibility and affordability remain a matter of opinion. The most prosperous country of the world and the world's only super power US has been failing to look after the health care needs of all its citizens. Those able to afford insurance are also only partially covered, exploited by insurance companies and subjected to unnecessary or excessive investigations and interventions and also administered medicines of doubtful value or outright toxic chemicals. (See Appendix 1 at the end of the book: Health is Wealth). India being a third world country with limited resources and poor governance is among the countries that provide poorest health care. Despite this statement none can deny that the country has many islands of excellence that offer world class health care at affordable prices, thus opening many opportunities for health tourism.

India's Health Care Scenario

There is a rise in both infectious and chronic degenerative diseases. While ailments such as poliomyelitis, leprosy, and neonatal tetanus have not been eliminated, communicable diseases once thought to be under control, such as dengue fever, viral hepatitis, tuberculosis, malaria, and pneumonia, have returned in force or have developed a stubborn resistance to drugs. This trend can be attributed in part to substandard housing, inadequate water, sewage and waste management systems, a crumbling public health infrastructure, and increased air travel.[1]

India is also grappling with the Diabetes Epidemic, AIDS as well as food- and water-borne diseases, etc. Diabetes is a life-long, incurable disease. And as Indians live more affluent lives and adopt unhealthy lifestyle, marked by high blood sugar levels. It is western diets that are high in fat and sugar. Almost 41 million Indians suffer from lifestyle diseases such as hypertension, cancer, and diabetes.

The incidence of diabetes is much higher in affluent urban areas of India than in villages, and the rates are increasing: In the 1970s, only 2.1% of Indians living in urban areas had diabetes. Today that figure is 12.1% for adults over the age of 20. The incidence is higher in the south than in the north, particularly in cities such as Chennai and Hyderabad, where about 16% of the population is diabetic. This form of the disease can be caused by genetics but also obesity, and it can lead to amputations, heart failure infections, and blindness. In addition to lifestyle changes that are causing diabetes—the dietary excess, reduced physical activity and increased stress associated with more affluence—Indians have a strong genetic vulnerability to the disease. As a result, Indians often contract diabetes a decade earlier than their counterparts in the developed world—a trend that is likely to have an enormous impact on India's working age population in the future.

Poor infrastructure

India's health care infrastructure has not kept pace with the economy's growth. The physical infrastructure is woefully inadequate to meet today's health care demands, much less tomorrow's. While India has several centers of excellence in health care delivery, these facilities are limited in their ability to drive health care standards because of the poor condition of the infrastructure in the vast majority of the country. After years of under-funding, most public health facilities provide only basic care. With a few exceptions, such as the All India Institute of Medical sciences (AIIMS), public health facilities are inefficient, inadequately managed and staffed, and have poorly maintained medical equipment. The number of public health facilities also is inadequate. For instance, India needs 74,150 community health centers per million population but has less than half that number. In addition, at least 11 Indian states do not have laboratories for testing drugs, and more than half of existing laboratories are not properly equipped or staffed. (Pandeya, Radhieka, "Outside the Sick Bay," *Business Standard*, June 28, 2007)

Private firms are now thought to provide about 60% of all outpatient care in India and as much as 40% of all in-patient care. It is estimated that nearly 70% of all hospitals and 40% of hospital beds in the country are in the private sector.

The health care divide

When it comes to health care, there are two India' : the country that provides high-quality medical care to middle-class Indians and medical tourists, and the India in which the majority of the population lives-a country whose residents have limited or no access to quality care. Today only 25% of the Indian population has access to Western (allopathic) medicine, which is practiced mainly in urban areas, where two-thirds of India's hospitals and health centers are located. Many of the rural poor must rely on alternative forms of treatment, such as ayurvedic medicine, unani and acupuncture. Among other things, the government launched the National Rural Health Mission, 2005-12 in April 2005. The aim of the Mission is to provide effective health care to India's rural population, with a focus on 18 states that have low public health indicators and/or inadequate infrastructure. These include Arunachal Pradesh, Assam, Bihar, Chhattisgarh, Himachal Pradesh, Jharkhand, Jammu and Kashmir, Manipur, Mizoram, Meghalaya, Madhya Pradesh, Nagaland, Orissa, Rajasthan, Sikkim, Tripura, Uttaranchal and Uttar Pradesh. Through the Mission, the government is working to increase the capabilities of primary medical facilities in rural areas, and ease the burden on to tertiary care centers in the cities, by providing equipment and training primary care physicians in how to perform basic surgeries, such as cataract surgery. (See Appendix 2: Tertiary health care system cannot sustain in isolation)

Collapsing system of family physicians and rise of specialist

Family physicians might have less knowledge than some of their specialized peers, but the tasks and ongoing demands of dedicated family practitioners are immense and worthy of the highest respect. Those of us who emulate these noteworthy practitioners deserve to be lauded; those who do not would do well to follow their example.

Lack of insurance

A widespread lack of health insurance compounds the health care challenges that India faces. Although some form of health protection is provided by government and major private employers, the health insurance schemes available to the Indian public are generally basic and inaccessible to most people. Only 11% of the population has any form of health insurance coverage. For the small percentage of Indians who do have some insurance, the main provider is the government-run General Insurance Company (GIC), along with its four subsidiaries. The New India Assurance Company, Oriental Fire and Insurance Co., National Insurance Co., and The United India Insurance Co. GIC is able to obtain funds for underwriting from other countries, although foreigners are not allowed to own insurance companies. Only 1% of the population was covered by private health insurance in 2004-05. Group insurance accounted for 35% of the total health insurance business during that period. India's first medical insurance scheme for the poor was launched in the 1996-97 budget. The "Janarogya Yojana" scheme is marketed by the four subsidiaries of GIC, and covers people between the ages of 5 and 70 for pre- and post-hospitalization expenses, for upto 30 and 60 days, respectively. The insurance coverage costs around $122 per annum.

More than four million policyholders were expected to enrol during the first year of operation, although reports suggest this was not the case. One problem is that the insurance is provided on a reimbursement basis: patients are required to pay for treatment out of their own pockets and then claim reimbursement—a process that can take upto six months, according to local reports.

While public sector health insurance has not fared well, the market for private health plans is expanding in India. In some cases, the government is partnering with the private sector to provide coverage at a low cost. For instance, the Yashaswini Insurance scheme, launched in 2002 in the state of Karnataka by a public-private partnership, provides coverage for major surgical operations, including those pertaining to pre-existing conditions, to Indian farmers who previously had no access to insurance. The premium is only Rs. 60 annually (roughly $1.50), which virtually all workers can afford, and the government contributes an additional Rs. 30 annually for each policyholder. While the Yashaswini scheme has been successful, it only provides coverage for approximately 50,000 farmers.

Because so little insurance is available to the population of India, out-of-pocket payments for medical care amounted to 98.4% of total health expenditures by households, as of the most recent (2001-02) census. Without insurance, the poor must resort to taking on debt or selling assets to meet the costs of hospital care. It is estimated that 20 million people in India fall below the poverty line each year because of indebtedness due to health care needs. Clearly there is an urgent need to expand the health insurance net in India. Among other things, that will require more state governments to pursue micro-insurance initiatives, such as the Yashaswini Insurance scheme in Karnataka, so that most or all of the population can afford to purchase at least a minimum level of coverage. The widespread availability of health insurance would help to drive demand for services and provide additional revenue to improve the quality of care. In recent years, there has been a liberalization of the Indian health care sector to allow for a much-needed private insurance market to emerge.

Due to liberalization and a growing middle class with increased spending power, there has been an increase in the number of insurance policies issued in the country. In 2001-02, 7.5 million policies were sold. By 2003-4, the number of policies issued had increased by 37%, to 10.3 million. The Insurance Regulatory and Development Authority (IRDA) eliminated tariffs on general insurance as of January 1, 2007, and this move is expected to drive additional growth of private insurance products. In the wake of liberalization, health insurance is projected to grow to $5.75 billion by 2010, according to a study by the New Delhi-based PHD Chamber of Commerce and Industry. The IRDA believes that eliminating tariffs will encourage scientific rating and adoption of better risk management practices, and lead to independent pricing for each line of business, so that premiums will be based on actual risks and costs. The implementation of the new policy also will encourage the development of innovative practices and customer-friendly options for policyholders, boosting penetration.

Removal of tariffs also will result in wider acceptance of individual health coverage. Health insurance will make health care more affordable to larger segments of the populace, boosting health care expenditures per household and driving the demand for quality care. Finally, the elimination of insurance tariffs will serve as a litmus test for further legislation, such as co-payments and hospital accreditations, which the government plans to implement over the next two to three years.

In the post-liberalization era, some companies have been licensed to act as third party administrators of health services. The objective is to strengthen the health insurance industry and increase its penetration by bringing more professionalism to claims management, facilitating cashless services to policyholders, and reducing the claims ratio. Currently, there are 25 licensed third party administrators in the Indian health insurance industry. In another effort to improve the insurance prospects for India, the IRDA is focused on standardizing medical definitions to ensure consistent pricing and products, and is providing incentives for stand-alone insurance companies. (Currently only Star Health exists as a stand-alone health insurance company.) In addition, government subsidies and tax incentives for health insurance are expected to attract key players to the industry. In response to liberalization, a large number of international private insurance companies are moving into India and forming joint ventures.

Two prominent examples are Max New York Life, a joint venture between Max India and New York Life, and ICICI Prudential Life Insurance, a joint venture between the ICICI Group and UK-based Prudential plc. Some companies are experimenting with more targeted forms of insurance coverage. For example, ICICI Prudential is offering plans designed specifically for diabetics. We can expect to see more innovations as the health insurance market evolves in the coming years.

While the liberalization of the health care sector will increase the penetration of insurance policies, the widespread use of health insurance in India could take many years. One reason is that insurance companies lack the data they need to assess health risks accurately. In addition, today's insurance products work on an indemnity basis—that is, they reimburse patients only after they have paid their health care bills. Since many people cannot afford such large payments, even if they are subsequently reimbursed, they will not choose to purchase medical insurance.

Thriving economy is pushing the demand for better health care

India traditionally has been a rural, agrarian economy. Nearly three-quarters of the population still lives in rural areas, and as of 2004, an estimated 27.5% of Indians were living below the national poverty line. Some 300 million people in India live on less than a dollar a day, and more than 50% of all children are malnourished. The Indian economy, estimated at roughly $1 trillion, is growing in tandem with the population. Goldman Sachs predicts that the Indian economy will expand by at least 5% annually for the next 45 years and that it will be the only emerging economy to maintain such a robust pace of growth. India's middle class, with more disposable income can now spend more on health care. A growing, 200-million-strong middle class of our own country is demanding world-standard quality in health care. While per capita income was $620 in 2005, over 150 million Indians have annual incomes of more than $1,000, and many who work in the business services sector earn as much as $20,000 a year. While this is a fraction of the income that their US peers earn, it is the equivalent of more than $100,000 per year when adjusted for purchasing power parity. More women are entering the workforce as well, further boosting the purchasing power of Indian households. Between 1991 and 2001, the percentage of women increased from 22% to 26% of the workforce, according to the latest Indian government census. Many of these women are highly educated: the ratio of women to men who have a college degree or higher level of education is 40:60. Today at least 50 million Indians can afford to buy Western medicines—a market only 20% smaller than that of the UK. If the economy continues to grow faster than the economies of the developed world, and the literacy rate keeps rising, much of western and southern India will be middle class by 2020.

Consumerism driving a change in health care marketing

It's actually the 28-year-old young woman who is contemplating whether to get a cosmetically fitting white ceramic crown versus a silver one for her dental treatment. It's also a 40-year-old man who can get his blood test at the local diagnostic centre or get the phlebotomist to come home and collect his sample while he still unwinds in the comfort of his house on a lazy weekend. These two examples illustrate the emerging trend of health care consumerism. Though the health care field is characterized by complexity, rapid change, evolving distribution, consumer-purchasing behaviour, and pricing and reimbursement pressure; awareness and technology now empower patients to make their own health care choices, rather than simply accepting the options lay down by a traditional health system.

The influence of health care consumerism today extends to every professional working in the health care system compelling providers to respond to consumers' evolving expectations, which are mainly based on choice, control, convenience, and customer service. Health care is now purchased from a wholesale and retail-oriented marketing model. Earlier, health care organizations did not need to market their services. The providers operated in semi-monopolistic environments. There was an almost unlimited flow of customers, and revenues were essentially guaranteed. This situation began to change. Increasing choice for consumers opened the door to competition. Health care organisations began to appreciate that to sustain in this new 'bad' world, they would have to introduce modern business practices into the health care arena and adopt concepts and methods long established in other industries. This led to the concept of direct marketing.

Unfortunately, in the early years health care professionals did not like the amalgamation of the words health care and marketing. Many misconstrued marketing for advertising, and, advertising on the part of health services providers was considered inappropriate. Though prescribed marketing activities became common early on among health care organizations like pharmaceuticals, medical equipments and medical supplies, targeting physicians and employers, marketing campaigns targeting health care consumers, i.e. patients were relatively rare. Health care service providers had long resisted the incorporation of formal marketing activities. They have been marketing under 'public relations, physician-relationship development, community services, and other activities,' but few health professionals equated these with marketing.

The use of marketing techniques have proliferated. Modern health care programmes, such as freestanding diagnostic centers and rehabilitation clinics, began using marketing as a means of luring patients from the already established sources of care. Health care marketing, however, initiated as an unstable concept. The marketing professionals that health care imported from other industries failed in their effort to adapt existing marketing techniques to health care uses. Marketing health care was not the same as marketing a soft drink! While few methods and techniques could be transferred untouched from other industries, most approaches had to be customized to health care. Furthermore, experienced marketers from other industries were not familiar with the health care market and, were therefore unable to appreciate the need for long-term initiatives in this industry.

The formal recognition of marketing as a suitable activity for health care providers represented an important milestone for health care. Health care organisations then saw the daybreak to a flurry of marketing activities and got into creating aggressive campaigns. Medical professionals using jargon like 'the market' along with 'angioplasty', 'arteries' and 'vitamins' became more common. The term 'marketing mix' is now heard commonly in boardroom discussions housed in the same building complex where patient care is provided, emphasizing on the 4 P's of Marketing: Product, Price, Place and Promotion. Today, the industry has matured into a sophisticated and competitive field, meeting the needs of knowledgeable consumers who are making their own health care decisions. The industry is now being compared to the hospitality sector, and is labeled as a service industry.

The acceptance of marketing by health professionals realised the need for the establishment of marketing budgets and the creation of numerous new positions within the organisations. This culminated with the establishment of a marketing department with its' own budget and staff. Positions like general manager and director for marketing came into existence in many organisations with responsibilities of contributing to the bottom line, just like any other department.

After years of reluctant acceptance, marketing has now become reasonably well established as a legitimate health care function. Though the industry still suffers from a lack of standardisation when comes to marketing, health care marketers now have a much better understanding of the market and their 'target audience'. New approaches have been developed specifically for the health care market and reasonably sophistical market research techniques have been put into place.

Health care professionals now appreciate their existence in a service industry and have in fact extended the marketing fundamentals to 7 P's, the addition ones being People, Physical Evidence and Process. A core of health care marketing professionals have now emerge along with the tools necessary to implement marketing initiative. These drive marketing approaches and consumer behaviour in health care. Market departments and marketing budgets are under increasing scrutiny in today' health care organisation. Developing a implementing communications and public relations program that meets the needs of both the hospital and diverse stakeholders is increasingly gaining popularity. From planning and executing an advertising campaign to analysing patient satisfaction data, evolution of health care marketing have been quite dramatic over the past years. Physician referral 'cuts' have been replaced by sophisticated terms like 'revenue sharing mode' and 'pan care' by 'customer focus'. Health care organizations are now using various means and tools for marketing their 'products'. Electronic media, print media, television, radio are just few of the many options health care providers are now opting for Hoardings and billboards now don't just carry favourite actor selling a car or toothpaste, but also a doctor-patient relationship.

It is now believed that when market planning, market research, and marketing communications come together; achieve planned strategic object: organizations succeed. Today, health marketing appears poised to play a greater role in the new health care environment. A few marketing methods are: Health education camps/awareness programmes for consumers, CMEs for physician relation building exercises, medical camps, website, marketing to various avenues like corporate, insurance companies, smaller health organizations, attracting international attention and promotional packages.

Over 4 millions of health sector employees

The health care industry employs over four million people, making it one of the largest service industries in the economy, reports a study by ASSOCHAM and Yes Bank (Health Care Services in India, 2009). There is a need for many more qualified people. Infrastructure spend is on a staggering growth clip, doubling in size and slated to reach Rs. 63,900 crore in 2013 (KPMG, 2009). In the metros, quality hospital beds are blooming, almost at par with the global benchmark of 35 beds per 10,000 people.

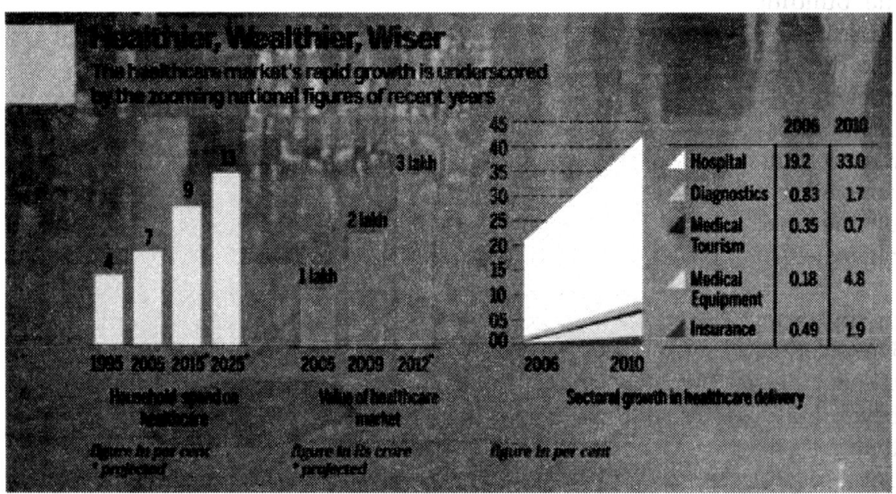

Source: Health Care Services in India: 2012, the path ahead. ASSOCHAM-YES Bank, 2009; McKinsey 2007.

Health care is the largest sector in terms of revenue and employment

During the 1990s, Indian health care grew at a compound annual rate of 16%. Today the total value of the sector is more than $34 billion. This translates to $34 per capita, or roughly 6% of GDP. By 2012, India's health care sector is projected to grow to nearly $40 billion. The private sector accounts for more than 80% of total health care spending in India. Unless there is a decline in the combined federal and state government deficit, which currently stands at roughly 9%, the opportunity for significantly higher public health spending will be limited. One driver of growth in the health care sector is India's booming population, currently 1.2 billion and increasing at a 2% annual rate. By 2030, India is expected to surpass China as the world's most populous nation. By 2050, the population is projected to reach 1.6 billion. This population increase is due in part to a decline in infant mortality, the result of better health care facilities and the government's emphasis on eradicating diseases such as hepatitis and polio among infants. In addition, life expectancy is rapidly approaching the levels of the western world. By 2025, an estimated 189 million Indians will be at least 60 years of age—triple the number in 2004, thanks to greater affluence and better hygiene. The growing elderly population will place an enormous burden on India's health care infrastructure.

Corporate investment in health care in the upswing: India Today

This year in 2010, about 15 major hospital projects with a total investment worth Rs. 3,415 crores are expected to be launched. There is now a trend of creating medi-cities which is a concept of integrating super specialty hospitals under one management. It is, however, easier to make the buildings and install the equipment than to find the able doctors, nurses and trained technicians to deliver better health care. Over the next two decades, India will need twice as many doctors, three times as many nurses and four times as many paramedics it has now. It is not all the game of numbers. More importantly it is the training, skill and experience of the medical and paramedics that is going to determine the quality of health care. After all, in the end the quality of care will depend on the competence of the medical professionals who come in contact with the patient regardless of how fancy the buildings may be.

The mega hospitals and super specialty medical centers are coming up in various parts of the country and offer hope of good medical care. However, cost to the consumer is a matter of concern. Also such centers fail to provide a cover of primary health care to the citizens of the area or beyond. However, it is opined that medi-cities can be planned in a manner that they not only provide a first class tertiary care to the critical patients, but also provide a holistic care and a comprehensive care to the community. Cleanliness is Godliness is an old saying. The new medi-cities differ from the older hospitals, in many ways, specially the typical stench of toilets is missing. At the Fortis La Femme in Delhi, the flavor of orange blossoms hangs in the air. At Bangalore's The Nest, the waiting area looks more like a bank, with wait-for-your-turn counters. Think twiddling your thumbs is your lot as a hospital visitor? At the Oyster and Pearl Hospital in Pune you can spend hours at the cyber café or the massage parlor. Worried about commuting to and from the hospital? At The Cradle, Bangalore, a luxury car will be at your beck and call.

The Pride of India's health care at a glance:

Fortis Hospitals
Locations: 62 hospitals across India.
Total Beds: 10,000
USP: Deep pockets, top doctors, specialized services.

Apollo
Locations: 50 hospitals across India.
Total Beds: 9,000
USP: The Apollo Heart Institute is one of the largest cardiovascular groups in the world.

Manipal Hospitals
Locations: Manipal and Bangalore.
Total Beds: 3,571
USP: Pioneering presence in medical education.

Narayana Hrudayalaya
Location: Bangalore
Total Beds: Over 3,000
USP: Subsidised cardiac surgeries.

Christian Medical College
Location: Vellore
Total Beds: 2,512
USP: Leveraging on highly skilled global network, high on charity, focused on the marginalised.

Max Hospital
Location: Delhi
Total Beds: 1,900
USP: Over 225 ICU beds, world-class physicians, 3,000 support staff and most advanced technologies.

SevenHills Health City
Location: Mumbai
Total Beds: 1,850
USP: Expertise in cardiology, emergency care, etc.

KLES Hospital
Location: Belgaum, Karnataka
Total Beds: 1,820
USP: Accident and emergency department compares with the best.

Medanta Medicity
Location: Gurgaon
Total Beds: 1,600
USP: Medanta has 45 operating theatres and over 350 critical care beds.

Arvind Hospitals
Locations: Madurai, Tirunelveli, Coimbatore, Puducherry
Total Beds: Over 1,500
USP: Traditional hospitality and low cost eyecare treatment. Known for service-oriented initiatives.

Kasturba Hospital
Location: Manipal
Total Beds: 1,475
USP: Service to the needy and poor people with care and compassion.

Yashoda Hospitals
Location: Hyderabad

Total Beds: 1,200
USP: Foremost centre for cancer treatment in the state using Asia's first Rapid Arc machine equipped with sophisticated 3D planning simulators.

Amrita Institute of Medical Sciences and Research Centre
Location: Kochi
Total Beds: 1,200
USP: Superspecialty with an attached medical college.

Lisie Hospital
Location: Cochin
Total Beds: 1,080
USP: Hospital recognised by the MCI for junior and senior House surgency.

Dayanand Medical College and Hospital
Location: Ludhiana
Total Beds: 1,000-bedded tertiary care teaching hospital in North India.
USP: The only institution in North India which has an entire floor of ICUs with 100 beds incorporating all the critical care areas.

Sri Ramachandra Medical Centre
Location: Chennai
Total Beds: 900
USP: International technology for Indian patients. Specialists in ortho. One of the key player in medical tourism.

Global Hospitals
Location: Hyderabad, Bangalore and Chennai.
Total Beds: 900
USP: Organ transplantation.

CARE Hospitals
Location: Hyderabad
Total Beds: 950
USP: Cardiology super specialty.

Little Flower Hospital and Research Centre
Location: Angamaly, Kerala
Total Beds: 800
USP: Registered not for profit health institution.

Kokilaben Dhirubhai Ambani Hospital
Location: Mumbai

Total Beds: 750
USP: Top of the line technology.

Sterling Hospitals
Locations: Rajkot, Baroda, Ahmedabad and Mundra SEZ.
Total Beds: 725
USP: Centre of excellence for cardiac care.

We shall deal with 'medi-city model of modern health care' later in another chapter.

New look and better quality

"A simple brief we recently received was that the hospital should not look like a hospital," said Dr. Sachin Wagh, a hospital planner. The spectrum of catering, food and dietetics have gone up, along with the processing of linen as an integral component of infection control. "Almost all newer hospitals opt to outsource support services—dietary, laundry, housekeeping and security," he adds. Apart from medical technology, hospitals are investing in electronic systems for hospital records. Shalby Hospital in Ahmedabad has invested heavily in IT infrastructure with Cisco and Nortel networking infrastructure. It has a fully integrated hospital management and information system, designed to manage every aspect of information flow and control across the hospital—right from vendor records to patient data—electronically. Shalby is also one of the first hospitals in the country to pioneer incorporation of infection control measures like HEPA Filters, Laminar Air Flow, Body Exhaust System, Plasma Sterilizer and Maquet Operating Tables.

An unintended consequence of the flourishing big hospitals has been a nation-wide "poaching" of human resources. Not only are people moving out of government hospitals, corporates are taking from each other too. "But these are market forces that you have no control over. You cannot make legislation to stop this. It's a free country, after all!" The prime driver is the compensation packages that corporate hospitals offer, often five to 10-times more than the market rate. "Some have 20 different scales and salary systems—with fixed and variable pay," he says. But not everyone would be eligible for the top slots. A doctor's field, his reputation capital and his finance-generating capacity will have to tally with the 'needs' of the health care corporate. "Someone in cardiology, for instance, will be able to dictate terms more than a skin specialist." "The private sector has not been able to take technology to the common man, although it has created phenomenal standards in the country," said a hospital planner. It is technology that forms the backbone of the paradigm shift in health care, but cost goes up as technology and treatment options increase. The constant evolution of life-support systems, diagnostics, expensive third and fourth generation medicines and greater number of devices-related surgeries—all come at a cost. "There are many hospitals which over equip them with technology," he says. "Where a 64-slice CT scanner is enough, people insist on buying 256-slice."

Indian doctors! Ham kisi se kam nahin

Whether it is in diagnostics, high technology or basic hospital services, urban India will no longer put up with shabby wards, outdated machines and endless delays, as seen in most public hospitals. Deteriorating standards and the rush of numbers in public health facilities are driving an increasing number of Indians to seek private medical care. This has encouraged new players from the private sector to get into the health care business and those who are already in it to upgrade or expand their facilities to offer better care. India is one of the largest health care markets in the world. It is estimated to be worth close to Rs. 200,000 crores. It is projected to reach Rs. 3,00,000 crore by 2012. The private sector controls 80 per cent of this and runs 60 per cent of India's 15,393 hospitals according to Arun Poorie of *India Today* (April 2010). According to a recent study, India's health care industry is growing at the rate of 16 per cent per annum. What adds more muscle to the industry is the increase of medical insurance to more people and the amount of investment that private equity investors are willing to put into expanding hospital numbers. A health care revolution is taking place in India. The new age Indian hospital now offers patients a clean environment, fewer queues and quality care along with the latest global equipment and drugs.

Bleeding-edge technology, wonder drugs and star facilities are now the hospital mantra. Health care systems are usually large, complex and slow to respond to change. But the surge of new ideas, approaches and institutions is melting away the age-old barriers to change. No doubt radical ideas are being implemented in hospital planning and design viz. picture windows to ward-off ICU psychosis, counselling areas for patients' relatives, cafeteria, convenience store, library, public booth, Internet access, and hotel-like front desk create a "healing experience"? A modern hospital focuses entirely on patient satisfaction.

A massive boom in private hospitals is changing the nation's health delivery landscape beyond recognition. New hospitals are mushrooming, even in smaller towns, and leading health care entrepreneurs with deep pockets are expanding their empires. The scent of big money is in the air. It's giving doctors the choice and option of moving from green to greener pastures.

15 MEGA PROJECTS IN 2010
Total: Rs. 3,415 cr

- Rs. 1,000 crore: SevenHills Health City, Mumbai. Multispecialty.
- Rs. 330 crore: Tata Medical Centre, Kolkata. Single specialty offering oncology services.
- Rs. 300 crore: Apollo Hospital, Bhubaneswar. Multispecialty.

- Rs. 250 crore: Fortis Hospital, Delhi. Multi-superspecialty hospital in Shalimar Bagh, Delhi.
- Rs. 250 crore: Rockland Hospital, Gurgaon. Multispecialty.
- Rs. 200 crore: People International Hospital, Bhopal. Multispecialty.
- Rs. 200 crore: Asian Institute of Medical Sciences, Faridabad. Multispecialty.
- Rs. 200 crore: Global Hospital, Mumbai. Super specialty.
- Rs. 175 crore: Fortis Hospital, Kolkata. Super specialty.
- Rs. 120 crore: AMRI, Bhubaneswar. Emami and Shrachi Group of Industries. Multispecialty.
- Rs. 100 crore: Narayana Hrudayalaya Health City. Multispecialty.
- Rs. 90 crore: ILS Hospital, Agartala. Multispecialty.
- Rs. 90 crore: Vikram Hospital, Bangalore. Multispecialty.
- Rs. 60 crore: Eternal Heart Hospital, Jaipur. Superspecialty.

Giant new projects

Be it pioneering cardiologist and health care entrepreneur Dr. Naresh Trehan's Medanta Medicity in Gurgaon, Mumbai's SevenHills, Apollo's 200-acre wellness hub in Lavasa or the technology paradise 'Kokila Dhirubhai Ambani Hospital' in Mumbai. Apollo is planning 32 hospitals in two years, Wockhardt is spending Rs. 400 crore in four super specialties, Columbia Asia is setting up 15 new hospitals in India, Shalby of Gujarat is opening OPDs across and beyond India, Narayana Health City is expanding to other states; DLF and Fortis are investing Rs. 3,000 crore on 15 hospitals; Kolkata's Ruby General has a Rs. 10-crore expansion plan; Global Hospitals of Hyderabad is charting a boutique hospital, health city in Chennai; Max is expanding by Rs. 243 crore; Hindujas are foraying into Rs. 50 crore: Aadhar Hospital, Kolhapur Superspecialty. The hospital growth saga is being written at a furious pace. Reddy of Apollo is once again navigating unexplored terrains, where healing, learning and rejuvenation get coupled with world-class infrastructure and modern medicine. "The market is booming because the demand completely eclipses capacity. He holds out the promise of numbers: India needs 1,00,000 beds each year for the next 20 years at Rs. 50,000 crore per year; double the number of doctors from 0.7 million to 1.5 million; triple the number of nurses from 0.8 million to 2.5 million; four times the number of paramedics from 2.5 to 10 million. "All of us can play this game, provided we keep the momentum going." What he forgot to add was : 'the growth of health care should maintain quality and ethics intact and make the cost less painful and more bearable.'

The Fortis Group truly shows the might of private players with the hospital buying binge it has entered into—Escorts Heart Institute in 2005 for Rs. 600 crore, scores of hospitals in Bangalore, Kolkata, Hyderabad and Mumbai, 10 Wockhardt hospitals for Rs. 909 crore in the year 2009 and 24 per cent of Singapore's Parkway holdings in March 2010. "That makes us the biggest hospital network in Asia," says Shivinder Singh, the man who heads the Fortis hospital network. The group initially focused on expanding aggressively pan-India through organic and inorganic growth. But its aspiration is clearly global. "I built Escorts two decades back because at that time there were very few places in India that offered world-class treatment and technology. But one can't possibly reinvent the wheel," he says. India may have moved up the health care delivery ladder, but there's still a very real gap in the market. "Even now, we don't have a single place that's at the cutting-edge not just of technology and treatment but of education and research too," he points out. Medicity is a new model where application and knowledge, cure and prevention, health and wellness, work and leisure, East and West can combine.

Reliance ADA Group has also joined the health care fray with the Kokilaben Dhirubhai Ambani Hospital, Mumbai. It's, in fact, a pleasure to come to this den of luxury—from high-end salons that even work out hair solutions for chemotherapy patients, to fine-dining restaurants, art not just on the walls but also on the floors, well-appointed rooms for patients, coffee kiosks everywhere. It's a hospital that houses the best of technology from intra-operative MRI suites to the high-end Trilogy radio-therapy equipment.

Max India boss Analjit Singh spoke about today's health care consumer—demanding and discerning, intelligent and interested in the services offered to him. His hospital chain offers both—service with a smile as well as the best of technology, especially in cancer care. Finally it's planning to branch out across North India—with 1,050 new beds across Dehradun, Mohali and Bathinda. "We intend to grow organically and through Greenfield expansions," says Singh.

Dr. Devi Shetty, who famously delivered cardiac care at Rs. 10, is busy perfecting a model that no one else has dared to venture into. "We are totally different from our competitors," he says. "As health care providers to the working class and the poor, we serve a market that no one else wants to touch." And Shetty's aim is to add 20,000 hospital beds in the next five years across states. To treat the rising tide of cancer patients, the group has created a Rs. 250-crore cancer hospital in association with Kiran Mazumdar Shaw of Biocon. How does the socially-inclusive model work? "We do over 10 per cent of all heart surgeries in India. So, we benefit from economies of scale," he says.

New Technology and Advanced medical equipment

Driven by the rising health care demands and spending power of India's affluent generation, medical technology looks set to enter a golden age. A new FICCI-Ernst and Young study predicts 15-20 per cent growth for the Indian medical equipment market, slated to grow from Rs. 9,000 crore now to Rs. 22,500 crore by 2012. Not surprisingly, private hospitals are taking the lead in introducing the latest technological wonders and creating milestones in treatment. In 2006, Asia's first high field strength intra-operative MRI (iMRI), the most advanced technology to treat brain tumors with utmost precision, was launched at the Institute of Neuroscience of the Max chain in Delhi.

New horizons in radio-imaging

Tele-radiology is the electronic transmission of diagnostic scans and X-rays from one location to another to facilitate their reporting. The idea struck Dr. Arjun Kalyanpur while working at the Emergency Room at the Yale School of Medicine, US. "During night shifts, we accessed scans from a hospital across towns which were transmitted electronically to us," he says. "I began to think that the same thing could be done from India, where it would be daytime." But the idea of starting a company came later when he met a radiologist friend in the US by chance. When he told his wife, Sunita Maheshwari, also a Yale medic, her response was instant: "That is a space-age concept." But the couple anyway put down their savings and started working from home through the Internet for US clients. Now with the Indian health imaging market expected to double from the existing Rs. 1,575 crore in the next five years, competition is brewing up. Wipro, Reliance and Apollo have recently joined the fray. But Telerad holds 90 per cent of the market share in the country, growing at 50 per cent year on year. Besides CT scan and MRIs now we have iMRIs. This is a great breakthrough in imaging medicine.

In the past, the difficulty in distinguishing between diseased and healthy brain tissue was addressed with a follow-up MRI scheduled a day or so after the surgery. In cases where residual tumor remained, a decision had to be made about whether another operation was a viable option. That delay between surgery and follow-up MRI could now be eliminated with iMRI. Surgeons could operate on a brain tumor, slide the MRI into the surgical suite for a scan and immediately assess whether more surgery is needed. By 2010, a host of private hospitals—from Medanta to Kokilaben Dhirubhai Ambani Hospital to the Asian Heart Institute—would have acquired the latest in neurosurgery innovation. Dr. N.K. Pandey, former head of surgery at Escorts has just started the Asian Institute of Medical Sciences (AIMS). "There is a huge demand-supply gap," he says. "There is a lack of good infrastructure and quality health care services here." AIMS is gearing up as the first super specialty focusing on cancer care in the area. From the cutting-edge Varian Trilogy machine—one of the very few hospitals in North India with such a device—Pandey has also brought in state-of-the-art systems—PET-CT, MRI, gamma camera, brachytherapy to mammography. His dream is to turn the 350-bed multispecialty tertiary care hospital into a flagship hospital in the field of oncology, minimal invasive surgery, urology and nephrology.

Robotic Surgery

A mechanical unit with arms and tiny hand-like instruments that the surgeon controls with joss-sticks from a console. The small incisions and extreme precision make it a patient-friendly procedure. Was introduced for cardiac surgery by Escorts in 2001. Today used widely across the country: Jaslok and Hiranandani hospitals in Mumbai, Narayana Hrudayalaya and Wockhardt Hospitals in Bangalore, Care hospital in Hyderabad, etc. Swarup Hospital in Kolhapur has an indigenous method of robotic laparoscopy; "intelligent robotics" for cancer—CyberKnife—was brought last year by the Apollo, Chennai. A Da Vinci robot costs about Rs. 10 crore, a cyberknife system 65-70 crore.

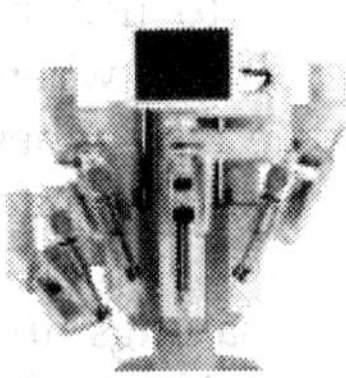
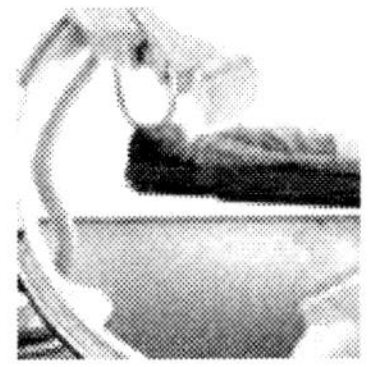
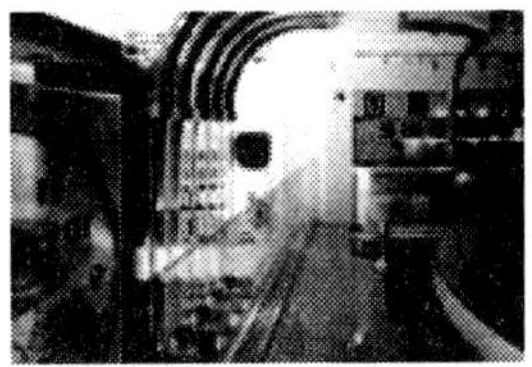

Flat Panel Digital Cath Lab

Cath labs have advanced imaging systems that allow doctors to see the workings of the heart and of tiny blood vessels around it. It's all live and doctors really rely on the images to make accurate decisions. The latest flat-panel digital detectors don't just capture distortion-free images but also bring the advantage of lower radiation dose to the patient, clinicians and technologists. A staple in all modern hospitals today.

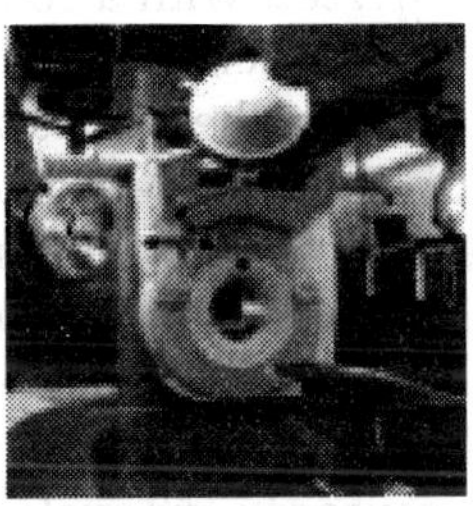

Pneumatic Chutes

They connect and serve hospital departments, transporting pharmaceuticals, lab samples and sensitive medical items at high speed. Done manually once, it ensures integrity of diagnostic processes, patient safety and service efficiency. Almost every specialty hospital in India has introduced the chute.

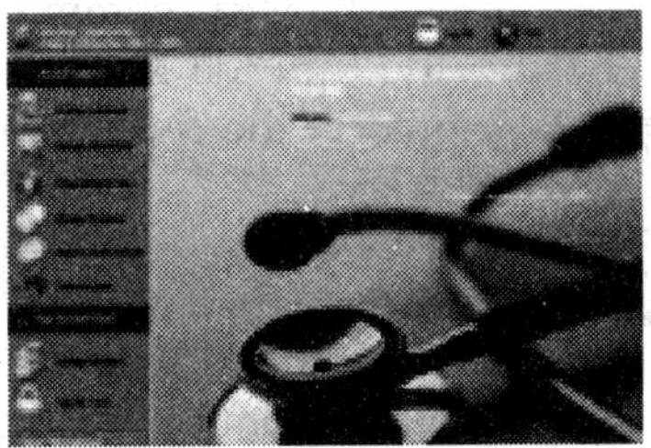

Paperless, Filmless

Scribbled notes, bills, prescriptions, large diagnostic charts, reports and even patient queues will soon be a thing of the past. Hospital workflows—from patient consultation, prescription, investigations, registration, doctor and nursing notes, billing, inventory management to discharge—are increasingly just a click away. Modern hospitals are now starting out with hospital information systems in place. Artemis Health Institute of Gurgaon, for instance, had an IT budget of Rs. 6.5 crore when it started in 2007.

IMRI and Brain SUITE

iMRI (intraoperative imaging) utilizes MRI during surgery to help neurosurgeons determine the success of a procedure by checking real-time images in complicated brain tumor and other brain surgery cases. A separate but fully-integrated operative area is named Brain SUITE. Max Health Care, Delhi, brought in Asia's first Brain Suite to India. Today, a number of private hospitals—Asian Heart Institute and Kokilaben Dhirubhai Ambani Hospitals in Mumbai, Medanta-Medicity in Gurgaon, Parvathy Hospital in Chennai—have introduced this fabulously expensive facility.

Hospitals are now finding ways to reach more patients and expand their business. Retail clinics like Manipal Cure and Care (MCC) in Bangalore are unique in that they complement the hospital business by providing feel-good, look-good care. A brainwave of the Manipal Hospital group, MCC offers a mix of world-class products and services in preventive, wellness and beauty—from health packages to skin care products, premium exercise machines, anti-snoring nasal devices to cosmeceuticals. "I am an active proponent of this integrated approach, especially the wellness to prevention route," says Dr. Ranjan Pai, Managing Director, Manipal Education and Medical Group, Bangalore. That makes perfect business sense in an age when Generation-X does not want to get into hospitals for services that can be rendered in a "non-sick" environment. "They prefer being served in boutique ambience, where service standards and the assurance of the genuineness of clinical care would be a significant pull," he adds.

Vaatsalya Model

"Improving the lives of billions of people at the bottom of the economic pyramid is a noble endeavor. It can also be a lucrative one," so says management guru C.K. Prahalad. New business models in Indian health care back up that theory. Ask Dr. Ashwin Naik, 37, and Dr. Veerendra Hiremath, 35, who grew up in Hubli, Karnataka, went around the world and returned to set-up Vaatsalya, a unique model of affordable hospital network in under-served tier II and III towns. "Doctors from rural districts rarely go back to their roots," says Naik. They decided to address this demand-supply gap. When Vaatsalya started, they tapped into their

NRI friends and family to chip in. "They gave easily because everyone wants to connect to their roots." Venture funds began contributing gradually, both with money and expertise. Vaatsalya runs in eight locations in the state, focusing on the mother and child, offers about 520 beds and sees 20,000 patients a month. Apart from full-time doctors, Vaatsalya also gets consultants from metros who want to go back to their roots or from local partners. What next? "Building up the chain in Maharashtra and Andhra Pradesh," they say.

Ayurvedic Hospitals

Alternative is the new normal now. Take Rajiv Vasudevan, founder and CEO of the new-generation AyurVAID Hospitals. That's because, he is applying contemporary business models to the ancient science of healing—ayurveda. AyurVAID operates exactly like a modern hospital—from a hub-and-spoke approach to insurance coverage, focus on chronic conditions, end-to-end medical management protocol. "We integrate ayurveda with modern medicine," says Vasudevan, who is hopeful that the business model will attract many more credible players to the industry. The 150-bed hospitals grew from three to seven centers across south and west India last year.

Aviation facilitates access; Air Ambulance

It is the most 'in' thing in the hospital circuit today with almost every super specialty hospital, over 24 in the NCR region alone, offering the service. With top-drawer emergency doctors on-board, it's a much-needed service for patients who can't reach hospitals easily or on time.

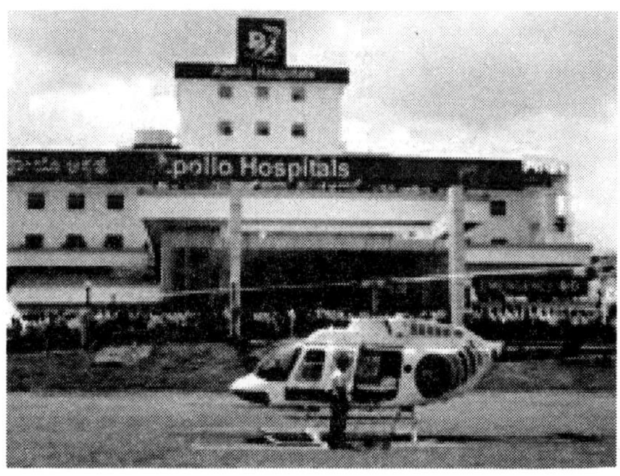

Escorts Heart Institute, Delhi, is no longer the only hospital flying critically-ill patients to and fro. Many hospitals like the Apollo, Hyderabad, and Akshaya Apollo, Ahmedabad, have their own helipads. The cost can run into lakhs depending on the distance. Every hospital worth its salt is dishing out air ambulance services these days. For a moment, he thought about the patient with abnormally fast heartbeat he had flown in from Ludhiana that afternoon. It was nearly touch-and-go, but they had managed to wheel him in to the OT safe and sound. For Chandra, head of air rescues at Escorts, it's all in a day's work. And it's that promise of being saved in the nick of time that's making more and more patients seek air ambulance despite the cost (Rs. 75,000 to Rs. 100,000 per hour) and lack of insurance cover. When Dr. Nitin Yende of Mumbai floated Vibha Lifesavers in 1996, calls came once in six months. "Today, we handle over 40 calls from across India and the world every month," he says. Older hospitals are tying up with private charter (Air Ambulance India lists up 24 hospitals in NCR, Tops Air Rescue 60 in Mumbai) or aviation companies (Deccan and now Religare Voyages). New hospitals are stealing the thunder by building roof-top helipads. Check out the 19-storied Kokilaben Dhirubhai Ambani Hospital in Mumbai. Not just the metros, they are all across—from the Aditya Birla Memorial Hospital in Pune to the Yashoda Hospital in Secunderabad, Akshaya Apollo in Ahmedabad, Pushpanjali Crosslay in Ghaziabad to Sri Hari Health Foundation in Bhiwani, Haryana.

Hospital Retail Clinics

Hospitals are now finding ways to reach more patients and expand their business. Retail clinics like Manipal Cure and Care (MCC) in Bangalore are unique in that they complement the hospital business by providing feel-good, look-good care. These clinics, a mix of world-class products and services in preventive, wellness and beauty, will offer everything—from health packages to skin care products, premium exercise machines to cosmeceuticals.

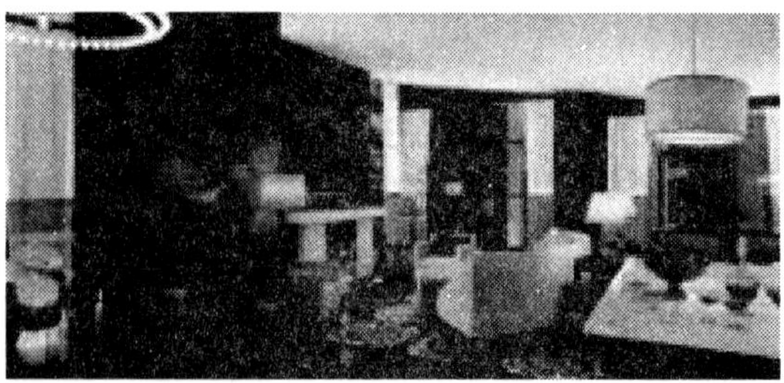

Boutique Hospitals

More money, more attention. Lavish personalized care was so long the fortÃ© of high-end birthing centres. Now Multi-specialties are entering that zone. Check out two upcoming hospitals of Mumbai—SevenHills in Marol Andheri and PD Hinduja at Khar—that are gearing upto offer this service—green sprawl, designer suites, spas, fine dining—to patients who expect country club facilities while in a hospital.

Presidential Suites

What's common between Fortis, Vasant Kunj, in Delhi, Kokila Dhirubhai Hospital in Mumbai, Artemis in Gurgaon, Sagar Apollo in

Bangalore or Ruby Hall Clinic in Pune? Well, they all have something that was so long associated with business travellers and five-star hotels: Presidential suites. Complete with patient and family rooms, separate bathrooms, microwave and refrigerator (sometimes a kitchen), computer stations, WiFi—there's enough room to accommodate personal staff as well. All clinical appendages are neatly tucked behind sliding artwork to complete the illusion. At Rs. 25,000-30,000 a day, it might just be possible to forget the reason for getting admitted to a hospital.

Bar-coded OPD card

Be it Paras Hospital in Gurgaon or the brand new Desun Hospital and Heart Institute in-Kolkata—bar-coded smart cards to track patient details are fast catching the fancy of hospital planners. These are issued the first time a patient visits a hospital. The unique computer generated registration number would not only hold good every time the patient visits, it would also give the hospital instant access to his/her profile. (*India Today*, April 2010).

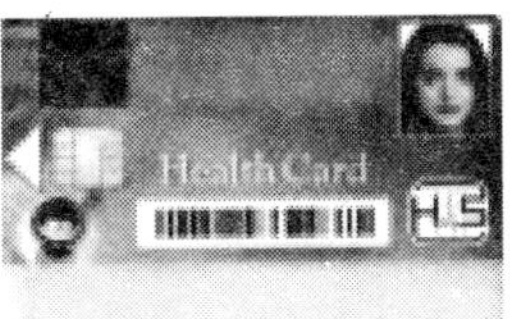

Leaders in India's health care Industry

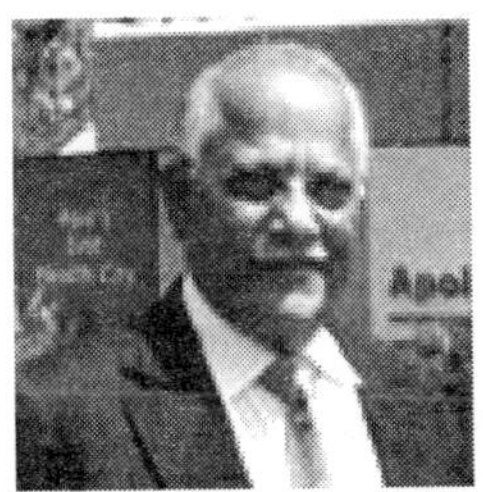

Dr. Prathap Reddy

His dream is taking the Apollo Group up along an unexplored trajectory where healing, learning and rejuvenation get coupled with world-class infrastructure and modern medicine. "The time has now come," says Reddy. That's because of the new churn in the market. He has been "playing the game" ever since he set-up India's first corporate hospital in Chennai in 1983. With an annual footfall of over seven million patients, 62,000 employees, 50 operational hospitals and 9,000 beds, today his group is a Rs. 4,500-crore company. Apollo has massive expansion plans—be it building medicities, moving into smaller towns with world-class facilities, or expanding internationally.

Dr. Prathap Reddy, is setting up an integrated health care facility at Lavasa Hill City, Pune. The state-of-the-art wellness centre will provide world-class facilities for rejuvenation, health education, research, multispecialty services. The wellness cluster will have facilities for complementary and alternative medicine, nutrition, preventive care, a medical and rejuvenation spa. Long-term care will include rehabilitation services for patients.

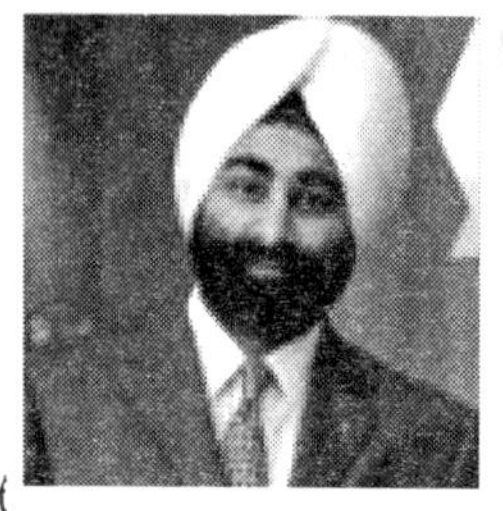

Shivinder Singh, FORTIS HEALTH CARE

"The health care industry is growing exponentially due to increasing per capita health care spending by consumers and investments by private players."

Sixty-two hospitals, 10,000 beds and a turnover of Rs. 4,500 crore—the Fortis group truly shows the might of private players. "That makes us the biggest hospital network in Asia," says Singh. Aggressive expansion, mergers and acquisitions have been the blueprint of growth. The aspiration is to be global leaders in health care eventually.

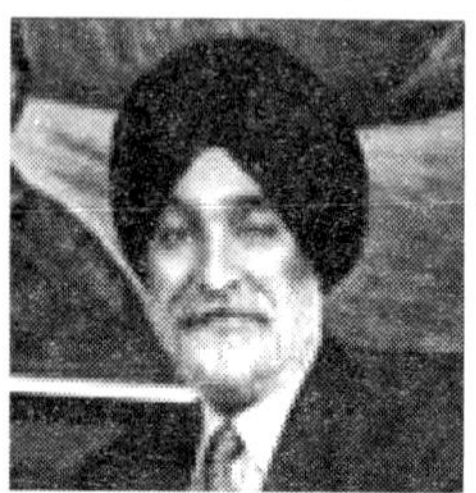

Analjit Singh, MAX INDIA LIMITED

"Health care cannot be franchised. We intend to grow organically and through Greenfield expansions." The NCR's very own hospital brand is ready to foray outside the Capital—from Dehradun to Mohali, Bhatinda to Shalimar Bagh. In the pipeline are 1,050 beds and superspecialties.

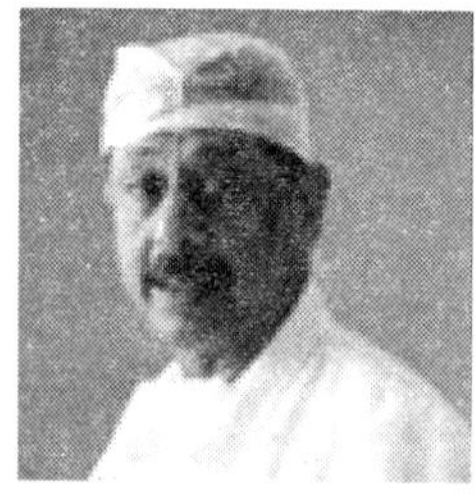

Dr. Naresh Trehan

Ace cardiologist and hospital builder, Trehan, had come up with Escorts to offer world-class treatment and technology in India. This time around, he has moved up the health care delivery ladder with Medanta, a medicity. The Rs. 1,000-crore medi-city is a new model where application and knowledge, cure and prevention, health and wellness, work and leisure, East and West combine. India's newest and largest medicity will have 1,250 beds, 45 OTs, over 1,000 doctors, 20 superspecialties and 48 clinical specialties. Medicity has acquired Rs. 300 crore worth of technology, including the BrainSUITE for neurosurgery, Da Vinci robotic system, a 256 slice CT scanner, molecular MRIS, among others. Wait for the medical college, research unit, wellness centre and other unique features.

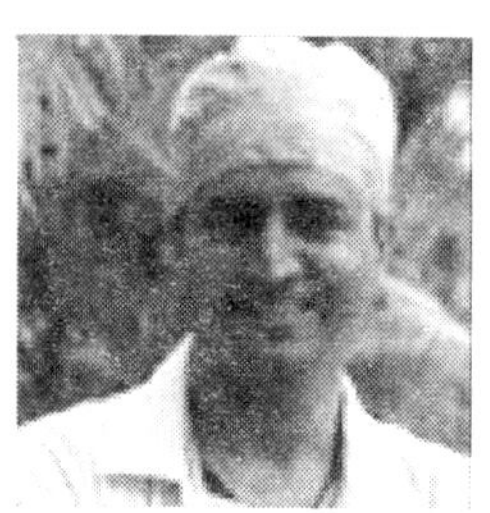

Dr. Devi Shetty, NARAYANA HRUDAYALAYA

"The biggest problem now is that the current health care players are too small. Unless a group has 20,000-30,000 beds, you cannot reduce the cost of treatment."

Dr. Shetty's blueprint remains essentially the same: health cities with advanced technological support at an affordable cost. "Our tele-medicine network has already treated over 53,000 heart patients and is now connected to 56 cities in Africa and Malaysia," he says. His Narayana Hrudalaya is the only centre in Asia to have invested heavily in the artificial heart.

Dr. Jitendra Das Maganti of Hyderabad-based SevenHills Health Care

SevenHills boasts of an infrastructure support from pneumatic tube system, HVAC, purified water system, tele-medicine, track and trace system using RFID and fully covered by WiFi. This hospital is being set-up in a public-private partnership (with Bombay Municipal Corporation) is setting up a hospital on 17-acre plot at Andheri near the Mumbai international airport, with a built-up area of 2 million sq. ft. The hospital has 16 blocks divided into 11 levels. The PPP model is premised on providing five-star hospital treatment at a lower price. It has 1,500 beds, 300 critical care beds, 120 outpatient clinics, 36 modular operation theatres, 30 specialties and an exclusive floor designed with 100 luxury suite rooms for international medical tourists and VIPs.

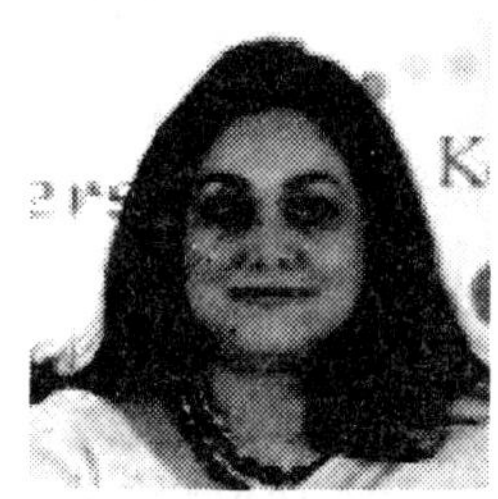

Tina Ambani

Kokilaben Dhirubhai Ambani Hospital and Medical Research Institute is a 19-storeyed building with two basements spread across one million square feet in the posh Four Bungalows area of Andheri, Mumbai. This is the only hospital in Mumbai to function with a full-time specialist system that ensures the availability and access to the best medical talent around-the-clock. The 750-bed hospital has over 103 full-time doctors, 520 nurses and about 200 paramedics, and growing. From high-end salons that even work out hair solutions for chemotherapy patients to stylish restaurants that offer fine dining, art not just on the walls but also on the floor, well-appointed rooms for patients, visitors and a lounge that's dotted with coffee kiosks.

Growth of Tele-medicine

Only 25% of India's specialist physicians reside in semi-urban areas, and a mere 3% live in rural areas. Rest all live in the cities. As a result, rural areas, with a population approaching 700 million, continue to be deprived of proper health care facilities. One solution is tele-medicine--the remote diagnosis, monitoring and treatment of patients via videoconferencing or the Internet. Tele-medicine is a fast-emerging trend in India, supported by exponential growth in the country's information and communications technology (ICT) sector, and plummeting telecom costs. Several major private hospitals have adopted tele-medicine services, and a number of hospitals have developed public-private partnerships (PPPs), among them Apollo, AIIMS, Narayana Hridayalaya, Aravind Hospitals and Sankara Nethralaya.

The early successes of tele-medicine pioneers have led to increased acceptance and proliferation of tele-medicine. Today there are approximately 120 tele-medicine centers throughout India. The Asian Heart Institute, Mumbai (AHI) is planning to establish 60 more tele-medicine satellite centers across the interiors of Maharashtra. The government has also made a major commitment to the growth of tele-medicine. The Indian Space Research Organization (ISRO) plans to establish 100 tele-medicine centers across the country. ISRO has already connected 25 major hospitals in the mainland and plans to link at least 650 district hospitals by 2008. The government also is reducing import tariffs on infrastructure equipment. And while India has yet to pass legislation on tele-medicine-related issues, the Ministry of Information Technology has developed "Recommended Guidelines and Standards for Practice of Tele-medicine in India," with the goal of standardizing digital communication in tele-medicine. The Medical Council of India has formed committees to explore this and other legal aspects of tele-health. There is a growing movement within India to establish a health grid that connects medical institutions and practitioners throughout the country. This would allow super specialists to exchange case studies, compare experiences, and hold virtual conferences to discuss critical disease patterns and provide treatment. Eventually, tele-medicine is likely to be practiced in the majority of Indian hospitals, initially in a separate department, and eventually, integrated into medical specialties.

Health care infrastructure expansion

An enormous amount of private capital will be required in the coming years to enhance and expand India's health care infrastructure to meet the needs of a growing population and an influx of medical tourists. Currently India has approximately 860 beds per million population. This is only one-fifth of the world average, which is 3,960, according to the World Health Organization. It is estimated that 450,000 additional hospital beds will be required by 2010—an investment estimated at $25.7 billion. The government is expected to contribute only 15-20% of the total, providing an enormous opportunity for private players to fill the gap.

Recently we have seen many new investments in health care infrastructure facilities in India. For instance, ICICI Venture, the country's largest private equity fund, has invested $8.6 million in a chain of diagnostics facilities, along with Metropolis Health Services Ltd. And in 2006, General Electric announced a $250 million investment in infrastructure and health care projects in India. With the advent of private insurance and the emergence of India as a medical tourism destination, there also has been a surge of growth in so-called "super specialty" hospitals, which have teams of specialists, sophisticated equipment, links to other medical centers, and the ability to treat a broad range of ailments. One example of an Indian public-private partnership is the Rajiv Gandhi Super Specialty Hospital at Raichur, Karnataka, opened in 2000. This facility is the product of a public-private partnership between the Government of Karnataka and the Apollo Hospitals Group, with financial support from the OPEC.

In addition to a deteriorating physical infrastructure, India faces a huge shortage of trained medical personnel, including doctors, nurses and medical specialists and support staff. The losses during the first three years of operation were borne by the Government. Approximately 30% of the profits from the fourth year onward are to be retained by Apollo, to meet modernization and expansion requirements. In the event there is no profit, the Government is liable to pay a service charge not exceeding 3% of gross billing. Separate monthly accounts are maintained for costs incurred on patients below the poverty line. These accounts are submitted to the Deputy Commissioner of Raichur for reimbursement.

Health insurance trend is on the rise

Time was when health insurance was not considered a safety net. The only insurance everyone knew and opted for was life insurance. That

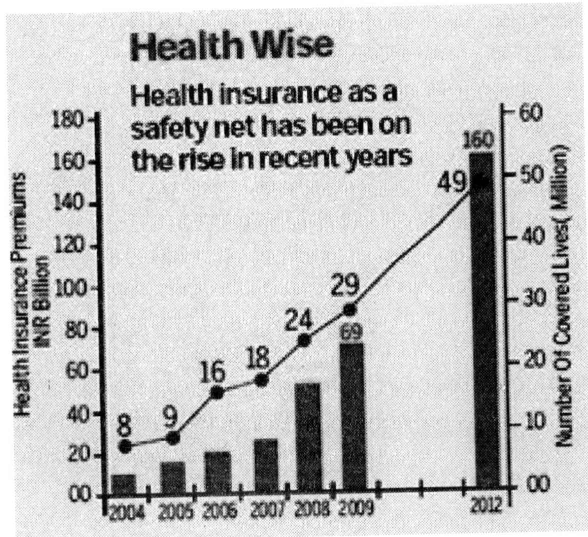

is increasingly a thing of the past. The health insurance business is growing at 50 per cent and is projected to grow to Rs. 25,875 crore by 2010, according to a study by the PHD Chamber of Commerce and Industry. Health insurance premium is also increasing by over 20 per cent every year and many stand-alone health insurance companies are coming into the field, apart from the general insurance companies focusing on health insurance. "This shows the important role played by insurance companies which has driven home the point that health insurance is becoming a very essential part in anybody's life," says V. Jagannathan, chairman and MD of Star Health Insurance, health insurance specialist.

Emerging trends show that today every middle income family feels that health insurance is a must for them, especially upper middle income groups. "Perhaps not to the extent of understanding every nitty-gritty of a policy, but they definitely insist on adequacy of the cover in most cases," he adds. "In the top 20 urban cities, the penetration of health insurance is 12 per cent," says Antony Jacob, CEO, Apollo Munich Health Insurance. Yet another trend is that executive health check-ups have become more common, especially among people above age 40, he explains. Health insurance is also being driven by group insurance covers, as most medium to large companies have group health insurance schemes.

Not just insurance, private equity (PE) funds are upbeat on health care and have invested in several health corporates. But how crucial a role are the PE firms playing in the health care boom in India? "PE firms invested Rs. 4,500 crore in Indian health care between 2006 and 2010," says Krishnakumar, executive director, private equity syndicator, Avendus Capital. Sandeep Singha, MD of Sequoia Capital India, which has invested Rs. 450 crore into health care, agrees: "PE is crucial. Health care requires capital and unless you have PE funding, the evolution of the sector will be slower."

Also, health care is a high-growth area that does not get impacted by an economic downturn. "It's a huge market," points out Singha, "that will be growing for the next 50 years and the market opportunity is staggering." Rs. 900 crore of PE has been invested into Indian health care companies in 2010. It's the surge of private equity in health care that's bringing in young entrepreneurs, often from unexpected backgrounds. Take Dr. Dharminder Nagar. He started work on Paras Hospitals, Gurgaon in 2005. The Rs. 70-crore venture required for this dream project was managed through a debt equity ratio of 1:1. "My father, Ved Ram Choudhary, was a philanthropist and the founder chairman of Paras Group of Industries," he says. From a humble beginning as the owner of a dairy, Paras, he became the largest milk producer and exporter, with interests in real estate across north India. Nagar worked as a doctor in the UK for a while and later joined the Imperial College, London, to study hospital and health systems. "It's this first hand experience as a practitioner in London hospitals that inspired me to bring international quality health care to India," he adds. Paras Hospitals started in Gurgaon in 2005. Within five years, the group has grown 30-40 per cent year on year and acquired a multi-specialty hospital in South Delhi. With easy access to visa facilities, medical tourism is turning out to be the other potential source of income for the health care industry. "It's a growing segment in India, with over 2 to 2.5 lakh annual travellers to India increasing at a rate of 30-35 per cent," says Charu Sehgal, head of life sciences and health care at Deloitte Touche Tohmatsu India. Most large health care providers are increasingly focusing on attracting medical tourists. "Apart from generating higher revenues for the hospital—to an Indian patient—a medical tourist also spends 2-3 times more than a normal tourist in the country." "It is definitely a segment that the big players have in mind as they make their expansion plans," says Sehgal.

Medical equipment market

The rebuilding of India's health care infrastructure, combined with the emergence of medical tourism and tele-medicine, will drive strong demand for medical equipment, such as X-ray machines, CT scanners and electrocardiograph (EKG) machines. Leading international companies market most high value medical equipment, while only consumables and disposable equipment are made locally. Many international companies have expanded their operations in the Indian market in recent years and established manufacturing facilities to assemble equipment for the domestic market and export sales. The competition is expected to intensify with the entry of more global firms into the medical equipment marketplace. The government is encouraging the growth of this market, through policies such as a reduction in import duties on medical equipment, higher depreciation on life-saving medical equipment (40%, up from 25%), and a number of other tax incentives.

Pharmaceutical industry opportunities

India has much to offer the leading drug makers. An increase in lifestyle diseases resulting from the adoption of unhealthy western diets, combined with a growing middle class that has more disposable income to spend on treatment, will provide new opportunities for global pharmaceutical firms.

India has emerged as a major supplier of several bulk drugs producing these at lower prices compared to formulation producers worldwide. The US Food and Drug Administration (FDA) already has approved 85 Active Pharmaceutical Ingredient (API) and formulation plants in India, the highest such number outside the US. India is poised to become a major exporter of pharmaceuticals, particularly generic and OTC drugs, to global markets. By 2010, India could be producing 15% of the world's bulk pharmaceuticals and drug intermediates. However, achieving that level of growth will require an estimated $1.2 billion investment in production capacity. Many multinational generics companies have been sourcing products from Indian manufacturers for some years. Some also use Indian contract manufacturers to manufacture the finished product. Contract manufacturing, currently estimated at $350 million, is expected to reach $1billion by 2010, according to CRISIL. Some companies-encouraged by the relaxation of the rules on foreign ownership and a favourable tax regime-have gone beyond contract manufacturing, setting up their own local manufacturing facilities. The financial incentive is compelling. Goldman Sachs estimates that the cost of setting up and running a new manufacturing facility in India is one-fifth of the cost of doing so in the West. Pharmaceutical research is one area that is expected to achieve tremendous growth in the coming decade, due to India's huge and growing population, low per capita drug usage, and increasing incidence of disease. Global pharmaceutical alliances with Indian drug firms are finally beginning to look like a two-way street, with major R&D deals being struck. For instance, Glenmark Pharmaceutical has teamed with Dyax to identify biological entities for its three targets in cancer treatment, and with Merck KGaA for its prospective diabetes molecule GRC 8200.

GlaxoSmithKline is working with Ranbaxy Laboratories to identify new targets and has partnered with TCS for data management, through a global drug development support center in Mumbai. India historically lacked the expertise to perform clinical trials, because most companies only tested different processes for producing copycat versions of Western products, and the rules were quite lenient. Several drug-makers have also been caught behaving unethically or even illegally.

However, in recent years, India has become a more attractive market for clinical testing. One reason is that in November 2004, the federal government amended Schedule Y of the Drugs and Cosmetics Act to make the rules on clinical trials more consistent with international practice. In addition, in January 2005 India became compliant with the Trade-Related Aspects of Intellectual Property Rights (TRIPS) Agreement and formally recognized product patents. This triggered growth in Indian clinical trial activity by contract research organizations, such as Quintiles, Omnicare, PharmaNet and Pharm-Olam, and by multinational corporations such as Novo Nordisk, Sanofi-Aventis, Novartis and GSK. Some multinationals, such as Pfizer and Eli Lilly, have been conducting tests locally for a while. Government taxation incentives are further boosting R&D in India. As a market for clinical testing, India holds other attractions as well. According to a study by Rabo India Finance, a subsidiary of the Netherlands-based Rabo Bank, the huge patient population offers vast genetic diversity, making the country "an ideal site for clinical trials." It has the largest pool of diabetic patients, the population is relatively easy to access, and many people are "treatment-naïve"; they have not been treated with medications being tested, which potentially could distort test results. Emerging Market Report: Health in India, 2007 (Price-water house Coopers). As a result of these favourable factors, the Indian clinical trials market, currently estimated at $120 million, is expected to reach $1 billion by 2010, according to Info-media. To achieve that level of growth, India will have to address a lack of skilled workers, high wage inflation, and inadequate infrastructure. For western companies that can navigate these obstacles, the rewards will be substantial: Clinical trials account for over 40% of the costs of developing a new drug, and Rabo India Finance estimates that a standard drug could be tested in India for as little as $90 million—60% of the cost of testing in the US.

There is a need to detect and circulate the information about the drug side effects. If this is not done, it can lead to many medical errors and consequent medical disasters. One such example is Rofecoxib (Vioxx). It was approved as safe and effective by the U.S. Food and Drug Administration (FDA) on May 20, 1999. On September 30, 2004, Merck withdrew it from the market because of concerns about the drug's potential cardiovascular side effects. The FDA estimates that in the 5 years that the drug was on the market, rofecoxib contributed to more than 27,000 heart attacks or sudden cardiac deaths and as many as 140,000 cases of heart disease. Rofecoxib was one of the most widely used medications ever withdrawn; over 80 million people had taken the drug, which was generating US$2.5 billion a year in sales. Today, it is reasonable to expect that after an FDA announcement of a drug's withdrawal from the market, patients will be informed and clinicians will immediately prescribe alternatives. However, similar drugs remain undetected indefinitely and continue to be used on and on.... Due to lack of circulation of the information to the doctors and others and also due to lack of stringent laws on this behalf.

Health tourism on the rise

Health tourism is one of the major external drivers of growth of the Indian health care sector. The emergence of India as a destination for health tourism leverages the country's well educated, English-speaking medical staff, state-of-the-art private hospitals and diagnostic facilities, and relatively low cost to address the spiraling health care costs of the western world. India provides best-in-class treatment, in some cases at less than one-tenth the cost incurred in the US. India's private hospitals excel in fields such as cardiology, joint replacement, orthopedic surgery, gastroenterology, ophthalmology, transplants and urology. According to a joint study by the Confederation of Indian Industry and McKinsey, Indian medical tourism was estimated at $350 million in 2006 and has the potential to grow into a $2 billion industry by 2012. An estimated 180,000 medical tourists were treated at Indian facilities in 2004 (up from 10,000 just five years earlier), and the number has been growing at 25-30% annually. India has the potential to attract one million medical tourists each year, which could contribute $5 billion to the economy, according to the Confederation of Indian Industries (CII). In addition to receiving traditional medical treatments, a growing number of western tourists are traveling to India to pursue alternate medicines such as ayurveda, which has blossomed in the state of Kerala, in southwestern India. The number of medical tourists visiting Kerala was close to 15,000 in 2006 and is expected to reach 100,000 by 2010.

Indian government is supporting an initiative by well known heart surgeon Dr. Naresh Trehan to build a "Medicity" in Gurgaon, on the outskirts of Delhi. The compound will include a 1500-bed hospital that supports 17 super specialties, a medical college and para- medical college. The project, on 43 acres of land, will cost an estimated $493 million. The Medicity will integrate allopathic care with alternative treatments, including unani, ayurvedic and homeopathic medicine, and it will provide tele-medicine services as well. To encourage the growth of medical tourism, the government also is providing a variety of incentives, including lower import duties and higher depreciation rates on medical equipment, as well as expedited visas for overseas patients seeking medical care in India.

Right to health, hasty and ill planned

India currently does not have any law to ensure health care to its people. The UK, Canada, Brazil, Thailand, Malaysia, Sri Lanka and the developed nations have such laws.

The Draft National Health Bill, 2009 was prepared on the recommendations of the National Human Rights Commission to recognize and operationalise the right to health care. The demand for such a right was led by the Jan Swasthya Abhiyan, the Indian chapter of the global Public Health Movement. The bill is important as India's health indicators are worse than its poorer neighbours. The country has one of the lowest public spending on health care. While the UPA government had committed to increase the spending to two-three per cent of the GDP, the increase has been from 0.96 per cent to 1.05 per cent. This places India in the league of Burundi, Sudan and Myanmar.

The bill is ambiguous on providing universal and free health care, experts said. It talks of providing free access to health care only for the vulnerable and marginalized. By this, the bill legitimizes a system in which the poor can't access free health care if they don't fall under the targeted sections. Those outside the purview of the targeted sections will have to cough up a fee to utilize these services. The fee will have to be "affordable", experts said. "Targeting vulnerable groups perpetuates and condones vulnerability rather than addressing the issue. Targeting programmes are no substitute for universal health care," Dr. K. Srinath Reddy from the Public Health Foundation of India, said. However, the bill can be used to generate demand for higher health spending. The concept can also be used to demand changes in other sectors, the experts added. For example, it is known that wider income disparity leads to an adverse impact on health—universal entitlement to health care can be used to file public interest litigations to demand an increase in minimum wages and decrease the income gap. Even a trade policy which would have an adverse impact on the right to health can be challenged if there is such a law, Reddy said. The bill also fails to prevent public health services being privatized. "It should assert the role of public sector health services. But, it does not talk about strengthening of the services," Colin Gonsalves, a human rights activist, said.

We may have to learn a lesson or two from Thailand's health care system, before we can provide right to health care. (See Appendix 3 at the end of the book: Health Care System of Thailand).

Sources

F. Mosteller, "Innovation and evaluation," *Science*, Vol. 211, pp. 881-86, 1981, doi: 10.1126/science.6781066.

J. Lind, A Treatise of the Scurvy (1753). Edinburgh University Press, reprinted 1953.

E.A. Balas, "Information Systems Can Prevent Errors and Improve Quality," *J. Am. Med. Inform. Assoc.*, Vol. 8, No. 4, pp. 398-99, 2001, PMID: 11418547.

A.C. Greiner and Elisa Knebel, Eds., Health Professions Education: A Bridge to Quality. Washington, D.C.: National Academies Press, 2003.

E.A. McGlynn, S.M. Asch, J. Adams, J. Keesey, J. Hicks, A. DeCristofaro, *et al.*, "The quality of health care delivered to adults in the United States," *N. Engl. J. Med.*, Vol. 348, pp. 2635-45, 2003, PMID: 12826639.

T.H. Davenport and J. Glaser, "Just-in-time delivery comes to knowledge management," *Harv. Bus. Rev.*, Vol. 80, No. 7, pp. 107-11, 126, July 2002, doi: 10.1225/R0207H.

B.S. Alper, J.A. Hand, S.G. Elliott, S. Kinkade, M.J. Hauan, D.K. Onion, and B.M. Sklar, "How much effort is needed to keep up with the literature relevant for primary care?" *J. Med. Libr. Assoc.*, Vol. 92, No. 4, pp. 429-37, Oct. 2004.

C. Lenfant, "Clinical Research to Clinical Practice—Lost in Translation?", *N. Engl. J. Med.*, Vol. 349, pp. 868-74, 2003, PMID: 12944573.

H.D. Noyes, Specialties in Medicine, June 1865.

3

Will the Indian Medical Cities Deliver Health Care and Promote Tourism?

India's health care delivery has been described as dismal to abysmal. It ranks low even among the third world countries. Poor resources and challenged governance both have been described as the main causes of the collapse of the health care system. While India is having low health care and hence low human development index, many developed countries like USA also lag behind in health care. It is a known fact that 'most developed nations regard health care as a fundamental right and quality health care services as an essential pre-requisite of development'. The finest example of National Health Service provision is the National Health Service (NHS) in the U.K. Developed by the government, the NHS soon became Britain's answer to the global search for an ideal health care model. Its inherent simplicity, being a government managed, socially driven model of equitable health care provision, led to its achieving "cult status" among health care professionals worldwide. Indeed, many countries around the world, especially those in the commonwealth, replicated it unquestioningly. Not only did this make health care provision very expensive for the State, it resulted in inappropriate health service utilization.

Government is unequal to the task

In India government delivered models of health care guarantee social equity; governments in general perform poorly in the service sector, airlines and hospitality being classic examples in the Indian context. Evaluated objectively, the argument that government supported health care initiatives should be exclusively carried through public investment, in public health care agencies, is backed neither by logic nor by experience. Health care delivery, unlike health policy development, is not an area of governmental "core competency." A measured and rational approach that explores various health care delivery models, pilots chosen models judiciously, finally adopting those that have both relevance and viability, is called for.

The citizen must bear a part of the cost

The citizen and the civil society must join the government in providing for an equitable health care for all. It cannot be entrusted to the government alone. We must accept that every health care intervention, from a consultation-interview-examination process, to the conduct of the most advanced investigations and procedures, has a "unit cost" appended to it, this being the cost incurred by the provider in delivering that intervention. The argument in health care must move from the conventional "should there be a unit cost?", to the more contemporary, "who will pay the unit cost?" The responsibility for "unit cost payment" may rest entirely with the state, as for the person below poverty line, or one who is disabled or otherwise disadvantaged; partly the individual and partly the state as in those from lower income groups, the unemployed, public and NGO service employees and other selected populations; and entirely with the individual or other parties contracted on his behalf as in the higher income group individual or private sector employee with employer cover. Any health care model that disregards this "unit cost" that every health care intervention attracts is doomed to fail, for sheer lack of sustainability or viability. Author's study during his recent China visit revealed that Health Care System is working satisfactorily. The citizens have to share a part of the cost of medical treatment.

It is important we acknowledge here that the majority of non-government health care services including health insurance are "for profit" enterprises, accountable to stakeholders and cannot on their own accord guarantee equity of care. Private providers also tend to marginalize those they perceive as "bad clients", people with chronic diseases, pre-existing medical conditions and those who cannot contribute to health care payments on regular basis. However, social responsibility dictates that all health care service providers participate in delivering health care to the have-nots in society and this is possible today in the context of government-driven health insurance schemes that cover families below the poverty line (BPL) for emergency and specialist treatments.

PPP models of health care

Can private and NGO providers step in to formally cover for the government in regions that lack health care provision; tribal areas and hill regions for example? To take the argument a step further, can we not envisage a time when one could walk into any registered health care provider (private, NGO or public) and expect a proportional health care cost subsidy based on one's ability to pay? Will this not guarantee "fair price health care" and thus greater health equity? These and many other questions beg answers in the contemporary context. PPP engagement must develop through a national health care blueprint, amalgamating government, private and NGO sectors in tripartite arrangements for health care provision, with the participation of all stakeholders, patient groups and health care professionals included. We must also engender the political will to legislate alongside for a "national health care guarantee" covering all Indian citizens.

Public-Private Partnership:

- Allocation of Land and Building by the State.
- Operation and infrastructure management undertaken by the private player.
- Profits are shared in an equitable ratio.
- Free of cost services to patients below the poverty line.
- Efficient solution to the lack of quality care in Government hospitals.
- Resolution of financial hurdles faced by private players.
- Elucidation of long-term funding problem.
- Increased ability to raise capital from developmental organisations.
- Successful Example: Rajiv Gandhi Super Specialty Hospital:
    - Partnership between the Government of Karnataka and Apollo Hospitals Group.
    - Financial support from the OPEC Fund for International Development.
    - Provides low cost specialty care to families below the poverty line.
    - Land and Building provided by the State, 30% of profits retained by Apollo.

Concept of Medical City

According to Dr. C.P. Kamle (quoted by Usha Holla), the concept of Medical City is based on such models already operating abroad. It entails "global standard multi-specialty tertiary health care centre, academic and research institution with rehabilitative centers for senior citizens affected with old age diseases like Alzheimers, etc. Such models are seen in Scotland, Boston, France, Algeria, etc." Thus Medicity—an integrated township of superspecialty hospitals, diagnostic centers, medical colleges, R&D, ancillary and subservient facilities, shopping malls, hotels, etc.,—is being tried in many states. There has been an attempt towards setting up of Medicity at Hyderabad a few years ago—which was promoted by NRI doctors from US. It was envisaged to be a Medical Sciences City at Medchal, about 35 kms from Hyderabad, complete with super specialty hospitals of international standards, ancillary and subservient facilities, academics and research institutions, health resort, rehabilitation centers, NRI housing, etc. on a 250 acres of land. But it has been found that after the setting up of two hospitals, the project failed to continue further with its objectives. Thus, the concept of medical cities is neither new, nor comprehensive and not even sustainable in all cases.

In India, the cost of medical/surgical treatment is high and is becoming even higher. Even the insurance companies have enhanced the cost of premium many fold. The cost of consultations, investigations and interventions is also rising rapidly. While the patients are enamored by the glamour of the medical cities, the cost is becoming unaffordable. Will it sustain? Utkarsh Palnitkar, partner, transaction advisory services, Ernst and Young, says, "The medical cities might even translate into higher costs of health care for the consumer." Dr. Rana Mehta, vice-president for health care at management consulting firm Technopak, agrees.

The great divide!

There is a huge gap that exists in the supply of health care to the haves and 'have nots' in our country. India has some of the finest health care facilities, comparable to the very best anywhere in the world, which offer services at a fraction of the cost in the west, yet most Indians can hardly access/afford these. The real challenge is how we bridge this huge divide. It is suggested to build a health care model based on Preventive, Primary, Secondary and Tertiary Health Care centers connected with each other through a hub and spokes system. Indian villages are filthy, people do not have any sense of public hygiene and children, who are most vulnerable, die of infections, which can easily be prevented if only one could improve sanitary conditions in our villages. Not many doctors wish to practice medicine in the hinterlands of the country. The quality of life that he expects for himself and for his family just does not exist in Indian villages as yet. The government has a fairly vast health care infrastructure at the district level. The district hospitals can easily serve as good secondary care hospitals provided they are managed efficiently and are held accountable for the quality of care they deliver. Tertiary health care costs can be significantly brought down if a hospital has a high turn out of patients. Thus, a tertiary hospital can amortize its fixed costs over a large number of patients, bringing the overall costs down. (See Appendix 2 at the end of the book: Tertiary Health Care cannot Sustain in Isolation).

Not for Profit institutions

In what could be the beginning of a medical renaissance, medical cities could change the way medical education and research and development is conducted in India, taking it from public to private to corporate. Interestingly, the turn of the wheel of thought has given birth to a unique concept of research in each mind. Where research at premier institutions like Harvard Medicine, Johns Hopkins and Mayo Clinic continues to redefine medical boundaries, the idea of directly copying therapies, cures and procedures from the West does not go down well with Indians any longer. Institutions like the Mayo Clinic have been modeled to be not-for-profit health care providers because the patients are being treated at a teaching hospital as also because of funds available from numerous foundations and grants.

Medical cities are marked by mammoth investment and long gestation periods. The gestation period can squeeze a lot of money out of the investor without offering much in return. "Here," explains Palnitkar, "the investor needs to look at a de-risking model. This could either be done through leasing or forming strategic alliances."

Commercial alliances have their plus points as well

Fortis thus signed an agreement with real estate developer Ansal API to set-up a 52-acre medical city in Lucknow at an investment between Rs. 500-800 crore (Rs. 5-8 billion). The project, owing to its proximity to the airport, hopes to attract medical tourism as well. Kunal Banerjee, vice president for marketing with Ansal API, explains, "The medical city will be complemented by a hotel and a country club, so there is enough infrastructure to promote medical tourism."

GE Health Care, a medical technology and equipment developer, also collaborated with Trehan's Medicity for developing diagnostic and R&D facility. But Max's Singh warns, "The question is who the stakeholders are and what their expectations are. As a profit-making proposition, it isn't a good model but if the motive is creating a talent and research pool, then it is excellent."

At the same time, industry insiders and analysts admit that there will be no shortage of consumers. "Growing urbanization, consumerism and accountability brought in by brand equity will make sure that private medical facilities continue to do good business because consumers now want facilities that are better than the best," says Mehta. The trend can be related with the growth in the health insurance market. At about 30 per cent CAGR in terms of collection of premium for health insurance, the growth is faster than anticipated.

Medical cities may be the next ideal step

It can be giant step towards building India's health care and medical expertise, but the numbers are still insufficient. More safeguards are needed to protect against greed. Even under the current, growing corporate set-up, a Technopak report points out that almost 90 per cent of the private health care is being serviced by an unorganized sector. The need is to take India's current ratio of 1.5 beds per 1,000 people to the world average of four beds per 1,000. Though this could be done through a trickle-down effect, Mehta believes that it would also require a bottoms-up approach, which would entail starting smaller medicity formats in tier-three cities. Trehan also admits that the way forward is by coming up with a new paradigm and newer cures, and "we will have a small role to play in it".

National Capital Region: Hot Destination for Mega Hospitals

After Delhi, it is now the turn of the National Capital Region (NCR), which includes Gurgaon, Noida and Faridabad to undergo a dramatic makeover in health care delivery. The satellite towns around Delhi have been witnessing a spectacular growth in terms of infrastructure and employment, propelled by MNCs which have set-up state-of-the-art offices here, thus bringing in a cosmopolitan culture.

However, as far as health care facilities are concerned the situation is not very satisfactory, barring a couple of hospitals in Noida and Faridabad. For instance in Gurgaon, which has been touted as the millennium city, there are no proper large hospitals to cater to the needs of the growing population and no proper health care. The projects like the Escorts/fortis Medi-City, Artemis Hospital (Apollo Tyres group) and Paras Health Care might change the health map of Gurgaon.

Artemis Health Institute

Apollo Tyres has forayed into the health care business with the launch of its Rs. 250 crore project Artemis Health Institute in Gurgaon. "The 500-bed multi-specialty tertiary level hospital has already been commissioned. The hospital will focus on three main specialties viz. cardiology, oncology (medical, surgical and radiation) and orthopaedics," says Somnath Chakravorty, CEO, Artemis Health Institute. "Talks are on with two universities in the US for forging an alliance/collaboration at medical and functional levels; there might be exchange programmes, technology transfer, etc." reveals Chakravorty. He adds that Artemis Health Sciences (AHS) seeks to transform India into a health care hub and mark its presence in 25 cities of India by 2015. AHS has four verticals, which include health care delivery (under which the 500-bed hospital is being constructed), research and development, medical education (both medical and paramedical education institutes) and manufacturing medical equipment.

Paras Health Care

The Paras group has also ventured into health care with Paras Health Care and in the first week of May the group is all set to launch

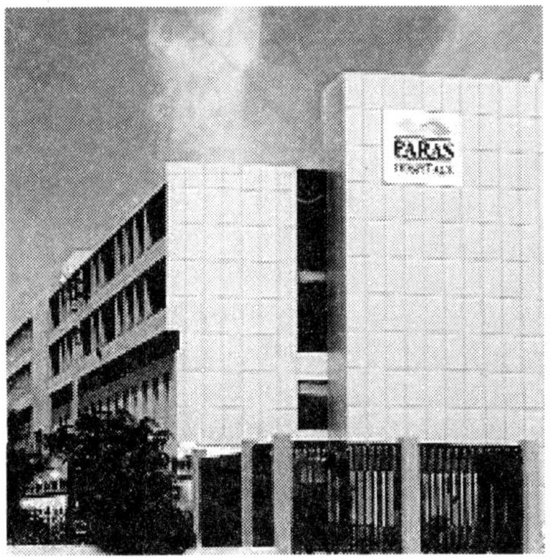

Paras Hospitals, a state-of-the-art 250-bedded, multi-specialty tertiary care facility with super specialty in neuro-surgery, trauma, orthopaedics, and mother and child, in Sushant Lok, Gurgaon. The total cost of the hospital, which is spread over an area of three acres, is over Rs. 100 crore. Paras Hospitals also offer specialised care in cardiology, gastroenterology, nephrology, paediatrics, urology and gynaecology and obstetrics. The seven-storey complex is spread over 2,50,000 sq. ft. and is slated to be one of the most sophisticated health care centres in the Southeast Asian region. Equipped with six state-of-the-art operation theatres, 48 critical care beds, special ICUs and NICUs, sophisticated diagnostics including a 1.5 Tesla MRI, and emergency, ambulance and pharmacy services, functioning round the clock.

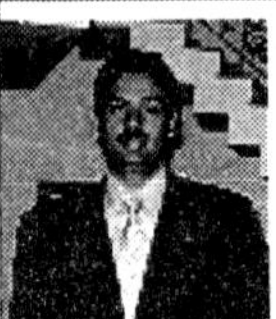

"The total cost of the hospital, which is spread over an area of three acres, is over Rs. 100 crore."

—Dr Dharmender Nagar
Managing Director
Paras Hospitals

According to Dr. Dharmender Nagar, Managing Director, Paras Hospitals can cater to the health care needs not only of Gurgaon, but the entire NCR region. The hospital has roped in reputed experts like Dr. Veer Singh Mehta (neurosciences) and Dr. J. Maheshwari (joint replacements and intricate orthopaedics).

"Gurgaon is our first hospital in the NCR, which has been designed by an architectural team RRP associates specialising in hospitals from Munich, Germany. Paras group's foray into health care is a decision backed not by market perception about health care market growth alone but also part a long-held vision of group chairman late Sh. Vedram Nagar.

Megapolis—the Medicity

Megapolis is strategically located next to fast growing business centers of Noida and Greater Noida and is easily accessible from the Capital of India. Megapolis is uniquely located next to 3 expressways and just 25 kms from the proposed second international airport thus enabling fastest connectivity to major towns and business districts. It is also near an 80 meter wide arterial road. Megapolis is also located in close vicinity to India's first formula one race track and next to (1 km) North India's largest railway terminal at Bootaki on the nation's most modern railway corridor. The township will be easily accessible by the linking expressways like NH 91, East-West Peripheral Express Way, upcoming Taj Expressway and Ganga Expressway.

Realizing the growing concern for health and fitness, Megapolis will have a dedicated medicity. The Medicity will have a large pool of trained, highly skilled and specialized doctors with an army of support staff. With a super specialty Medicity, Megapolis will cater to the growing medical tourism in the country thus attracting many patients from the developed and developing countries. This Medicity will have renowned hospitals, a series of hi-tech medical healing centers with ultra modern health care facilities to take care all of all health related needs. The various facilities in Medicity include full body pathology, comprehensive physical and gynaecological examinations, dental checkup, eye checkup, diet consultation, audiometry, spirometry, stress and lifestyle management, pap smear, digital Chest X-ray, 12 lead ECG, 2D echo colour doppler, gold standard DXA bone densitometry, body fat analysis, coronary risk markers, cancer risk markers, carotid colour doppler, spiral CT scan and high strength MRI.

Medanta—the medical city

It is one of India's largest projects in multi-specialty tertiary care medical treatment is envisioned as an institute that will redefine standards of excellence in health care delivery by bringing together the best of infrastructure, technology, training, education and medical intelligentsia. With an investment of over $350 million, Medicity aims to create a world-class education and training centre backed by remarkable infrastructure, futuristic technology and extraordinary vision of eminent cardiac surgeon, Dr. Naresh Trehan - Chairman and Managing Director of Global Health Private Limited. Located across 43 acres in the new international business-destination in the National Capital Region of New Delhi-Gurgaon, Medicity is a 1600 bed medical institute of world standards. The objective of Medicity is to bring in global health care delivery standards at affordable prices while firmly placing India on the international roadmap as premier destination for health care services, medical research and high-end medical education. Besides offering the best of preventive and curative medicine, Medicity also offers to explore integrating the knowledge of traditional and alternative medicine with modern medicine. Medicity will provide integrated primary, secondary and tertiary care services spanning over 20 super-specialties and high-end services in:

- Cardiology and cardiovascular surgery
- Oncology (including medical, radiation and surgical oncology services)
- Neurosciences (neurology and neurosurgery)
- Musculo-skeletal (advanced orthopedics, joint replacements, rheumatology and physical medicine)
- Transplant services
- Minimal access surgery including robotic surgery
- Advanced pediatrics, neonatology, gynecology and obstetrics
- Ophthalmology
- Internal medicine and respiratory medicine

- Plastic and reconstructive surgery
- Gastroenterology and hepatology
- Dermatology
- Dental and oral health (including oral and maxillofacial surgery)
- Endocrinology

Medicity will have a state-of-the-art research and development centre integrated with the hospital and the teaching establishment. It is planned to be one of the best funded, staffed and managed medical R&D centre in the country. Its Research Advisory Committee will consist of 12 members from amongst the best-known names in modern medicine. (0091-124-42603135/39/42)

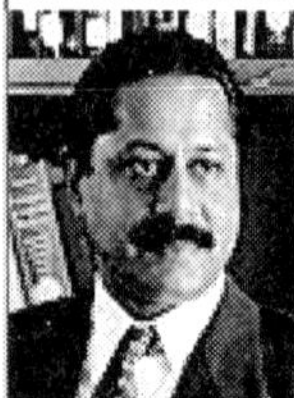

"The hi-tech medical facility will see different streams amalgamating to find a holistic treatment solution for modern ailments."

—Dr. Naresh Trehan
Executive Director
Escorts Heart Institute

Besides a state-of-the-art hospital, there will be research centres, residential areas and hotels. MediCity will have a 1,500-1,800-bed world-class hospital with 20 super-specialties, 40 hi-tech air-conditioned operation theatres equipped for robotic surgery and so on. There will be a medical college and a paramedical college along with a diagnostic and R&D facility in the MediCity campus. "Designed on the lines of the John Hopkins Institute and Mayo Clinic, MediCity is the beginning of a new era of medicine, which will find solutions to make health care affordable and reach the neglected sections of the society," says Dr. Trehan.

Other eminent doctors to join Medanta are several from Fortis and Max, including Dr. Ajay Jha, head of Neurosurgery at the Max Institute of Neurosciences; Dr. Ashok Rajagopal, Dr. Vijay Kher and Dr. Rajesh Ahlawat from Fortis. Sources said they were also likely to bring in their teams. Other doctors who have joined are Dr. Rakesh Khazanchi, head of the Plastic Surgery department at Sir Ganga Ram Hospital and from AIIMS Dr. Sumit Singh, Neurology, Dr. Aditya Gupta, Neurosurgery, and Dr. K K Handa, ENT.

The hospital will have 1,250 beds with 45 operating theatres. It will have eight special departments—the Heart Institute, Critical Care and Anesthesiology, Neurosciences, Bone and Joint Institute, Cancer Institute, Liver and Gastroenterology Sciences, Kidney and Urology Institute and Transplant and Regenerative Medicine.

Dr. Trehan was the Executive Director and Chief Cardiovascular Surgeon of the Escorts Heart Institute and Research Centre for 20 years. He graduated from King George's Medical College, Lucknow and completed his internship at Safdarjung Hospital, New Delhi. He subsequently obtained a diplomat from the American Board of Surgery and the American Board of Cardiothoracic Surgery in the United States at New York University Medical Center. After obtaining his degrees, Dr. Trehan was in private practice at N.Y.U. Medical Center from 1979 to 1988, when he returned to India to set-up Escorts Heart Institute and Research Centre. Dr. Trehan has received many prestigious awards, including the Padma Shree and the Padma Bhushan Award, by the Government of India.

This new global centre will help integrate and explore the new frontiers in the field of medicine and health care on the lines of a Mayo, Cleveland, Harvard and Johns Hopkins in its basics and will go where no conventional medical institute has gone before.

Haryana Urban Development Authority (HUDA) had allotted 43 acres of land for the project. The project will also provide for a cluster of buildings each for a super specialty facility. Research laboratories, education, residential facilities and attendant accommodation facilities will be an integral part of the city.

The proposed project will cater to well-heeled Indians as well as foreigners who would be drawn by the comparatively lower price of treatment.

Fortis International Institute of Medical Sciences

Fortis Health Care Ltd., a local hospital chain, unveiled a Rs. 800 crore investment plan to set-up a 950-bed medical city in Gurgaon, funded by debt and equity in equal parts. To be called Fortis International Institute of Medical Sciences (FIIMS). The first phase of the Fortis venture, to be operational shortly, will require an investment of Rs. 300 crore to set-up 350 beds and initially provide treatment in areas such as oncology, trauma, paediatrics, mother and child, and cosmetology. "FIIMS is going to be our flagship hospital and will contribute significantly in setting new health care standards," said Shivinder M. Singh, Fortis' managing director. Gurgaon will also be the location for a Fortis medical college and a small hospital to treat the poor, added Singh. Fortis, like all other corporate hospitals, is betting on the rising purchasing power and health insurance penetration.

Rockland Hospital

The Rockland Hospital, which started off in 2004, has in its agenda five more hospitals in Delhi and the NCR within the next seven years. Already the group has acquired land plots of five acres each in Greater Noida and Gurgaon. Funding for these projects is through a consortium of banks and the hospital has also collected funds by external commercial borrowing, adds Dr. Das. The hospitals are operational since 2008.

Spread over 52 acres, the Fortis project in Lucknow will see an investment between Rs. 500 and Rs. 800 crore. It will have an 800-bed hospital, a medical college offering undergraduate, postgraduate and post-doctoral courses, a dental college, nursing college, college of physical medicine and rehabilitation, college of rehabilitative medicine and a college of allied medical science.

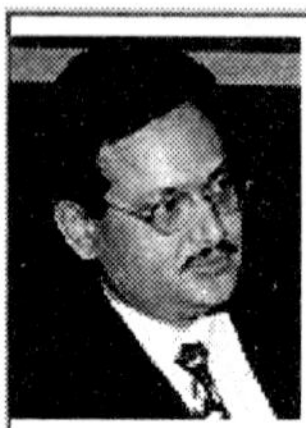

> "The size of the each multi-specialty facility will be 250-300 beds and construction will start simultaneously in June-July this year."
>
> —Dr. Bidhan Das
> Director, Operations
> Rockland Hospital

Apollo Health City

At an investment of Rs. 1,000 crore, this 33-acre project in Hyderabad will not impart undergraduate education. However, it has a postgraduate college for doctors, a nursing school and college, college of physiotherapy, institute of hospital administration, institute of medical informatics, institute for emergency medicine and an institute for paramedics. The hospital has 500 beds and almost 200 more will be added over the next six months

CMC Ajit Singh lottey medicity

A sister concern of the famous CMC, Vellore, the Christian Medical College and Hospital at Ludhiana has initiated a Rs. 50 crore (Rs. 500 million) medicity project in Ludhiana. The project will have a general and speciality hospital and an education institute. However, lack of funds and other hurdles have currently stalled it.

Chettinad Health City

An emerging centre of excellence in health care education, research and patient-care, the Chettinad Health City (CHC) is located in Kelambakkam, about 30 kms from Chennai. Promoted by the prestigious Rajah Sir Muthiah Chettiar Charitable and Educational Trust. The 100 acre, state-of-the-art campus, fast moving to completion, integrates a 600 bed* charitable hospital, superspecialty units and world-class colleges for Undergraduate and Postgraduate studies. CHC also has modern diagnostic labs, emergency facilities and support services.

Kovai Medical Center and Hospital COIMBATORE

It has embarked on a Rs. 200 crore project to establish a Medi City that will comprise a 300-bed cancer hospital, a 100-bed pediatrics wing, an eye hospital and institutions for graduate and postgraduate courses in medicine, paramedical sciences and hospital administration. The project is to be implemented in three phases and expected to be completed in June 2010, to mark 20 years of KMCH's presence in the health care sector, Chairman of the hospital Nalla G. Palanisami said on Friday. The hospital was opened with 250 beds, with an investment of Rs.15 crore, he said. In the first phase of expansion, a 150-bed block would be built to meet the immediate demand for more in-patient bed facility. This would take the total bed strength to 500. Five well-equipped operation theatres, a 20-bed modern intensive care unit and an advanced dialysis facility would also be established. The cancer hospital with seven operation theatres would be built in the third phase of the expansion project, Dr. Palanisami said. It would also have all modern diagnostic and treatment equipment. The construction of the cancer hospital was expected to be over by June 2010. This wing would take the total health care facility area in the KMCH from five lakh to 10-lakh sq.ft.

Apart from the eye and pediatrics hospital, the KMCH would establish a medical college. When completed, this would be the third medical college in Coimbatore and the second in the private sector. The Coimbatore Medical College was being run by the Government and another medical college was being planned on the premises of the Employees' State Insurance Hospital in the city. Dr. Palanisami said separate buildings would be constructed to house a multi-cuisine cafeteria, a nursing hostel, a convention centre with two conference halls, a library and 400-seat auditorium and a food court. High speed internet connectivity for international conferences was among the expansion programme.

The hospital is into efforts to get accreditation from the National Accreditation Board for Hospitals and Health Care Institutions.

It had tied up with Iyer Clinic of London, Gounder Clinic of Chicago and Payal Associates based in Fiji Islands to promote medical tourism and tele-medicine.

Medical City Cochin

This Medical city is from D.M health care group. The group is having plans of establishing various medical firms throughout Kerala. The Medical city at Cochin will be a 500 crore project. The group is having plans of investing 800 crores in the Medical field of India. Along with the medical city Cochin the group will establish a medical college at Wayanad. The new plans were announced by the chairman of the group Dr. Asad Muppan. The Medical city will be constructed in 35 acres of land. The project will be constructed in 2 phases. In the initial stage hospital with 500 beds, convention centre, Hotel facility for Guests and relatives of patients, accommodation facility for doctors and staff will be constructed. In the second stage expert facilities for specialized branched will be established. This includes modern treatment facilities for specialties as eye, heart and cancer. The group is also conducting several social service activities in the medical field.

CMC Vellore

Milestones

1948 - First reconstructive surgery on leprosy patients in the world.
- First Eye camp.

1961 - First Successful open heart surgery in India.
- First middle-ear microsurgery for deafness in India.

1966 - First Rehabilitation Institute in India.

1971 - First kidney transplant in India.

1976 - Artificial kidney Unit.

1977 - Rural Unit for Health and Social Affairs.

1986 - National AIDS Reference and Surveillance Centre.
- Bone Marrow Transplant.

1990 - Infant Open Heart Surgery.
- 1000th live donor Kidney transplantation.

1992 - 10,000th open heart surgery.

1996 - First carotid bifurcation stenting procedure in India.
- First trans-septal carotid stenting procedure in the world.
- First trans-jugular mitral valvuloplasty procedure in the world.

1998 - First Bone Marrow Transplant in a 6 month old baby.

2003 - Palliative Care Unit.
- Vellore-Bombay Artificial Limb.
- India's Best Employer Award.

2005 - First live donor liver transplant.
- First Surgical Ventricular Restoration (SVR).

Quality and Training

What is of utmost importance to CMC is the fact that in all its activities, quality takes precedence. Ideas like the constitution of an infection control committee, audits and documentation have been in practice for long. An infection control committee was set-up as early as 1970, testing for hepatitis, models and guidelines for antibiotics, quality control measures, *et al.*

CMC reported the first case for HIV/AIDS in India. Recalls Dr. G. Chandy, "Nobody believed the reports at that time. But looking at this case, we knew that few years down the line, this is going to wreak havoc in the country." In the aspect of education also, CMC has been bestowed with the highest rating by the NAAC of UGC for its quality courses. The strict quality control measures are reflected in the innumerable firsts it has to its credit. The first open heart surgery, the first kidney transplant surgery, the first home care system in a mental hospital were all initiated by CMC. It is believed that former Principal Dr. Jacob Chandy had said, 'If there is anything in the world that is good and advanced in the field of health care, it must be at CMC.'

Updated technology and high-end surgeries requires skilled employees. It imparts regular training to employees. A formal five-day training programme is held for all trainees. Three days are allotted to teaching trainees and the remaining two days for these trainees to practice with senior employees.

Genesis

Genesis of CMC has its roots to a divine intervention. The story goes that on an evening in 1894, when the young Scudder was sitting in her study a Brahmin knocked at her door requesting her to help his wife deliver their baby. Considering that her father (who was a doctor) was not in. Scudder presumed she could be of little help. The rigid social structure in those times prohibited a man from playing mid-wife, the Brahmin was adamant that Scudder do the delivery. He was sent away. Half an hour later, there was another knock at the door saw a Muslim come with a similar plea. Scudder sent him away rejecting his plea. Half an hour later, another Hindu came to her seeking help but was refused and sent back. All the three women died that night. Narrates Dr. George Chandy, Director, CMC, Vellore, "In a span of two hours, three women died and all this because of a lack of women doctors at that time. For the young Scudder, this was God sending out a message to her." After graduating as a doctor from the Cornell University in the USA, Dr. Scudder came back to Vellore and in 1900 started her first one-bed clinic. In 1902, she built a 40-bed hospital and four years later started a roadside clinic. In 1909, she started the School of Nursing, and in 1918, the School of Medicine—built on the lines of the 'gurukul' system. She travelled regularly to villages, taking medical care to the doorstep of poor villagers living in a famine-struck country with no food and medical help.

Medical Tourism and International Tie-ups

For CMC, medical tourism has a different connotation altogether. Over the years, CMC has seen myriad patients coming in mainly from the North and North-East. "Medical tourism is not new to us. For the past 50 years, even before it became a concept, people from across the country come in for treatment and then visit areas like Tirupati and Sabrimalai," adds Dr. G. Chandy. Dr. Chittaranjan says, "Patients come in from Jharkhand, West Bengal, North-East even Andhra Pradesh and Karnataka." CMC has MoUs with around 20 top-notch universities like the Cornell University, USA, John Hopkins University, University of Adelaide, University of South Australia, University of California and three universities in Europe. Exchange programmes of students as well as teachers are held for research, training education and teaching purposes.

The Future

It is setting up a medicity. "The area will be enlarged to make Vellore a medical city and we have purchased 100 acres of land for the purpose," says Dr. G. Chandy. In fact, CMC has various technology-savvy challenges to face. We have been doing the balancing act of bringing in the latest available technology and at the same time making it available in a country largely predominated by a middle-class society. To be relevant in an industry dominated by international and corporate groups is one of the target aims for CMC. Till then there is never a full stop to the principles of care and commitment services to its clientele.

Even during pre-Independence, founder Dr. Ida Sophia Scudder sought innovative ways to teach students to distinguish between nerves, veins and arteries through various colours. She then graduated to using the Global Positioning System (GPS) to track medical histories of people in rural India. She set-up the Medical College in 1918 and started the MBBS course in 1942. Unusual methods has been one of the reason how the college has managed to establish its name as a not-for-profit organization, and creating a name with innumerable firsts to its credit, while providing surgeries at a subsidized cost to its large middle-class clientele. Today, CMC is a 2,340-bed hospital, a stupendous growth from a 40-bed hospital, housing 5,910 employees and looking after the needs of at least 4,000 outpatients per day.

Brand

According to a report by the US Department of State, Bureau of South and Central Asian Affairs, about 28 per cent of the Indian population lives below the poverty line, but there is a large and growing middle class of 325-350 million whose need requires looking into, as they have the maximum amount of disposable income. CMC aims to cater to this growing populace without plunging into concepts like branding and marketing, as it is understood today. Says Dr. Samuel Chittaranjan, Professor, Department of Orthopedics, CMC, Vellore, "We do not wish to identify ourselves as a marketing brand. We have been here for almost 107 years to serve people and have a strong sense of commitment. That has already established CMC as a brand." "We get large number of patients every day. Many patients paying Rs. 10 can be termed equivalent to one patient paying Rs. 4,000," says Dr. George Chandy, Director, CMC. Even the students pay a mere Rs. 3,000, which is nominal as compared to other medical colleges. Says Dr. Mammen Chandy, Professor, Department of Hematology, CMC, "We do not function as a capitation medical educational centre. Our income is utilized towards medical education."

"A large number of patients paying Rs. 10 is equivalent to one patient paying Rs. 4,000."

—Dr. George Chandy
Director
CMC, Vellore

CMC's philosophy focuses on the poor, the marginalized and the underprivileged, to provide them low cost, effective care with the help of money raised by looking after paying patients.

"We don't need to compete with anyone. We provide the best care to all our patients. As long as we maintain that excellence, competing will not be our strategy," points out Chandy. Chandy says, "Our forte is all our disciplines under one roof. A patient can expect accurate diagnosis because all the disciplines work hand in hand."

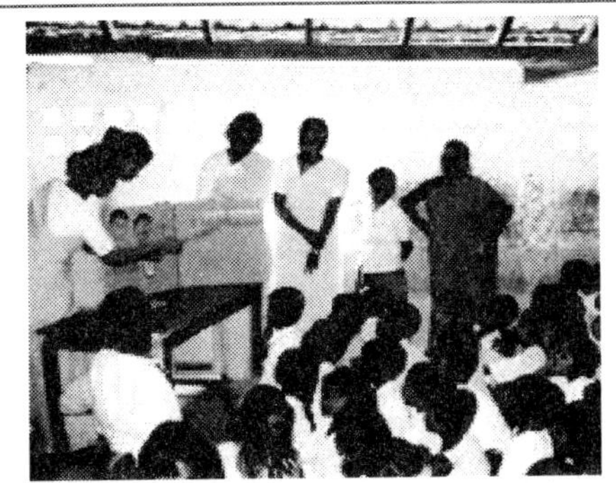

CMC focuses on social outreach programmes for the marginalized section

Hard work has indeed paid-off. Last fiscal, CMC's turnover stood at Rs. 225 crore. This is then utilised for noble causes. "Of Rs. 225 crore, Rs. 42 crore was spent on community outreach programmes and helping poor patients, while Rs. 24 crore went into educational subsidies," adds Dr. G. Chandy.

CMC offers education courses for MBBS, postgraduate diploma courses in 11 specialties, postgraduate degree courses in 21 specialties, nursing courses upto Ph.D. level and 27 allied health science diploma programmes, as well as a distance education programmes. Around Rs. 24 crore is regularly spent on education alone. The growth graph altogether has also been astounding where in the last four years saw a rise from 50 per cent to 200 per cent.

Community Health and Development (CHAD) Programme

Based at Bagayam, about five kilometre from Vellore, CHAD is a part of the Community Health Department of CMC. It provides primary health care for nearly 2,50,000 people in nearby rural, urban and tribal communities and provides training in the principles and practice of community-based health care for medical, nursing and paramedical students, postgraduates and staff from CMC itself. Dr. G. Chandy says this programme has been in practice for the last 50 years. "In fact, The National Rural Health Mission that the Government is planning to implement, is based on the lines of this programme." Outpatient services include special clinics for antenatal patients, high-risk infants, tuberculosis, leprosy and ENT diseases, in addition to daily general clinics. On an average, doctors at the OPD see 180 patients a day. "Nurses from CMC go out, visits homes, conduct regular check-ups and bring people to the hospital," says Dr. Chandy. Regular services such as maternal and child health clinics, morbidity clinics, school health and mothers' programmes are also a part of this. Periodic dental and eye check-up clinics are conducted with the help of the dental and ophthalmology departments of CMC. The LCECU, set-up in 1982, meets the health needs of the urban poor, especially in the slum areas of Vellore. The treatment cost is kept low without compromising on the quality of care. Available technology is used for simple but appropriate tests. The emphasis is placed on 'clinical acumen' and the use of relatives in the nursing care to keep the costs down.

Cuttack Medical City

Sahyog Foundation, a city-based non-profit organization, would invest Rs. 1100 crore in setting up a medicity spread over 300 acres at Jagatpur near Cuttack as well as a medical college and hospital at Keonjhar. The amount will be raised by the foundation through a mix of debt and contributions from the promoters and Non-Resident Indians (NRIs). The Keonjhar project which is being taken up on the public-private partnership (PPP) mode at an investment of Rs. 200 crore will have a medical college with an intake of 50 seats to begin with and a 300-bed hospital.

Construction work on the proposed medical college and hospital at Keonjhar is set to take off in April this year and the first batch of students for the MBBS course will be admitted in 2011. "While the hospital at Keonjhar will offer treatment in various super specialties, the focus will be on malaria and tuberculosis. Seventy per cent of the beds in this hospital will be reserved for the BPL (Below Poverty Line) families." ... The medical college and hospital at Keonjhar will offer direct employment opportunities to 3000 people.

For its Rs. 900-crore medicity project at Jagatpur, Sahyog Foundation has started the process of land acquisition. The medicity project is expected to be operational by 2014. Besides a 150-seater medical college and a 700-bed hospital, the medicity will have a homeopathic college, an Ayurvedic college and other public amenities like a shopping mall, gymnasium, swimming pool and food court.... Apart from generating around 5000 direct jobs, the medicity will also create indirect employment for 150,000 people.

Apollo Medicity, Pune: Focus on Ayurveda

With an eye on foreign patients, Apollo Hospitals is setting up a medicity near Pune that will offer "first rate ayurveda treatment". The hospital has signed an agreement with Hindustan Construction Co (HCC), a real estate firm, to set-up the medicity inside the upcoming hill station named Lavasa in Maharashtra.

"It's a joint venture between HCC and Apollo. The medicity is coming up over an area of 200 acres," said HCC chairman and managing director Ajit Gulabchand.

"It would be a state-of-the-art health and wellness centre, including hospitals, research and development labs, long-term care centres. We (HCC and Apollo) have pegged Rs. 2 billion as the initial investment," Gulabchand told IANS.

The concept of medicity is a holistic health centre where one can find high-end hospitals, rejuvenation centres, research and development labs and facility for medical education as well. Rajgopal Nogja, president of the Lavasa project, said: "Apart from the regular treatment in which Apollo has done very well over the years, the major focus would be ayurveda." This medicity would be a huge wellness centre rather than just a tertiary hospital," Nogja said. "There would be adequate facilities for ayurvedic healing of various diseases and complete rejuvenation. There would be various types of massage facilities as well. The effort will boost the medical tourism scenario in the country.

"Besides ayurveda, the medicity will do extensive research on cancer and heart related issues. We will have a full fledged R&D lab," he said, adding the medicity would be an hour's drive from Pune.

HCC is building a hill station over 12,500 acres near Pune at a cost of Rs. 440 billion ($11 billion). Nestled in the picturesque Sahyadri mountains along a 20-km long lake, the Lavasa hill station will have all kinds of facilities, including five-star hotels, a library, a golf course and a convention centre. The authorities said looking at the picturesque setting, nearly two million tourists would be expected to visit the township after the completion of the entire project. "These tourists can avail themselves of both health care and rejuvenation at our medicity," he said.

Oxford University is also setting up a business research centre inside the hill station.

Fortis Medicity, Lucknow

Ansal Properties and Infrastructure Ltd has announced that the Company has signed an Agreement with Fortis Health Care Holding Ltd, (Fortis) for setting up a world class Medicity at its Project, Sushant Golf City, located in Lucknow (U.P). In terms of the said Agreement, Fortis shall, set-up Fortis facility for medical treatment and teaching at the Sushant Golf City, Lucknow. The Medicity is planned to be spread over 52 acres of land and to be completed in about 7 years. It will have an 800 bed ultra modern hospital along with teaching facilities. The Medical College is to offer undergraduate medical courses, specialized postgraduate and post-doctoral courses. The Dental College is to provide both undergraduate and postgraduate dental education. The Nursing College in the Medicity will offer graduate, postgraduate and post-doctoral nursing education. Moreover, the Medicity will have a College of Physical Medicine and Rehabilitation, a College of Rehabilitative Medicine, and also a College of Allied Medical Science offering Para medical and technical training.

There will also be a College of Pharmacy which will offer graduation, postgraduation and doctoral education. The entire facility will be based on the norms set by Medical Council of India, Dental Council of India, Indian Nursing Council, Rehabilitation Council of India and Pharmacy Council of India.

Rapid Rescue Services

Gurgaon-based Rapid Rescue Services has launched an emergency medical rescue service across the Capital and Gurgaon. Colonel (Retd.) Rahul Pandey, in-charge of operations and HR said: "In case of an emergency, registered members in both Delhi and Gurgaon will be attended to by doctors within a time span of 30 minutes. We aim to provide fast, effective and reliable medical service. To help the team reach the patient faster, the company has bought 30 modified bikes, which have Global Positioning System (GPS) installed and blink-lights mounted on them. This will not only help the doctor find the exact location of the patient, but will also make sure he reaches the patient as fast as possible even during peak traffic hours. The service will be available 24×7, 365 days a year, to all customers signed into a plan, in Delhi and Gurgaon."

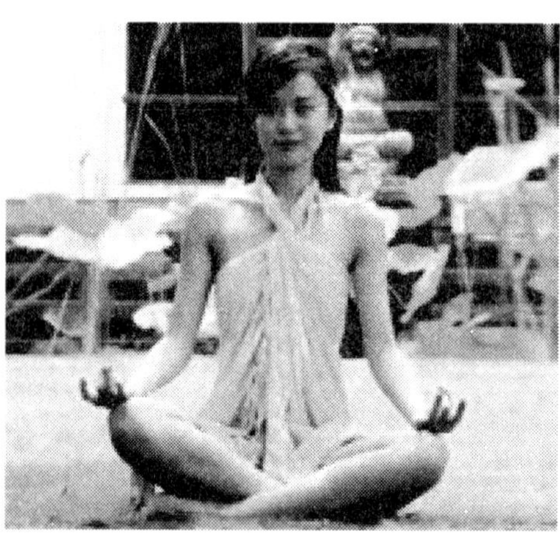

The team at present comprises 30 bikes and a team of 30 MBBS doctors and riders. "Other than these doctors, we have the facility of three general physicians at our customer care centre for members who want by-phone consultation. Members are also free to call any number of times," said Pandey. The company has floated two types of memberships—Gold and Silver. The annual subscription charge for the gold membership is Rs. 15,000 per person; any additional membership will cost Rs. 7,500. "Gold members will be located using a GPS key ring. In the event of an emergency, the customer has to press a predefined number on their mobile phone. This will send a message to the customer-care centre, who will inform the nearest team." Silver membership customers need to call the toll free number—1800 102 3005.

They would be given medical treatment at the incident scene and, in case of a life-threatening emergency, can be taken to the nearest or desired hospital in an ambulance. The annual subscription fee for two members of a family is Rs. 10,000 per year. Additional membership costs Rs. 2,000. Apart from patients' preferences, the company is also in the process of tying up with prominent hospitals across the two cities—Max Health Care, Moolchand Hospital, Apollo and a few government hospitals.

Ayurveda: The Indian system of medicine in upswing

If your normal perception about Ayurveda is limited to spas and some herbal treatments from Kerala, then its time to rethink. The boardrooms of most corporate health care players are now reverberating with plans to set-up huge medicities solely dedicated to Ayurveda. The pioneers of private health care—Apollo Group will also be a pioneer in this segment. This medicity is coming up near Pune that will offer ayurvedic treatment. It has signed an agreement with real estate firm, Hindustan Construction Co. (HCC), to set-up the medicity inside the upcoming hill station, Lavasa in Maharashtra. "It's a joint venture between HCC and Apollo. The medicity is coming up over an area of 200 acres. We (HCC and Apollo) have pegged almost Rs. 2 billion as the initial investment," says Ajit Gulabchand, Chairman and Managing Director, HCC. "It would be a state-of-the-art health and wellness centre, including hospitals, research and development labs and long-term care centres," says Raghav Rao, Vice-President—Projects, Apollo Hospitals. Now, if a giant like Apollo is investing so much in Ayurveda treatment, it is indication enough about how bullish health care providers are about this segment. On the same lines of Apollo, another big player to tap this market is Hinduja Group who will foray into wellness by setting up the World Knowledge Centre (WKC). WKC will be built on the philosophy of multi-disciplinary approach to health care wherein traditional Indian system like Ayurveda, yoga and meditation would be integrated with modern medicine, so as to provide comprehensive health care to treat complete range of illnesses, whether they are chronic, stress-oriented or lifestyle related. To authenticate its therapies, WKC would also be upgraded with a clinical R&D setup wherein the ayurvedic preparations would be clinically tested. The project would take 36 months to complete and the Group plans to spend almost $ 270 million that is approximately Rs. 1200 crore, in this mega project. Says PC Sood, Project Head, WKC, "WKC will provide quaternary care health, have three hospital premises with a capacity of 900 beds, 200 suit, five to seven residential facilities for dependents with service apartments, modern plaza with lavish food courts, wellness centers and clubs, convention centre, R&D for advanced medical research, e-library and a helipad." It would be equipped with state-of-art diagnostic centre and modern spas and wellness clinics. Initially, the Group will have only one such centre and subsequently more such models would be setup in each region in India. After the concept matures over a period of time, the Group plans to franchise it overseas.

Evolving Market

It is estimated that the total market size of the Indian Ayurvedic market is Rs. 500 crore and it is growing substantially between 8-10 percent, with the same growth rate targeted for the next five to 10 years. "The current market is estimated at US $ 1 billion. But the potential for growth is immense as we interact with consumers at the confluence of wellness and natural healing. The market is pushing the boundaries across the board with Ayurveda at its core," states Jitu Mehta, President, Katra Group—Kerala Ayurveda, a health care service chain which provides Ayurvedic products, therapies, resort experiences, and an academy learning mode. The Group has aggressive expansion plans locally as well as globally. It plans to roll out 50 clinics across India. Kerala Ayurveda currently has 30 clinics, predominantly in south India which are being revamped and modernised. In the US the company has three clinics and four academies that offer courses in Ayurveda. In the next two years, it intends to have a total of 10 units in US and would also look at entering Europe later. "We have infinite scope. Our touch points include 300 plus products and a national clinic network that is expanding rapidly. We opened clinics as far apart as Pondicherry and Delhi within six weeks, resorts, hospitals and centres across the US. Hundreds of students are trained in our academy in India and US," adds Mehta. Kerala Ayurveda's resort format, Ayurvedagram, will also be replicated in other locations within India initially. Mehta intends to make Kerala Ayurveda a global brand and introduce Ayurveda as a way of life. "I brought in a colored, carbonated drink into the country (Pepsi). If I can do that, I am much more comfortable propagating a healthy way of life. If I have brought in international brands into India, now I intend to make an Indian brand global," he states passionately.

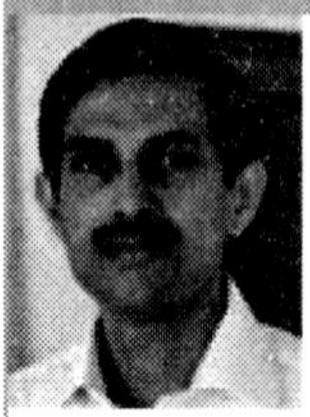

"We plan to set-up 40 hospital chains across India. We will position our services across the value spectrum, ranging from BoP patients to high-end patients."

—Rajiv Vasudevan
Founder and CEO
AyurVaid

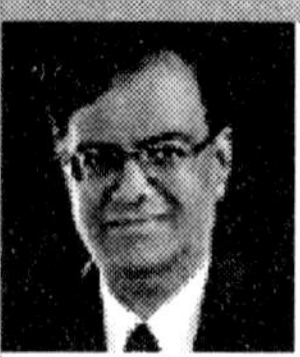

"The current market is estimated at $ 1 billion. The market is pushing the boundaries across the board with Ayurveda at its core."

—Jitu Mehta
President
Kerala Ayurveda

The company has also tied up with Manipal Cure and Care (MCC) wellness centre at Pune to provide Ayurvedic services. "We are the only full spectrum, listed Ayurveda company in the world. We are integrated from herb farms to clinics in the US. We are a one stop wellness solution. MCC is a unique, very important route to reach urban, up market consumers," adds Mehta.

Cardiac Rehabilitation Centre

Madhavbaug is a rehabilitation centre focusing only on cardiac diseases which is establishing itself all across Maharashtra and other states.

"We have already covered almost whole of Maharashtra with centres in Mumbai, Nashik, Pune, Jalgaon, Sangli, Aurangabad, Kolhapur and many more to come in Maharashtra itself. Next states to be targeted will be Gujarat and Goa," informs Dr. Rohit Sane, MD, Madhavbaug Cardiac Rehabilitation Centre, located in the outskirts of Mumbai. The list of groups looking for setting footprints across India does not end here. Kerala based AyurVaid Hospitals has a highly aggressive plan of setting up 40 ayurvedic hospitals across India from the current strength of two hospitals in Kochi. For its ambitious growth plans it has already attracted investment from the Private Equity firm Acumen which has announced an initial investment of Rs. 4.5 crore. "We are one of the few chains that will focus on bottom of the pyramid with 70 per cent of its capacity focused on poor patients. There are two hospitals in Aluva and Cochin, Kerala that are functional and around 40 more will come up across India based on the hub and spoke model," beams Rajiv Vasudevan, Founder and CEO, AyurVaid. AyurVaid plans to leverage Acumen investments to expand its footprint and pioneer the development of a low-cost health care delivery system that focuses on preventive and curative care, as an alternative to the highly capital intensive and curative system presently used to treat chronic ailments. Acumen's initial equity investment will support AyurVaid's plan to open six more hospitals across the country in the next 12 months, including two 'AyurVaid Seva' (AV-Seva) hospitals that would exclusively focus on low income group (BoP) patients. AyurVaid has set itself the goal of 60 per cent of its bed capacity for patients from the middle and lower socio-economic classes. "AyurVaid's health care delivery model for chronic illnesses can be positioned across the value spectrum ranging from BoP patients to high-end patients from India and abroad, permitting a viable and profitable business model," believes Vasudevan.

Growth Drivers

The reasons for so many groups flooding for ayurvedic health care are manifold. The growth drivers for this industry are not only the yawning gap of demand supply but the rising incidences of chronic diseases. The PWC Study for World Economic Forum's 'Working towards Wellness' programme highlights that deaths from chronic diseases will register a sharp increase from 3.78 million in 1990 to 7.63 million in 2020 accounting for 66.7 per cent of all deaths. Chronic diseases would be the number one killer in India. "The current growth rate of Ayurveda can be attributed towards lifestyle related disorders only, other disorders will obviously increase the count in the future," says Dr. Sane, who solely focus on cardiac diseases.

The ayurvedic health care providers view this as a huge opportunity to grow as currently there is no cure available for such ailments as far as conventional medicine go. Agrees Vasudeven, "Modern health care delivery system has done a great job in diagnosis and cure of most illnesses. But chronic illness is one area where its advantages pale in comparison to traditional systems like Ayurveda. By infusing modern medical practices we are creating a reliable and replicable system akin to allopathy which will make Ayurveda the choice of millions with chronic illnesses over the next decade."

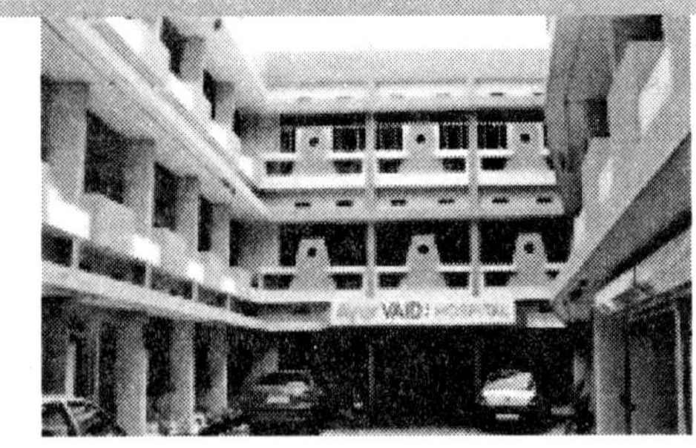

Private Equity firm Acumen has invested Rs. 4.5 crore in AyurVaid for its pan-India expansion plans

The second reason for alternative medicine to flourish is the paradigm shift of health care from curative care to preventive care. It is in this segment that systems like Ayurveda score well. The 'wellness trend' is also gaining momentum in the health care, firstly, because of the new aged well-informed consumer who is becoming health-conscious. Secondly, due to inflation and ever-increasing cost of high-end medical care, people are ready to invest more time and energy in preventive health care products and practices. "This is causing a rapid increase in the demand for value-added wellness products particularly the nutritional supplements (both in India and abroad). In India, lifestyle disease is already the prime killer mainly in cardiovascular disease and diabetes. Hence, health care is becoming expensive and Indians are taking to wellness and preventive health care practices in droves," agrees Ashutosh Garg, Chairman and Managing Director, Guardian Lifecare.

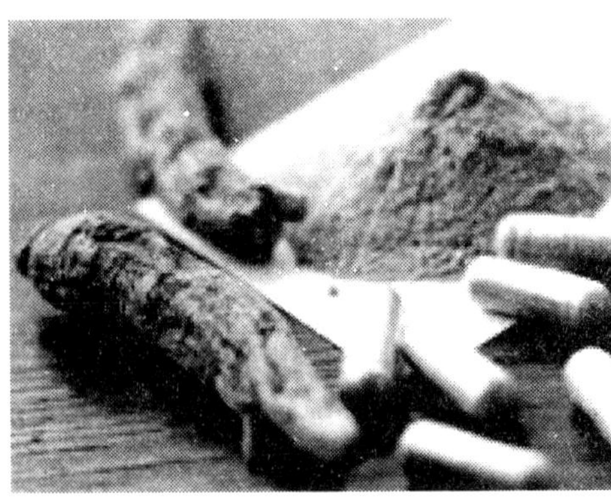

Business Models

Since the health care Ayurveda market is yet at nascent stage, the groups are experimenting with almost all kinds of models for expansion. Be it the hub and spoke model or joint ventures, tie-ups or franchisees—all the expansion routes are on the radar, depending on the target audience.

AyurVaid Hospitals will be establishing through the hub and spoke model, trying to reach maximum audience as possible. "We just opened a hospital in Bangalore and within a few months will be establishing a hospital in the city of Mumbai. The demand for such health care is huge with a population of 18 million people and not a single Ayurvedic hospital available. Hence, we are confident that we would survive well," informs Vasudevan. Since it is targeting the middle and lower-income groups by offering subsidised health care, the Group has tied up with leading insurance players to make the model economically sustainable by generating volumes. AyurVaid Hospitals is accredited by 12 of India's leading medical insurance service providers facilitating cashless Ayurveda medical management, subject to the terms of the underlying insurance policy. "In tying up with leading insurance players and standardising a low-cost and cross-subsidy model, it is a pioneering way to bring affordable services to low income communities, increasing both the quality and the accessibility of treatment available", says Acumen Fund Country Director, Varun Sahni.

Talking about tie-ups, leading Ayurveda health care services provider, Kerala Ayurveda is looking for expansion through a multi-pronged strategy. The tie-up with MCC is to target upmarket consumers. "Our current focus is large urban centres. The franchised clinic model has a potential for deeper penetration we have Dehradun and Vadodra on our map. The need for wellness is global. Wellness naturally has a very strong resonance. Our delivery skills at a local level are formidable. We will not be limited by geography—rather, we will be led by consumer pull. The description of our market is in integrated consumer reach. Wellness naturally can be within driving distance of 250 million consumers within five years. The products strategy will make us ubiquitous," reveals Mehta. As for Madhavbaug Group which has plans to open new centres all across Maharashtra and nearby states like Goa, it will expand on a stand-alone basis as well by the franchisee model. "Initial investment for opening a clinic is around five lakh (if the space is rental and not owned)," informs Dr. Sane.

The companies also plan to increase their reach by complementing instead of competing with the allopathic doctors. It is the concept of integrated medicine that is catching up. "We heal patients referred to by hospitals, and it helps the hospitals to reduce their occupancy time," informs Dr. Issac Mathai, Founder, Soukya, a holistic centre in Bangalore. They receive patients from Manipal Hospital, HOSMAT Hospital, MS Ramaiah Hospital and NIMHANS, Bangalore.

Re-Branding

Whilst the opportunity is immense so are the challenges. The number one challenge this traditional health care system is facing is its brand value. Most people still associate Ayurveda with rejuvenation and relaxation instead of a preferred module for hardcore 'treatment' option. "As Ayurveda is marketed as a preventive therapy by the wellness industry, people hardly know that it has got a great power to cure. The doctor themselves have hammered that it takes time to cure in case of Ayurveda. All these notions have been proven faulty at Madhavbaug, where a fatal disease like heart disease is treated in mere six days. We have been educating the masses how Ayurveda is helpful for the mankind in case of severe and chronic diseases," reacts Dr. Sane. This feeling is unanimously echoed by all the Ayurvedic treatment providers who still feel that because of the way it has been marketed by tourism and hospitality industry, people still find it hard to believe that Ayurveda can be a first line treatment option. "It is the number one challenge the industry is facing. Because spas and wellness resorts are just a part of Ayurveda. It has to move beyond being a 'massage industry.' Also even in North India, the perception is limited to 'jadi-bootiwalas' and it is definitely beyond that. It is a matter of time that people would be aware of the curative powers of Ayurveda and who knows in the future that it may be a first line therapy treatment," believes Vasudevan. Too ambitious we may think, but fast forward a few years and maybe it would indeed be a preferred health care modality and no more it would be a case of Allopathy *vs.* Ayurveda but indeed Allopath vis-à-vis Ayurveda. It's ultimately the 'new' consumers who will decide the fate of the 'oldest' form of medicine.

Himalayan Institute Hospital and Medical City

The Himalayan Institute is one of the first accredited medical schools in India, integrating both modern and traditional medicine. Adjacent to the school is a 700-bed hospital, serving approximately 10 million people from the neighbouring towns and villages. A range of inpatient and outpatient services, including a "combined therapy program" (CTP) forms a vital part of the institute. Services include biofeedback, yoga, nutrition, counselling, breathing, relaxation, meditation, and self-awareness techniques. With its integration of different medical systems, especially with respect to such illnesses as heart disease, hypertension, diabetes, and age-related disorders, the CTP has become the focus of current research at the institute. Specific programs are also being developed to study the various pharmacologic agents used in traditional medical systems, such as ayurveda (Indian science of medicine), to treat women's illnesses, arthritis, and neurologic and chronic respiratory conditions. With the focus on physical, mental, and spiritual dimensions of health, this institute continues to attract international attention for its unique therapeutic and educational health care initiatives.

Rural Development Institute

The most impressive aspect of the institute's work is its rural outreach program that serves about 100,000 people living in the Garhwal region of northern India. People in these rural and remote mountainous areas have little or no access to medical care. Travel is difficult, and those in need of medical attention die before reaching a hospital. With initial funding from the Canadian International Development Agency, the Rural Development Institute (RDI) project was started in 1991 and today, through its 16 remote centers, serves approximately 300 villages with basic health care services, education, and income-generation programs, all installed at the village level. The health care component of the RDI is provided by mobile medical clinics run by general practitioners, specialists, and paramedics.

Basic health care services and information about areas such as appropriate shelter, externally ventilated stoves, clean water, effective sanitation, child care, immunization, and prenatal care are emphasized. Ongoing projects on women and child health, health fairs, school health, and water and environmental sanitation are described. Because women who know more about health promotion are more likely to make better decisions on matters affecting their own and their family's health, the RDI has made women and children's health care an important focus.

The women and children health care project, funded by Indian national and state governmental agencies, currently runs 12 clinics that disseminate information, education, and counselling, all implemented at the village level. The "bottom-up approach" is encouraged, where village health committees choose local people to be trained as health service providers. These village health workers enable the community to assume responsibility and ownership for sustaining health care services in the future.

Through partnership with the Government of India's Department of Health and Family Welfare, the RDI provides six health fairs throughout the state of Uttar Pradesh. In 1996, the RDI started a school health project that provides health screening and services to primary school children. Innovative audio-visual aids, such as puppetry, debates, and quiz games, are used to teach health and hygiene to children. The water and environmental sanitation project forms an essential part of health promotion (surveys show that three out of five people in developing countries do not have access to safe drinking water). With partial funding from the World Bank, this project is currently being carried out in 50 villages in the hill districts of northern India. Water purification and storage practices are taught to avoid the spread of water-borne diseases, such as dysentery, cholera, and hepatitis. Self-reliance and community involvement in planning, constructing, and maintaining proper sanitation is encouraged. Approximately 10% of the costs of the project are carried by the community.

The education component of the RDI includes ongoing health education for nurses, certification programs for village health workers, and traditional birth attendant training in safe deliveries. A reduction in maternal and infant deaths has been observed over the last few years as a result of these programs. Other positive outcomes include awareness of better nutrition, family planning, protection against sexually transmitted diseases, and respect for female children. Recent reports show an increase in immunization rates by 35% over the last 5 years.

As women's education and incomes are important factors in the use of health care services, RDI's income-generation programs were introduced to provide women members of rural families with opportunities for self-employment viz. stitching, embroidery, tailoring, typing course; courses in beekeeping; and training in incense stick and chalk-making.

Vibrant Gujarat; Health Care and Health Tourism in the upswing

Gujarat, being an economically stable, industrially and agriculturally developed state has become one of the most favoured medical destinations too.

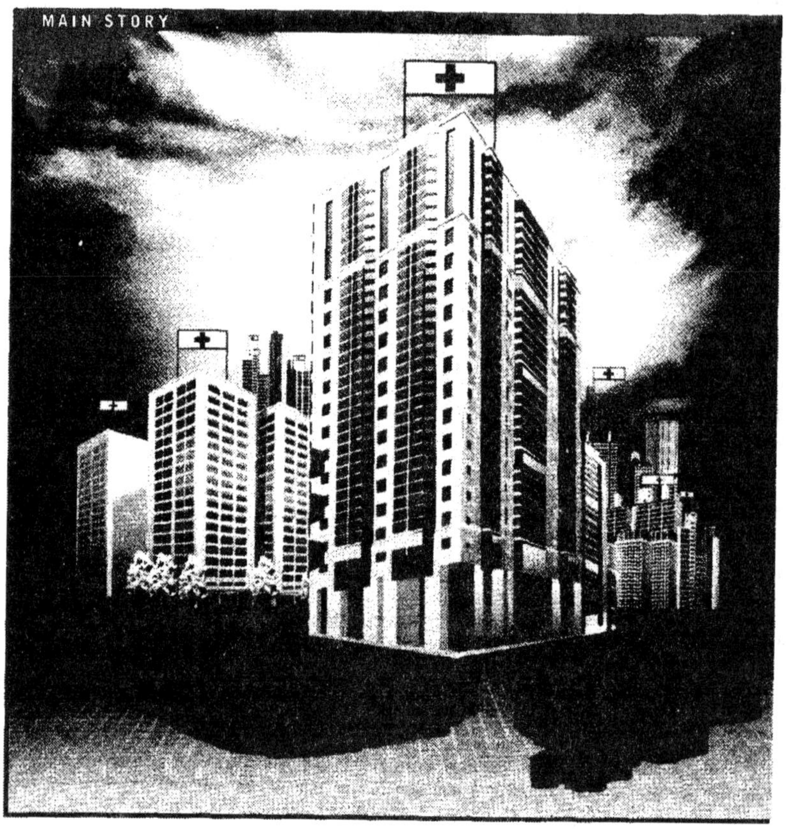

Gujarat, a state which has achieved a stupendous 12.5 per cent industrial growth rate from 2002-07, a GDP growth of 10.2 percent and a contribution of almost 20 per cent of Indian exports, has a similar success story to share when it comes to health care. (Sonal Shukla, Express Health Care)

From Strength to Strength

This land of Mahatma has always played an important role in the economic history of India. Today, Gujarat is believed to be fast transforming into a health care hub with the focused Government-led health care initiatives with leading corporate health care groups entering this market.

The state currently has 13 medical colleges, 1,072 PHCs; 7,274 sub-centres, 273 Community Health Centres (CHC) and 85 mobile health care units. Experts agree to the fact that the health care landscape in Gujarat has been changing rapidly. "The State Government has undertaken several initiatives to make Gujarat a global health care destination. Gujarat is fast evolving in terms of number of hospitals, health care centres and beds and is expected to continue a positive trend in future," snares Pradip Kanakia, Head of Health Care, KPMG, India.

The available medical infrastructure and easily accessible health care facilities have remarkably improved the health index of the population over the last few years. Well developed ports, roads, airports, rails are also said to be responsible factors. Gujarat, being an economically stable, industrially and agriculturally developed state, has therefore become one of the most favoured medical destinations. From dominance of small nursing homes, 25-years back, today Gujarat has made a rapid progression to the state-of-the-art tertiary care corporate hospitals getting established in major as well as two and three-tier cities. Experts give credit for this rapid development to the changing mindset of the patients who have become quality conscious and more aware of their health care needs. Besides, growing per capita income and want of specialized and sophisticated health care has given further impetus to this health care boom. "Currently, Gujarat health care market is standing on a verge of great take-off. Medical tourism, enhancement of existing medical infrastructure, involvement of state Government in improving other facilities has significantly boosted health care market in Gujarat," says Dr. Praful Pawar, CEO, Apollo Hospitals, Ahmedabad.

Land of Opportunities

Other major private players in this market are Shalby Hospitals, SAL Hospital, Medisurge hospital, Krishna Heart Institute.

Sterling Addlife India Limited that owns and manages the largest chain of corporate hospitals in Gujarat, in terms of bed strength and markets covered, under the brand name of Sterling Hospitals, today boasts of 725 operational beds in Rajkot, Baroda, Ahmedabad and Mundra SEZ. "We are coming up with three more hospitals in Surat, Bhavnagar and Baroda, which will further ramp up the capacity to more than 1,000 beds by the end of this year. We plan to build a chain of corporate super-speciality hospitals in Gujarat. We strongly believe that we are operating in an underserved market and outstanding opportunity for private health care delivery exists in every city in Gujarat in which we have entered and planning to enter to deliver best in class health care," according to Rajiv Sharma, CEO, Sterling Addlife India Limited. Sterling Hospitals Group plans to invest close to Rs. 200 crore in various green field and O&Ms in the state. "We are going to leverage our brand to workout a sustainable model by charging for it," he adds further.

Ahmedabad-based 240-bed Shalby Hospitals, which started as a single speciality hospital giving orthopaedic care, is also on an expansion spree. The hospital is coming up with three new multi-speciality hospitals—two in and around Ahmedabad and one in Surat. "We are planning to add 600-700 beds together in all these three hospitals. The construction will start in a couple of months and we plan to complete it within 15-18 months," shares Dr. Vikram Shah, Chairman, Shalby Hospitals, Ahmedabad.

Artemis Health Science

It has been reported that Artemis Health Science is planning to set-up a Rs. 500 crore medical education hub on the Baroda-Ahmedabad highway in Gujarat. The medicity envisions a research centre, a medical college, nursing college, pharmacy college, medical administration college and a hospital which will have over 500 beds. Bombay Hospitals has signed an MoU to establish an Under Graduate and Postgraduate Medical institute with MS Hospital. Twenty-five-year-old and 210-bed Rajasthan Hospital, which is a major trust hospital, has plans to expand its bed strength to 250 beds. The hospital is planning for a separate cardiac wing, new ophthalmic centre, bone marrow transplant and stem cell unit. "Ahmedabad is a big city and we would like to start two-three OPD and emergency management city centres in Ahmedabad. We see a big opportunity in critical and emergency care management," shares Dr. Nitin Shah, Director, SAL Hospital, Ahmedabad.

The State Government is also reported to be joining hands with private players to set-up medical education facilities in the State. According to Dr. M.M. Anchalia, Medical Superintendent, Civil Hospital, investment is happening from both private and Government. "Our State budget has doubled in the last two years for health care sector. We are getting aid from Central Government and state Government.

In the year 2009-10, the health department of Gujarat Government has planned to extend the services and start new medical colleges. "One such college is likely to come next year in Patan. The plans are on for four medical colleges in Ahmedabad, Gandhinagar, Vadodara and Valsad. Hopefully one or two should start next year," adds Dr. Anchalia.

Narayana Hruduyalaya, Fortis Health Care, and Artemis Group of Hospitals are planning to set-up medical colleges in the State. The Chiranjeevi Scheme, which has been touted as one of the few PPP success stories in health care, has significantly reduced the rate of maternal and infant mortality.

Care with Quality

It won't be an exaggeration to say that the health care sector in Gujarat has come in the limelight by adopting global practices to deliver seamless patient care of quality. "Gujarat's medical expertise and the strength of its facilities are arguably better than those of some of the South-East Asian Nations and Gujarat hospitals are trying to do a lot more hard

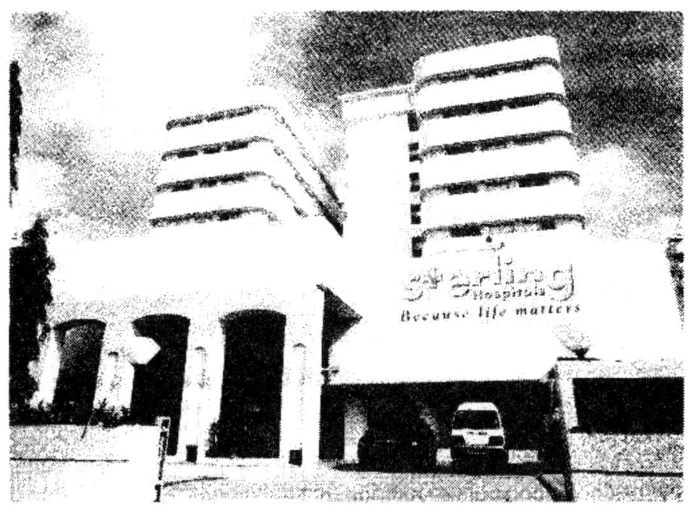

Sterling group is coming up with two more hospitals in Bhavnagar and Baroda

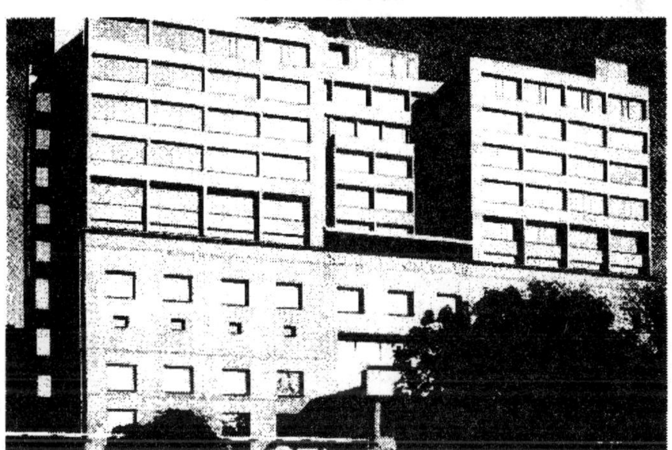

Shalby Hospital is coming up with three new multi speciality hospitals—two in Ahmedabad and one in Surat

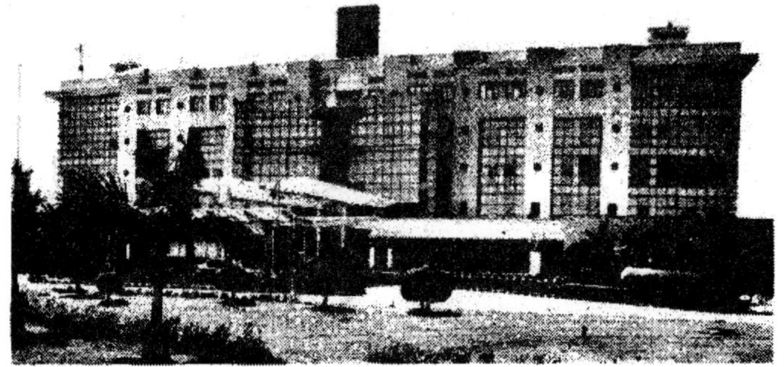

Apollo is exploring opportunity to start Reach Hospitals in Gandhidham, Kutch, Rajkot, Baroda and Surat

selling abroad," says Kanakia. They are seeking to achieve this by measures such as creating centre of excellence in respective fields, developing a network, customising packages and providing a stamp of quality through accreditation from global certification agencies such as JCI. Not only corporate hospitals like Sterling, Medisurge, Apollo, Shalby but also major trust hospitals like Rajasthan Hospital and 2,040-bed Civil Hospital, which is also known as Asia's largest hospital, are in the process of getting either NABH or JCI accreditations in the next one or two years span. Civil Hospital has done first round of accreditation for its blood bank and is now going for final accreditation. It has plans to go for its lab accreditation and finally accreditation of the entire hospital. Today, hospitals like Shalby is known for its joint replacement surgeries and dental care. Krishna Heart Care Centre has established its name in the area of cardiac care. After getting a strong backing from HCG Global group, Medisurge group is trying to establish its presence in cancer care by establishing three cancer care hospitals. HCG Global acquired Medisurge Hospital, a local hospital in 2007.

Gujarat in Medical Tourism

In tune with the national goal to promote India as the most favoured medical tourism destination, Gujarat has aggressively pushed the concept of medical tourism by using its well known 'Vibrant Gujarat' annual event. Government and private health care organisations have come together to attract patients from abroad with measures such as creating accredited centres of excellence in the respective fields and by aggressively promoting Indian systems of medicine specifically, Ayurveda, naturopathy and yoga.

Apollo Hospitals, Ahmedabad attracts high number of foreign tourists for various kinds of surgeries and health checkups. The hospital is planning to ramp up its platinum wing meant for international patients by total 26 beds in the coming few months. "People are now aware of the quality of health facilities being provided in Gujarat, helped by English-speaking doctors and staff and an almost zero waiting period," says Kanakia. The major factor for increasing medical tourists to the state is the low cost of cardiac surgery, angiography, joint replacements, radiation and other medical services, which is a fraction of what they would have to incur abroad.

Shalby Hospitals, known for its joint replacement, has witnessed 10-15 per cent increase in the medical tourism patients since its inception. The hospital has an international patient co-ordinator especially roped in and fully dedicated to its international clientele. Besides, the other major reason for medical tourism in Gujarat to flourish is the increasing number of NRGs or Non-Resident Gujaratis settled abroad are preferring their homeland not just as a treatment option but also for putting investments to establish hospitals.

Krisha Heart Care Centre is one prominent example of NRG-led speciality care hospital. "Around 6.5 million Gujaratis are NRGs. They visit their native place, especially in the month of November and December. This is the period when besides vacationing, they also prefer getting treated. However, the repeat cases only come through word-of-mouth publicity," says Dr. Pawar.

Challenging Grounds

Today, one of the key challenges faced by all the health care players wishing to penetrate this market is the shortage of trained manpower especially when they are planning to expand in tier two and tier three cities. Gujarat health care is also believed to a 'doctor driven market. Experts agree that physician is a key link in the success of corporate health care in this market. Says Dr. Shah, "It is a 100 per cent doctor-driven market and is a difficult one to penetrate and sustain if you have not involved the well known doctors." Agrees Dr. Pawar, "Gujarat is still a doctor-driven market and not institution driven and this poses a huge challenge for corporates who are willing to enter this market. Doctors also do not prefer to join as full-time consultants in the hospital."

The ever increasing real estate and electricity costs are the other major deterrents. "We need to have deep pockets. As real estate prices will impact the per bed cost, therefore the kind of infrastructure built and technology brought in will impact the break-even and profitability. One needs to invest prudently and manage cost well and be prepared to invest for long-term in this market, "shares Sharma.

Future

The fledgling health care industry in the state of Gujarat is set to become a leading sector, which other states can look upto replicate. "We are witnessing a change in this market which will soon shift its focus from doctor-centric to patient centric. Gradually, we shall also see nursing homes disappearing and corporates gaining a stronghold in this market," quips Dr. Bharat Gadhavi, CEO, HCG Medisurge Hospitals. Gujarat, thus, with all its right growth enablers and strong building blocks can become a serious global health care hub in India. However, this would call for serious continuing transformation efforts on the part of the Government and private players to change mindsets of foreign investors and patients in order to attract global capital, talent and business flow.

D.M. Medicity, Kochi

The beautiful port city Kochi, dubbed as the 'Queen of the Arabian Sea', also happens to be the commercial and industrial hub of the state of Kerala. The city with a population of 2.2 million attracts foreign tourists by the drove for its scenic backwaters, coconut-fringed beaches, Chinese finishing nets, multi-hued historical past and its cosmopolitan culture. So, a mega health city of global standards becomes a project of national significance. The health city—DM Medicity—is coming up in a sprawling 35-acre land on the banks of Periyar river. This is the second upcoming

Greenfield project of DM Health Care Private Limited, a JV between Dubai-based Dr. Moopand's Group and private equity firm India Value Fund Advisor. DM Health Care is also constructing Aadhar Hospital, another 150-bed Greenfield project in Kolhapur district of Maharashtra. In September 2009, the Indian arm of DM Health Care Commissioned its first hospital—the 150-bed Malabar Institute of Medical Sciences (MIMS), Kottakkal in Mallapuram district of Kerala. DM Health Care, by dint of its majority stake in Dr. Moopand's Group, also manages the 600-bed MIMS, Kozhikode.

Location

The DM MediCity is coming up at Cheranellur, North West of Kochi, with close proximity to NH 17 and 47. Located around 25 kilometres from the airport, the site is close to the proposed Container Terminal Road, the project that would lead to expansion of the port and would also reduce the distance from airport to the site. Said Dr. Azad Moopand, Chairman, Dr. Moopand's Group and DM Health Care,

Project Details

The first phase of DM MediCity with 500 beds would consist of one million square feet built up space. This phase having privileges like hotel, medical convention centre and residential apartments is built at an estimated cost of Rs. 500 crore (exclusive of land cost) and is expected to be commissioned by 2012.

Explains Anupam Verma, CEO, DM Health Care, India, "MediCity will be woven around an anchor tertiary/quaternary care institute supported by several centres of excellence in clinical and allied services. Acclaimed and established national and international health care players would be invited for association in the centres of excellence. Medicity will forge partnership with international health care bodies to bring in global accreditation, systems and protocols, technical expertise and acceptance."

The project, when completed, would have two million square feet built-up area. "The total cost of the project will be 1500 crores of rupees.

DM Health Care is in the process inking an MoU with an US-based internationally-acclaimed health care architectural firm to design, plan and execute this project. There shall be employment opportunities for about 5,000 people in the first phase and 15,000 people in the completed project.

"Kochi has been gaining recognitic world-wide due to its improving coi nectivity. It has witnessed remarkab progress in areas like tourism and I sector. A similar enhancement an facelift of health care delivery system the need of hour and demands since effort from concerned entities. The emanates from historical recognition Kerala for health tourism with the healing nature, requirement of health value travel in illness related area; availability of well trained health care professionals in the state and NRI professionals wanting to relocate helpin a reverse brain drain. These positive drawn from geographical location, global recognition, consumer demand availability of supportive service makes Kochi a preferred destination."

Advantage Medicity

A medicity scores over a mega hospital project in more ways than one "There are many good hospitals in the state, but still there are many treatment modalities that are not available here. This points to the requirement foi an institution which can be on par with any internationally renowned health care institutions in advanced treatment facilities. There is a growing population in India looking for state-of-the-art facilities provided by international health care standards. Medicity would establish a suitable platform to bring in international health care brands to India and assimilate that knowledge locally," says Dr. Moopand. Medicity will provide suitable resources to bring in international brands to conduct clinical and equipment research and manpower training, besides being an integrated platform where specialised brands of world can come in and add to the 'attractiveness' of India as a preferred medical destination.

Carestream Health India; Innovative Radiology Imaging Solutions

At the recently concluded 63rd Indian IRIA 2010 Congress, Care stream Health India showcased its latest digital imaging products and solutions which help health care providers improve quality and operational performance. The company announced state-of-the-art systems for the capture, processing, printing and storing of images for diagnostic applications. The four-day annual Radiology Congress, organized by the Indian Radiological and Imaging Association (IRIA), was held in Ahmedabad recently.

At the Radiology Congress, Carestream Health had developed its products showcase around the theme 'Our focus is your success'. According to Mr Prabir Chatterjee, Managing Director of Carestream Health India, "Our products are designed to make life easier for the radiology community. Our radiology imaging solutions increase efficiency, integration and backup by our world-class professional services group bring total peace of mind. The radiologist gets to concentrate on patients, not problems." Mr Chatterjee emphasized that Carestream Health has evolved technologies that provide support to the needs of radiologist in the digital world of tomorrow, with paths forward that protect the radiologists investments today.

The centerpiece of Carestream Health's product show at the IRIA was the DRX-1, world's first cassette sized wireless digital DR detector, which fits in to existing systems. An extremely cost-effective digital solution, the current X ray rooms can shift to digital radiography without a complete revamp of their existing system. The DRX-1 system delivers high-quality preview images in less than five seconds, which significantly improves productivity, even for users of computed radiography (CR) systems.

Being a wireless DR detector, the DRX-1 system provides flexible positioning that enhances both efficiency and patient comfort. Its extreme compact size and light weight further enhance convenience and throughput for radiology professionals. The innovation—the Carestream DryView5850 high-image quality Laser Imager—which brings tabletop convenience and outstanding reliability with extra-sharp 508 pixels-per-inch resolution that makes it ideal for medical imaging applications and digital mammography. The new DV5850 laser imager addresses the need for affordable laser-quality film output from full-field digital mammography (FFDM) and CR-based mammography systems. With a simplified user panel and capability to change films in full room light, it is easy to operate. Moreover, the DryView technology does not use thermal print heads thereby requiring minimal maintenance.

"The compact nature and simplicity of use of the machine will be extremely helpful for imaging centers, hospital departments, and clinics alike. Besides, the high-quality of output will result in accurate and better diagnosis and treatment," informed Prabir Chatterjee.

Carestream also demonstrated its product model CR Classic, Point-of-Care CR 360 and the DryView 6800 laser imager. The extremely convenient Kodak Point-of-Care CR360 system enables even smaller health care facilities to provide best-in-class digital imaging diagnostics to patients. Being compact, robust and affordable, the CR360 is a lightweight system that can be mounted on tabletop, enabling instant diagnosis at the patient location.

Kodak Point-of-Care CR360 system has a capacity to handle through put of over 60 plates per hour (1 per minute) and the option for high-resolution scanning modes, the technician is able to customize the output depending upon the type of examination/diagnostics needed. The Point-of-Care CR 360 comes with DICOM 3.0 capabilities, making it seamlessly compatible with a broad variety of printers, modality equipment, RIS and PACS systems.

Snaring some of his plans for the Company, Mr Prabir Chatterjee who has recently assumed charge as the MD of Carestream Health India, informed, "We will continue to introduce innovative new products and bring the latest technology to India as fast as possible. Understand their needs and develop solutions that meet those needs." Carestream Health, Inc. markets a broad portfolio of CR and DR. systems that equips hospitals, outpatient imaging centers, orthopaedic practices and other health care providers with digital image capture for X-ray imaging studies. Care stream Health's laser imagers range from desktop systems designed for imaging centers, small hospitals and clinics to fully featured units designed for high volume, multi-modality output at hospitals of all sizes. These imagers offer output from CR, DR, CT, MR, US, NM, and Digital Mammography and other gray scale imaging applications.

The company originated as a business unit within Eastman Kodak Company and brings from its former owner a proud history of innovation, more than 110 years' experience in health imaging, and over 1,000 patents in digital and film imaging and information technology. As a result of its innovative product portfolio and broad global sales, service and distribution capabilities, products from Carestream Health can be found in approximately 90% of hospitals and dental practices around the world.

In India, the Company's Indian subsidiary Carestream Health India commenced independent operations in May 2007. Since then, the business has grown to over Rs. 220 crore in 2009. Carestream Health India has a comprehensive portfolio of medical imaging and health care IT products, services, and solutions, as well as the latest in X-ray films, laser films, computed radiography (CR) systems, digital radiography (DR) systems and medical laser printers.

About Carestream Health, Inc.

Carestream Health, Inc., is a worldwide provider of dental and medical imaging systems and health care IT solutions; molecular imaging systems for the life science research and drug discovery/development market segments; and X-ray film and digital X-ray products for the non-destructive testing market.

Shalby Hospitals, Gujarat

Shalby Hospitals has transitioned from a joint replacement centre to a full-fledged multispecialty hospital, offering care in over 25 specialties. Today, health care in Gujarat is developing at a rapid pace with many corporate groups trying to grab a significant pie of this emerging market. In such a competitive market, there are few hospitals who have carved a niche in a particular specialty and now moving towards multi-specialty status at a lightening speed. One such group is Ahmedabad-based Shalby Hospitals, the 240-bed multi-specialty private hospital. Shalby Hospitals transitioned from a small 15-bed single specialty unit established in 1993 to a technologically-advanced 200-bed multi-specialty hospital in 2007.

The Origin

The hospital was started by Dr. Vikrarn Shah, a well known joint replacement surgeon. After returning to India, Dr. Shah started Shalby Hospitals offering for the first time in the city. Total Knee Replacement (TKR) surgery. The hospital near Vijay Cross Roads was commissioned in 1993 with six beds, one operation theatre, five staff, three level building and a small built-up area. The hospital offered only joint replacement and his dental surgeon wife Dr. Darshini Shah practiced high-end dentistry with oral implantology. In a short time it became an acclaimed joint replacement centre. Over 20,000 TKRs. were performed during the period 1993-2009 by the joint replacement team spearheaded by Dr. Shah. The hospital today is globally renowned for TKR and hip replacement surgeries.

"We consider ourselves as our competitor. The hospital has grown 60 per cent over last 15 years. We have achieved a growth of over 60 per cent (CAGR) each year. Where we had performed 15 operations during the first year, it grew to 600 about five years ago, but last year alone, we performed around 3,000 operations," shares Dr. Vikram Shah, Chairman and Managing Director,

The Trendsetter

The hospital always had an eye for innovation, implementing the green building concept in the hospital or reducing the time in joint replacement surgery. The hospital building is environment-friendly with features like fire brick construction to reduce energy loss, dual reflective vacuum spaced glasses, rain harvesting for reduced water requirement and cooled compressed air for air-conditioning.

The hospital took efforts in bringing in efficiency by adopting process driven approach in areas required. The surgical time in the hospital has been dramatically reduced from 1 : 20 : TKR in 1994 to approximately 22 mins, thereby reducing the infection rate.

The hospital offers more space per patient for increased comfort and at home feeling with the patient area of over 900 square feet. It has also incorporated infection control measures viz. HEPA filters, laminar body exhaust system, plasma sterilizer and Maquet operating tables. The hospital initiated cardiac stem cell transplant, ozone therapy for non-invasive and painless uterine fibroid embolism, and Kyphoplasty to treat progressive vertebral compression fractures in the Western region.

Tech Savvy

Keeping abreast with the globally developing technologies is an integral part of Shalby's mission, says Dr. Shah. The hospital has invested heavily in IT Infrastructure with Cisco and Nortel networking infrastructure. It has a fully integrated Hospital Management and Information System which is designed to manage every aspect of information flow and control across the hospital. Right from vendor records to patient record, everything is electronically managed. "This will eventually help achieve the goal of a paperless office," shares Dr. Shah. Imaging technology is enhanced further by incorporating a mini PACS radiology viewing system. This enables doctors to view patient's scans online, saving time taken for reporting.

"At Shalby, we try to indigenize technology to suite the changing requirements of the patients and ensure that we deliver at affordable costs," states Dr. Shah. The hospital took few steps towards adapting new technologies by recently acquiring plasma sterilizer, 5-part blood cell counter, Vitros 250 dry chemistry analyzer, ECQI, immunology analyzer and fully-automated urine analyser-U411.

Productivity Personified

The hospital has dedicated patient relations officers for each floor and encourages patients to give feedback of their stay during the treatment. There is a systematic follow-up system that the hospital follows for each patient discharged from the hospital. "We believe that patient feedback is not just important, it is critical for us to amend/improve the systems in the hospital," quips Dr. Shah.

The hospital has been a profit centre right from its inception; it is currently operating at EBIDTA margins of 20-22 per cent. To ensure its focus on medical excellence, the hospital has outsourced ancillary patient care services like laundry, kitchen, housekeeping and security.

The patient is not shifted from one bed to the other. The same electronically controlled bed will take the patient through the hospital whether it is a X-Ray, CT or even surgery preparation," says Dr. Shah.

Socially Inclined

Dr. Virkam and his wife Dr. Darshini Shah have formed a trust to effectively contribute to the society. The trust activities involve extending financial aid to the needy patients. "The Vijay Cross Roads unit of Shalby Hospitals extends support to the underprivileged by performing surgeries at a low cost," says Dr. Shah.

The trust also publishes a monthly magazine 'Shalby Times' with an intention to spread awareness about well-ness, which is distributed to all its in-patients. Free camps and public outreach programmes at various locations across India are organized at regular intervals.

Shalby Hospitals today is also proving to be a substantial contributor to the booming medical tourism in the state of Gujarat. Since last year, the group has been focusing more on medical tourism and has seen 10 to 15 per cent increase in medical tourism patients.

The first foreign patient was operated in the hospital for TKR way back in 1994. The hospital has been receiving patients from over 16 countries, especially for joint replacements. Dr. Shah agrees that even though his contacts with fellow doctors and the representatives of Gujarati community abroad helped him propagate his skills at the initial stages, but what has acted as a catalyst for Shalby is word-of-mouth publicity.

"Patients who have taken treatment at Shalby have always referred patients. We keep our patients informed (especially international) about the addition of new facilities, enhancement of services, etc. and the patients always respond to us in a positive fashion," says Dr. Shah. The hospital has specially recruited an international patient coordinator dedicated completely to the international patients wing.

The hospital has been getting a large pool of patients from destinations within India too, including Kolkata, Jaipur, Chennai and strongly feel that there is enough scope to grow even if we just focus on treating our fellow Indian friends," shares Himanshu Sharma, Senior Manager, Strategic Initiatives, Shalby Hospitals.

Challenging the Odds

The biggest challenge faced by Shalby Hospitals is creating awareness about new upcoming technologies which it is incorporating to help its patients. It took almost 15 years for joint replacement to establish itself in Gujarat, in spite of the state being techno-sawy. According to Dr. Shah, same is the situation for propagating Kyphoploasty and Ozone Therapy. The hospital is therefore using outreach programmes and CMEs to propagate the concepts.

Paving the Way

The modern hospital, which currently has seven OPDs (clinics) in different cities of the country, is adding 10 more to provide facilities in tier II and III towns, informs Wing Commander Arun Kaul (Retd.), Executive Director. The group is investing Rs. 450 crore in the next five years to set-up OPDs in eight cities of the world and 10 more clinics in the country to expand its reach to patients. It will fund its expansion plans through internal accruals. The outstation centres would coordinate between foreign patients and the Ahmedabad-based hospital which plans to rope in travel agencies to offer the patients travel-*cum*-treatment package. The group will add another 600 beds in the State within next one and an half years. Two units of 150 bed each are coming up at distinct locations in Ahmedabad city and a 300-bed unit in Surat. All the three hospitals will be multi-specialty units offering global class health care facilities. A total of Rs. 300 crore would be pumped in for the upcoming projects. All our upcoming units will be designed for medical tourists.

4

The Advent of Medical and Health Cities in South India

While South India took a lead in providing good care in private set-up, north is also taking steps in 'Public-Private Parnership' (PPP) to improve health care. The battle for providing cutting-edge, integrated health care delivery system, replete with international standard benchmarking and patient-centric approach, which was so far limited to the urban landscape, is all set to move to a newer turf. World-renowned health care powerhouses such as Apollo Hospitals, Fortis Heath Care, Max Health Care and Rockland will clash for a bigger pie in the health care services, away from the swanky metros to the dust-laden villages of four districts of Uttar Pradesh, where the management, upgrade, operation and maintenance of public health service facilities have been opened up for the private sector. This is for the first time in the country that any state government has opened up the public health care service infrastructure at the district level to the private sector. (Deepa Jainani)

The four health care powerhouses have been short-listed out of 12 companies, for the request for proposal (RFP) stage for far-flung Basti, Allahabad, Ferozabad and Kanpur districts. The project, which envisages an estimated investment of Rs. 200 crore, will entail the upkeep of four district hospitals, eight community health centres, 23 primary health centres and 210 sub centres. While Apollo Hospitals has emerged as the strongest bidder, having bid for all the four districts, Rockland has bid for Ferozabad and Kanpur City, Fortis for Basti and Kanpur and Max for Kanpur only. "The selected developer would upgrade the hospitals, to bring them on par with the prescribed standards, and would manage, maintain and operate them for 33 years," an official of the state health department told the newsmen. After the private partner is identified through the competitive bidding process, it will form a special purpose company (SPC) with the

Uttar Pradesh government holding 11% and having one of its nominees on the board of directors, in lieu of the infrastructure that the state would allow the SPC to use. The eligibility criteria for a private partner is a turnover of Rs. 100 crore for the last three years and a networth of Rs. 100 crore with experience of running a 100-bed hospital. This has brought a paradigm shift in the approach to public health care and opened vistas for public private partnership (PPP). This may herald a new era in massive investment in the health care sector, which is the need of the hour.

Demand outstrips the supply

From a pan-India perspective, presently there are more than half a million doctors employed in 15,097 hospitals. Additionally there are 0.75 million nurses, who look after more than 870,000 hospital beds. During the previous decade, the number of doctors has increased by 36.6 per cent. An estimated 30 per cent of medical practitioners hold specialist qualifications. A survey by NCAER, an independent economics research agency, suggests that per-capita expenditures on health care rise with higher education levels. Households that have higher education levels tend to spend more per illness than households with lower education levels. Rising literacy in India is improving health awareness, especially about lifestyle-related diseases—which tend to be more costly to treat than infections.

While rising incomes and growing literacy are likely to drive higher per- capita expenditures on health care, the shift in disease profiles from infectious to lifestyle-related diseases are expected to raise expenditures per treatment. Lifestyle-related diseases are typically more expensive to treat than infectious ones. In 2001, the average inpatient cost for lifestyle-related diseases (cardiac problems, digestive issues, etc.) was US$ 658 compared to US$ 91 for infectious diseases. India's disease profile is expected to follow the same pattern as in developed economies. Based on demographic trends and disease profiles, lifestyle diseases—cardiovascular, asthma and cancer have become the most important segments, and in-patient spending is expected to represent nearly 50 per cent of total health care expenditure. In the inpatient market, the share of infectious diseases has declined from 19 per cent in 2004 to 16 percent in 2008.

As per an earlier report, the number of cardiac-disease-related treatments in India is expected to grow from 1.5 million to 1.9 million per year over 2004-08, which would constitute 5.1 per cent of all treatments, The spend share of inpatient cardiac treatment is estimated to grow to 19 per cent of the total in 2008 from 16 per cent in 2004. This would drive a 13.4 per cent CAGR in the inpatient cardiac care market from US$ 1.2 billion in 2004 to US$ 2.04 billion in 2008. The average realization per inpatient for cardiac related treatment is much higher than for other disease segments. Increased life expectancy and an ageing population to play a role as well. In the domestic market, health spending will be sustained by two demographic trends: increased life expectancy and an ageing population.

Life expectancy, which averaged 63.3 years in 2000-04, is expected to increase to 65.1 years in 2005-09 and to 66 years in 2006-10. The proportion of the population aged 65 years and over is also on the rise, and will increase from 4.7 per cent in 2000 to 5.3 per cent in 2005 and 5.8 per cent in 2010. Although the rate of ageing in India is slower than the developed world, the large population makes any increase significant in terms of absolute numbers, and therefore also in terms of market potential. Rising share of the private health care sector. The majority of health care services in India are provided by the private sector. In 2002 fee-charging private companies accounted for around 82 per cent of overall health care expenditure, with various levels of government covering the remaining 18 per cent.

HYDERABAD

Hyderabad took a lead in 80s to set-up a medical city

As mentioned in the previous chapters, state-of-the-art corporate hospitals are fast becoming an integral part of the Indian health care landscape. And as major metros compete with each other to become the country's leading health centers, corporate groups like Apollo and fortis are leading the way with a mix of superspecialty and single-specialty hospitals, well-reputed doctors as well as competitive prices. It was not until the mid-'80s, when the Nizam's Institute of Medical Sciences (NIMS) became an autonomous institution and Apollo health city, Hyderabad was set-up, that medical care in Hyderabad grabbed national attention. This set off a chain reaction, and today Hyderabad boasts of the largest number of hospitals in the private sector in the country. Bangalore, Mumbai, Chennai, Ahmedabad, Delhi are not lagging behind.

Hyderabad has several medical cities

"Every city in India is becoming a self-sufficient medical centre. It's because at a certain stage, government hospitals were not able to provide the requisite infrastructure, these were lagging behind," says Dr. B. Somaraju, a cardiologist at Care Hospital, Hyderabad, who headed the team of doctors at NIMS in 1985 that performed the country's first angioplasty. Today, he and his team routinely perform coronary angioplasties, mitral valvuloplasties (procedures for removing artery blockages), intercoronary stent implants, rota-blators. First he established Mediciti hospital as the foremost centre for cardiac care in the country. Mediciti was conceived by Dr. P. Sudhakar Reddy, a professor of cardiology at the University of Pittsburg, with funds raised from fellow doctors in the US. (After Gujarati doctors, Andhraites form a large proportion of Indian doctors in the US.)

In fact, while many hospitals like Mediciti, Apollo and the L.V. Prasad Eye Institute (LVPEI) have been established by Andhraite doctors from the US keen to return home, others have been set-up by doctors with entrepreneurial intentions. "The trend now has shifted from government to private hospitals, from smaller nursing homes to superspeciality hospitals and from curative to preventive medicine," says Dr. C. Dayakar Reddy, an anesthetist who heads the successful CDR group of hospitals that has diversified into allied fields like a school for hospital administration.

Happily, these superspeciality hospitals are doing their bit to reverse the brain drain, inspiring Indian doctors abroad to return home. Little wonder then that Hyderabad is emerging as a leading medical care centre. In fact, the city is considered way above other metros in areas like cardiology, urology, nephrology and ophthalmology; its hospitals offer young doctors challenging opportunities. Says Sangeeta Reddy, managing director, Apollo: "We can prevent young doctors from going abroad."

Besides superspeciality hospitals like Apollo, CDR, Mediciti, Medwin and Kamineni, there are single speciality hospitals like Dr. Ram Bhoopal's Satya Kidney Centre (where one of the country's top nephrologists, Dr. S. Sahariah, performs kidney trans-plants), Dr. Ramesh Ramayya's Pramila Kidney Hospital, Dr. Mamta Deendayal's Infertility Institute and Research Centre (where 2,500 childless couples have already been treated and two babies delivered by the IVF method) and Dr. Y. Chiranjeev Reddy's Amrutha Diabetic Centre. Recently, Reddy has also set-up the Amrutha Holiday Hospital, the country's first health spa where diabetics, hypertensives and those suffering stress-related problems recoup in idyllic surroundings. Nearly 500 diabetics have stayed here and almost all have gone back on a reduced dosage of insulin.

And so, while not long ago Hyderabad residents would go abroad for angioplasties or bypass surgeries, today they are being referred back by doctors abroad to hospitals like Care, Mediciti for cardiac complications and the LVPEI for ophthalmological problems. LVPEI, set-up by Dr. Gullapalli N. Rao (associate professor of ophthalmology at the University of Rochester where he was director of the Corneal Research Bank) achieved a breakthrough when one of its doctors, Dr. Taraprasad Das, performed the world's first transplant using tissues from a human foetus to restore five per cent vision to a blind man.

Hyderabad is also emerging as an important centre of training. Dr. D. Nageshwar Reddy, an endoscopic gastroenterology specialist and visiting professor at the Boston Medical University and the Harvard Medical School in the US, not only has patients coming from India and abroad with gall bladder or intestinal problems, but even doctors from well-known hospitals across the world visiting him for training in diagnostic and therapeutic endoscopy. And the medicare boom seems nowhere near an end. Because of rising real estate costs in the metros, Hyderabad has emerged as a viable option for setting up new hospitals and expanding existing ones. For instance, while Delhi and Madras both houses Apollo's prestigious hospitals, it is only in Hyderabad, notes Sangeeta Reddy, that there's an opportunity for expansion because of the 30 acres of land Apollo Hyderabad is built on. Besides, it is the cheapest in terms of medical services offered. Even otherwise the cost of medical care in Hyderabad is less than half of what it is in Bombay or Delhi, and less than a tenth of the cost abroad. For instance, bypass surgeries at Mediciti cost Rs. 1 lakh, angiography Rs. 8,000-9,000, a lithotripsy between Rs. 7,000 and Rs. 15,000, and a simple cataract operation Rs. 2,700-Rs. 10,000.

Confirming this, Uma Nath, administrator, LVPEI, says that recently a group of Swiss citizens on a tour of India came to them for cataract operations because not only is such surgery cheaper here, but the institute compares with the best in Europe; it is already the best in South-east Asia.

Apollo Health City

Apollo Hospitals, Jubilee Hills, Hyderabad was formally inaugurated by the then President of India, His Excellency R. Venkat Raman on 27th August, 1988. Today, Apollo Hospitals, Hyderabad has risen to be on par with the best in terms of technical expertise, deliverables and outcomes. Apollo Health City, Hyderabad covers the entire spectrum to illness to wellness and is thus a health city and not a medical city. Institutes for Heart Diseases, Cancer, Joint Diseases, Emergency, Renal Diseases, Neurosciences, Eye and Cosmetic Surgery are all centers of excellence and are positioned to offer the best care in the safest manner to every patient.

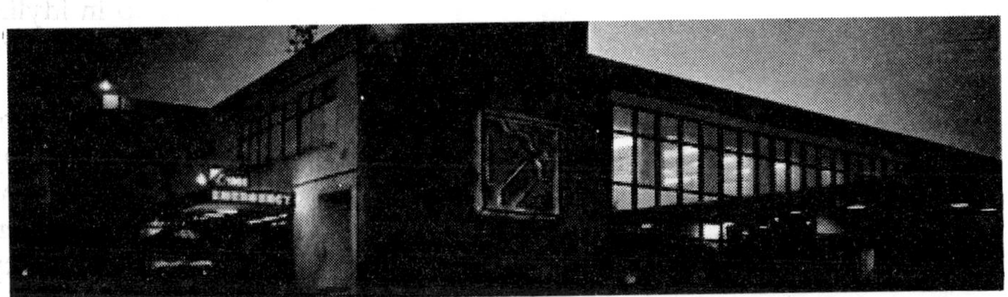

Apart from patient care, each of these centers of excellence spends a significant amount of time in training and research essentially aimed at preventing disease and improving outcomes when the disease does occur. From the moment one arrives at Apollo Health City, Hyderabad he or she becomes part of a tradition of distinguished health care. We strive to lead the world in the diagnosis and treatment of disease and to train tomorrow's great physicians, nurses, and scientists. Above all, we aim to provide the highest quality health care and service to all of our patients with an additional intervention called the tender loving care.

Apollo Health City, Hyderabad thus strives to go beyond good medicine towards good health. Being the first city in Asia, it provides the impetus for more such institutes to develop and places Hyderabad on the global map of quality health care.

EMERGENCY SPECIALIST—Hyderabad today has the nation's first pre-hospital emergency network consisting of 12 fully-equipped ambulances manned by trained personnel

APOLLO HEART INSTITUTE—Prevention and treatment of heart disease has led to the achievement of better outcomes, and improved quality of life for thousands of cardiac patients who visit Apollo Hospitals each year.

APOLLO CANCER INSTITUTE—The institute provides world-class comprehensive cancer care with dedicated professionals and state-of-the-art equipment and facilities with a tumor Board and now PET CT (a powerful imaging technique that holds great promise in the diagnosis and treatment of many diseases, particularly cancer) addition which is first of its kind in the country.

APOLLO INSTITUTE OF NEUROSCIENCES—The department is headed by world-renowned consultants backed by outstanding clinical staff and sophisticated equipment. Stroke is the clinical term for acute loss of circulation to an area of the brain, resulting in a corresponding loss of neurologic function and even death.

Apollo Hospitals Hyderabad is the FIRST HOSPITAL IN THE WORLD to be accredited by the Disease or Condition Specific Care Certification (DCSC) for Acute Stroke by JCI. The average length of stay reduced from 11 days to 4.5 days for Acute Stroke patients.

APOLLO INSTITUTE FOR AMBULATORY CARE (Lazer and MIMAS Surgi Center)—We provide high-quality health care at affordable costs because we focus only on one aspect: treating ambulatory patients efficiently so that these patients get back to their work or home the very next day

APOLLO INSTITUTE OF JOINT DISEASES—The institute provides the most competent and professional treatment of trauma of the musculo-skeletal system

APOLLO INSTITUTE FOR COSMETIC SURGERY—Whether it's a nose that's too big, breasts that are too small, or wrinkled, sagging skin, it is a problem that can often be solved with cosmetic surgery. There are procedures available that help people not only look better but feel better as well

APOLLO INSTITUTE OF RENAL SCIENCES—Paediatric nephrologists is a part of the Nephrology team at Apollo, which is missing in many other hospitals. All facilities required for Nephrology patient is available under one roof with necessary medical and diagnostic support and guidance round the clock.

APOLLO EYE INSTITUTE—With advanced methods to treat eye conditions Holistic Health

APOLLO INSTITUTE OF LIFESTYLE MANAGEMENT and PREVENTIVE CARE—Apollo Hospitals have been astute enough to have tailor-made packages for all age groups. A proper health check-up scans the bio-history, interprets signals and provides the opportunity for the proverbial "stitch in time".

APOLLO INSTITUTE FOR REHABILITATION and REJUVENATION—Paralysis, stroke, trauma, cancer, heart disease, surgery....can all leave behind some form of disability....physical, physiological, psychological and/or social disability. A structured multi-disciplinary approach will bring down this disability and will help the individual get back to normal at the earliest. Rehab Rejuvenation unit at Apollo Hospitals is the first unit in the country offering comprehensive multi-disciplinary care under one roof.

Ayurveda rejuvenation is a time tested program to top up energy levels and re invigorate you, your body, your mind and soul. The centre also offers a self contained Ayurvedic wing that caters to total therapy and rejuvenation needs. India home to Asia's largest hospital network

Apollo Hospital, Chennai

In 1983, the Apollo Hospitals Group founded India's first corporate hospital in Chennai. With a network of over 35 hospitals, 6,400 hospital beds, 30 primary care clinics and more that 120 pharmacies, Apollo is today the largest private hospital network in Asia and has treated over six million patients and performed over 750,000 major surgical procedures since it was established. The Group has an integrated business model that, in addition to hospitals, includes clinics, diagnostic services, pharmacies, tele-medicine, and health care education and training. It has a network of over 2,000 doctors, around 2,000 nurses and 1,000 paramedical personnel on its payroll. The Group's aggregate turnover is around US$ 111.1 million. The company, helped by a first-mover advantage, is well ahead of other organised private players on geographic reach and breadth of services. Apollo is the only private hospital group in India with a national footprint and presence across most disease segments, which allows it to cater to a large population.

Indrasprastha Apollo in New Delhi is the largest private hospital outside the United States and the fourth largest corporate hospital in the world. The 700-bed JCI accredited hospital offers over 50 medical specialities and has 92 ICU beds, the largest number of ICU beds in India. The hospital has 19 operating theatres, five hi-tech cardiothoracic operating theatres, dialysis units and transplant facilities. It provides 24 hour emergency and trauma care and includes facilities for burns treatment, head injuries, acute cardiac emergencies, fractures and poisoning.

Apollo Hospitals is looking to enhance its presence in the secondary health care segment by setting up 'First Med' hospitals, each operating 100-120 beds in mini-metros and smaller towns. These hospitals are designed to focus on specific services such as emergency medicine, maternity and general surgery, and would be scalable to 200 beds. They could potentially be scaled upto tertiary-care hospitals. The company is setting up three such hospitals, and is expected to have seven such facilities overthe next three years. These hospitals are expected to be a significant growth driver for Apollo over the next few years given that there are more than 30 towns in India that offer opportunities for setting up secondary-care hospitals such as 'First Med'. Apollo is also looking at increasing its presence in the high-return cardiac-care segment, and is targeting a 5 per cent market share. The company already has a reasonable presence in the segment, having performed over 50,000 cardiac surgeries so far, across its various facilities. It plans to set-up two specialty secondary-care hospitals in the cardiology segment over the next three years.

Kolkata Health City

The Association of Hospitals in Eastern India has decided to set-up a Rs. 20,000-crore Health City at Sonarpur in West Bengal's South 24 Parganas district. It made a presentation to the Chief Minister Buddhadeb Bhattacharjee on the issue. On the latter's instruction, the health and urban development department is now carrying out a feasibility study of the project. The proposed Health City, which may take five years to come into being, will be spread over 800 acres and contain about 100 hospitals with a bed strength of 50,000. Other components of the whole concept include a hospital management school, ayurveda and naturopathy centers, nursing colleges, shopping malls, guesthouses, banks and Internet cafes. Foreign investors will fund half of the project's cost. Meanwhile, the Global Hospitals Group of Hyderabad will set-up an organ transplant centre in Kolkata, the city's first and the country's biggest, thanks to the efforts of the Bengal Chamber of Commerce which persuaded K. Ravindranath, GHGs managing director, to opt for the Bengal metropolis rather than Mumbai as originally thought of. The complex will be spread over a 10-acre plot off Rajarhat area near Salt Lake with the project cost estimated at Rs. 125 crores. Once ready, it will have 750 beds (10% of them for the poor) and 150 full-time specialists in the field of liver diseases, gastro-enterology, heart and kidney. NRI doctors as well as those from AIIMS, New Delhi and PGI, Chandigarh are likely to be part of the faculty. Patients from South-East Asia and the West are expected to come for treatment.

Narayana Health City, Bangalore

The Rs. 16 billion group, which currently has two hospitals in Bangalore and Kolkata, plans to invest Rs. 50 billion over next five years in expanding its operations to six other Indian cities. Speaking at the inauguration of the health city, Bangalore, Dr. Shetty said the aim of the health city is to provide affordable high quality health care to the masses. The target would be to reduce the cost of health care by 5 per cent every year. According to him, the number of cardiac surgeries performed should be 50 to 60 in a day to reduce the cost of the surgery.

Dr. Shetty said that every state capital should have a health city with a 3,000 to 5,000 bed hospital and every district headquarters should have a 1,000 to 2,000 bed hospital. Currently, the Narayana Health City has 3,000 beds and in two years, it is planning to expand to 5,000 beds. It also aims at catering to 10,000 out-patients and 5,000 in-patients in a day.

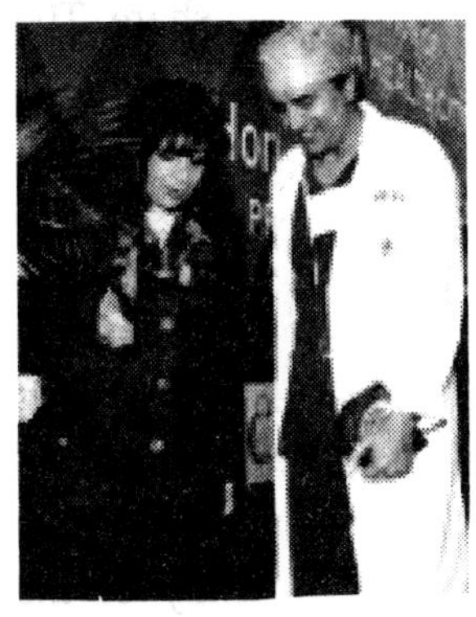

Narayana Hrudayalaya

Narayana Hrudayalaya, a 1000-bed heart hospital, started in 2001 A thrombosis research institute started in 2002. Sparsh, a 500-bed hospital for orthopaedic and trauma in 2005 Narayana Netralaya, a super speciality eye hospital with 300 beds, in 2006 Narayana Multi-Speciality and Mazumdar-Shaw Cancer Centre with 1,400 beds in 2009.

Apart from Bangalore and Kolkata, the group runs 16 hospitals across Dharwad, Hyderabad, Jaipur, Jamshedpur and Assam. Narayana Hrudayalaya, the hospitals conglomerate promoted by Dr. Devi Shetty, said it has signed an MoU with the Gujarat Government to set-up a 5,000-bed Health City in Ahmedabad. Narayana Hrudayalaya, which plans a Health City in every State, will initially invest Rs. 480 crore in a 1,000-bed heart hospital, to be operational by June 2010. This will be followed by cancer, kidney, neurosurgery and women and child welfare hospitals of 1,000 beds each, apart from a nursing college and paramedical training centers. The facility is expected to receive 15,000 outpatients a day. The facility will be built on a 37-acre area at Monogram Mills in Bapunagar, Ahmedabad. When built, it would be Asia's longest hospital spread over half a kilometre and measuring 12.5 lakh sq. ft., the health care major said.

Dr. Devi Shetty said the Ahmedabad project was meant to make medical services and technologies affordable to the masses. "This project will generate direct employment for 2,000 people and indirect employment for 5,000 people in the State," he said.

Dr. Shetty plans to set-up a health city in Mexico that will also cater to patients from the US. "Our next project will be a health city in Mexico. We may tie up with some American hospitals for this project," said Devi Shetty, eminent cardiologist and chairman of the Narayana Hrudayalaya group of hospitals. Shetty was addressing a news conference here to announce the setting up of a health city—a multi-specialty hospital with research facilities—in Hyderabad on the lines of the group's famous facility in Bangalore. "The health city in Mexico will be a 3,000 to 5,000-bed facility and we are looking for joint ventures," he said adding that the government of Mexico had requested the group to set-up a large health facility. Sources said the health city would come up either in Mexico City, the capital of Mexico or at Guadalajara, the second largest city in Mexico.

"We foresee health care delivery problems in the United States. They also have problems in undertaking a 20-hour journey to India for heart and other surgeries. As Mexico is closer to America, they will find it easy to undergo treatment there," he said. The chain of hospitals, which has already built one of the world's biggest cardiac hospitals in Bangalore and is planning similar facilities in other cities, is reportedly in talks with the US-based Sutter Health for the Rs. 10 billion health city project in Mexico.

Health City, Kochi

The Kozhikode-based Baby Memorial Hospital (BMH) has finalized plans to establish a Rs. 1,200-crore 'Health City' in Kochi. The project, coming up at Kakkanad and 2 km away from the Seaport-Airport Road, will incorporate the guidelines and standards prescribed by the Joint Commission International of the US, according to Dr. K.G. Alexander, Chairman and Managing Director, Baby Memorial Hospital. According to the plan, a hospital of international standards, costing Rs. 450 crore, will be set-up in the first phase of the project. With a built-up area of seven lakh sq. ft, the hospital will have 700 beds and 30 operation suites and 2,000 employees.

Global Health City, Durgapur

The steel city of Durgapur in West Bengal will soon get the country's first dedicated 'Knowledge and Health City'. Christened 'SPS Synergy Knowledge and Health City', the proposed city will include a 500-bed hospital-*cum*-private medical college, super speciality clinics, medi-care centre, nursing college, dental college, pharmacy college, paramedical college, international residential school, media and management college, technology colleges, indoor sports complex, outdoor sports complex, apartments, shopping malls, a health hotel, etc. To be developed by SPS Synergy Foundation (a joint enterprise of SPS Group and Synergy Group), at a cost of Rs. 600 crore, the project will be completed in three phases over the next seven years. The ceremony to lay the foundation stone for the first phase of the project was held recently in Durgapur. Speaking on the occasion, Nirupam Sen, the West Bengal Commerce and Industries Minister said, "Several leading health and educational institutions have evinced keen interest to set-up their projects in the city." He added that though 60-odd private engineering colleges have been set-up in the State, private medical colleges have not come up in the State due to strict regulations and restrictions of the Medical Council of India. "But I am happy to note that a private medical college-*cum*-hospital is coming up within the city."

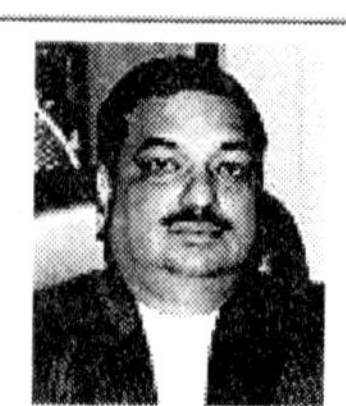

Bipin Vohra

The first phase of the project will entail an investment of Rs. 150 crore and is likely to be completed in the next two and half years. Bipin Kumar Vohra, Chairman and Managing Director of SPS Group and promoter of the project said, "A 500-bed hospital-*cum*-medical college, a nursing college, a paramedical college, an international residential school, apartments, a sports complex and a shopping mall will be built in the first phase."

The Asansol-Durgapur Development Authority (ADDA) has handed over 100 acres of land for the first phase. Another 200 acres will be acquired in phases. The first phase is expected to generate direct employment for more than 2,000 people. The three phases together have come with a job promise for over 7,000 people and is expected to generate indirect employment for 10,000 others.

In the third phase, an old-age home, homeopathy, naturopathy, pharmacy units and a medical mall and a health hotel will be constructed, Vohra said.

Chettinad Health City (CHC)

An emerging centre of excellence in health care education, research and patient-care, the Chettinad Health City (CHC) is located in Kelambakkam, about 30 kms from Chennai. Promoted by the prestigious Rajah Sir Muthiah Chettiar Charitable and Educational Trust. The 100 acre, state-of-the-art campus, fast moving to completion, integrates a 600 bed charitable hospital, superspecialty units and world-class colleges for Undergraduate and Postgraduate studies. CHC also has modern diagnostic labs, emergency facilities and support services.

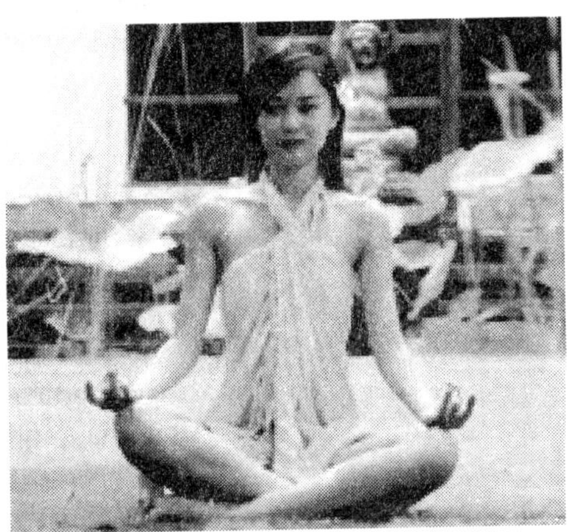

The focus is on professional excellence and community engagement draws an increasing number of patients, bright students and young researchers. It will be upgraded to 1200 beds over the next four years

Ayurvedic Health Care Cities

Ayurvedic Health Care is witnessing an exciting transition phase with organized health care players entering this market. Nancy Singh analyses the changing market dynamics of Ayurveda treatment. If your normal perception about Ayurveda is limited to spas and some herbal treatments from Kerala, then its time to rethink. The boardrooms of most corporate health care players are now reverberating with plans to set-up huge medicities solely dedicated to Ayurveda. The pioneers of private health care—Apollo Group will also be a pioneer in this segment. This medicity is coming up near Pune that will offer ayurvedic treatment. It has signed an agreement with real estate firm, Hindustan Construction Co (HCC), to set-up the medicity inside the upcoming hill station, Lavasa in Maharashtra. "It's a joint venture between HCC and Apollo. The medicity is coming up over an area of 200 acres. We (HCC and Apollo) have pegged almost Rs. 2 billion as the initial investment," says Ajit Gulabchand,

Chairman and Managing Director HCC. "It would be a state-of-the-art health and wellness centre, including hospitals, research and development labs and long-term care centres," says Raghav Rao, Vice-President—Projects, Apollo Hospitals. Now, if a giant like Apollo is investing so much in Ayurveda treatment, it is indication enough about how bullish health care providers are about this segment. On the same lines of Apollo, another big player to tap this market is Hinduja Group who will foray into wellness by setting up the World Knowledge Centre (WKC). WKC will be built on the philosophy of multi-disciplinary approach to health care wherein traditional Indian system like Ayurveda, yoga and meditation would be integrated with modern medicine, so as to provide comprehensive health care to treat complete range of illnesses, whether they are chronic, stress oriented or lifestyle related. To authenticate its therapies, WKC would also be upgraded with a clinical R&D set-up wherein the ayurvedic preparations would be clinically tested. The project would take 36 months to complete and the Group plans to spend almost $ 270 million that is approximately Rs. 1200 crore, in this mega project. Says PC Sood, Project Head, WKC, "WKC will provide quaternary care health, have three hospital premises with a capacity of 900 beds, 200 suit, five to seven residential facilities for dependents with service apartments, modern plaza with lavish food courts, wellness centers and clubs, convention centre, R&D for advanced medical research, e-library and a helipad." It would be equipped with state-of-art diagnostic centre and modern spas and wellness clinics. Initially, the Group will have only one such centre and subsequently more such models would be set-up in each region in India. After the concept matures over a period of time, the Group plans to franchise it overseas.

Evolving Market

It is estimated that the total market size of the Indian Ayurvedic market is Rs. 500 crore and it is growing substantially between 8-10 percent, with the same growth rate targeted for the next five to 10 years. "The current market is estimated at US $ 1 billion. But the potential for growth is immense as we interact with consumers at the confluence of wellness and natural healing. The market is pushing the boundaries across the board with Ayurveda at its core," states Jitu Mehta, President, Katra Group—Kerala Ayurveda, a health care service chain which provides Ayurvedic products, therapies, resort experiences, and an academy learning mode. The Group has aggressive expansion plans locally as well as globally. It plans to roll out 50 clinics across India. Kerala Ayurveda currently has 30 clinics, predominantly in south India which are being revamped and modernised. In the US the company has three clinics and four academies that offer courses in Ayurveda. In the next two years, it intends to have a total of 10 units in US and would also look at entering Europe later. "We have infinite scope. Our touch points include 300 plus products and a national clinic network that is expanding rapidly. We

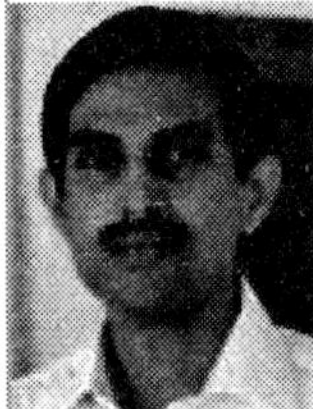

"We plan to set-up 40 hospital chains across India. We will position our services across the value spectrum, ranging from BoP patients to high-end patients."

—Rajiv Vasudevan
Founder and CEO
AyurVaid

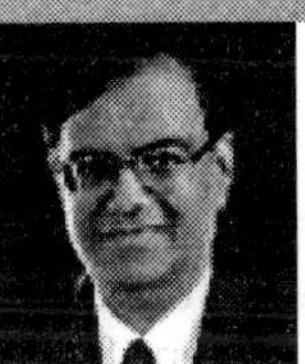

"The current market is estimated at $ 1 billion. The market is pushing the boundaries across the board with Ayurveda at its core."

—Jitu Mehta
President
Kerala Ayurveda

opened clinics as far apart as Pondicherry and Delhi within six weeks, resorts, hospitals and centres across the US. Hundreds of students are trained in our academy in India and US," adds Mehta. Kerala Ayurveda's resort format, Ayurvedagram, will also be replicated in other locations within India initially. Mehta intends to make Kerala Ayurveda a global brand and introduce Ayurveda as a way of life. "I brought in a colored, carbonated drink into the country (Pepsi). If I can do that, I am much more comfortable propagating a healthy way of life. If I have brought in international brands into India, now I intend to make an Indian brand global," he states passionately.

Manipal Cure and Care (MCC) Wellness Centre, Pune

The company has also tied up with Manipal Cure and Care (MCC) wellness centre at Pune to provide Ayurvedic services. "We are the only full spectrum, listed Ayurveda company in the world. We are integrated from herb farms to clinics in the US. We are a one stop wellness solution. MCC is a unique, very important route to reach urban, up-market consumers," adds Mehta.

Madhavbaug Cardiac Rehabilitation Centre is a rehabilitation centre focusing only on cardiac diseases which is establishing itself all across Maharashtra and other states. "We have already covered almost whole of Maharashtra with centres in Mumbai, Nashik, Pune, Jalgaon, Sangli, Aurangabad, Kolhapur and many more to come in Maharashtra itself. Next states to be targeted will be Gujarat and Goa," informs Dr. Rohit Sane, MD, Madhavbaug Cardiac Rehabilitation

Centre, located in the outskirts of Mumbai. The list of groups looking for setting footprints across India does not end here. Kerala-based AyurVaid Hospitals has a highly aggressive plan of setting up 40 ayurvedic hospitals across India from the current strength of two hospitals in Kochi. For its ambitious growth plans it has already attracted investment from the Private Equity firm Acumen which has announced an initial investment of Rs. 4.5 crore. "We are one of the few chains that will focus on bottom of the pyramid with 70 per cent of its capacity focused on poor patients. There are two hospitals in Aluva and Cochin, Kerala that are functional and around 40 more will come up across India based on the hub and spoke model," beams Rajiv Vasudevan, Founder and CEO, AyurVaid. AyurVaid plans to leverage Acumen investments to expand its footprint and pioneer the development of a low-cost health care delivery system that focuses on preventive and curative care, as an alternative to the highly capital intensive and curative system presently used to treat chronic ailments. Acumen's initial equity investment will support AyurVaid's plan to open six more hospitals across the country in the next 12 months, including two 'AyurVaid Seva' (AV-Seva) hospitals that would exclusively focus on low income group (BoP) patients. AyurVaid has set itself the goal of 60 per cent of its bed capacity for patients from the middle and lower socio-economic classes. "AyurVaid's health care delivery model for chronic illnesses can be positioned across the value spectrum ranging from BoP patients to high-end patients from India and abroad, permitting a viable and profitable business model," believes Vasudevan.

The reasons for so many groups flooding for ayurvedic health care are manifold. The growth drivers for this industry are not only the yawning gap of demand supply but the rising incidences of chronic diseases. Chronic diseases would be the number one killer in India. "The current growth rate of Ayurveda can be attributed towards lifestyle related disorders only, other disorders will obviously increase the count in the future," says Dr. Sane, who solely focus on cardiac diseases.

The second reason for alternative medicine to flourish is the paradigm shift of health care from curative care to preventive care. It is in this segment that systems like Ayurveda score well. The 'wellness trend' is also gaining momentum in the health care, firstly because of the new aged well-informed consumer who is becoming health-conscious. Secondly, due to inflation and ever-increasing cost of high-end medical care, people are ready to invest more time and energy in preventive health care products and practices. "This is causing a rapid increase in the demand for value-added wellness products particularly the nutritional supplements (both in India and abroad). In India, lifestyle disease is already the prime killer mainly in cardiovascular disease and diabetes. Hence, health care is becoming expensive and Indians are taking to wellness and preventive health care practices in droves," agrees Ashutosh Garg, Chairman and Managing Director, Guardian Lifecare.

AyurVaid Hospitals will be establishing through the hub and spoke model, trying to reach maximum audience as possible. "We just opened a hospital in Bangalore and within a few months will be establishing a hospital in the city of Mumbai. The demand for such health care is huge with a population of 18 million people and not a single Ayurvedic hospital available. Hence, we are confident that we would survive well," informs Vasudevan. Since it is targeting the middle and lower-income groups by offering subsidized health care, the Group has tied up with leading insurance players to make the model economically sustainable by generating volumes. AyurVaid Hospitals is accredited by 12 of India's leading medical insurance service providers facilitating cashless Ayurveda medical management, subject to the terms of the underlying insurance policy. "In tying up with leading insurance players and standardising a low-cost and cross-subsidy model, it is a pioneering a way to bring affordable services to low income communities, increasing both the quality and the accessibility of treatment available", says Acumen Fund Country Director, Varun Sahni.

Wellness naturally can be within driving distance of 250 million consumers within five years. The products strategy will make us ubiquitous," reveals Mehta. As for Madhavbaug Group which has plans to open new centres all across Maharashtra and nearby states like Goa, it will expand on a stand-alone basis as well by the franchisee model.

Re-Branding Ayurveda

Whilst the opportunity is immense so are the challenges. The number one challenge this traditional health care system is facing is its brand value. Most people still associate Ayurveda with rejuvenation and relaxation instead of a preferred module for hardcore 'treatment' option. "As Ayurveda is marketed as a preventive therapy by the wellness industry, people hardly know that it has got a great power to cure. The doctor themselves have hammered that it takes time to cure in case of Ayurveda. All these notions have been proven faulty at Madhavbaug, where a fatal disease like heart disease is treated in mere six days. We have been educating the masses how Ayurveda is helpful for the mankind in case of severe and chronic diseases," reacts Dr. Sane. This feeling is unanimously echoed by all the Ayurvedic treatment providers who still feel that because of the way it has been marketed by tourism and hospitality industry, people still find it hard to believe that Ayurveda can be a first line treatment option. "It is the number one challenge the industry is facing. Because spas and wellness resorts are just a part of Ayurveda. It has to move beyond being a 'massage industry.' Also even in North India, the perception is limited to 'jadi-bootiwalas' and it is definitely beyond that. It is a matter of time that people would be aware of the curative powers of Ayurveda and who knows in the future that it may be a first line therapy treatment," believes Vasudevan. Too ambitious we may think, but fast forward a few years and maybe it would indeed be a preferred health care modality and no more it would be a case of Allopathy *v/s* Ayurveda but indeed Allopath *vis-à-vis* Ayurveda. It's ultimately the 'new' consumers who will decide the fate of the 'oldest' form of medicine.

Eye surgery in India

With 10,000 eye doctors in India, the status of eye care and surgery in India is impressive. India has well-qualified doctors and well-equipped eye care centres in smaller towns and metropolitan cities of the country to offer minor to highly specialized eye care treatment. For instance, there are more Lasik centres in India than in some developed countries. Cost-effectiveness and quality are the two factors driving the flow of foreign patients to the eye care centres in India. India has state-of-the-art eye care centres like Sankar Nethralaya, Chennai; All India Institute of Medical Sciences (AIIMS), New Delhi; Aravind Eye Hospital, Madurai and L.V. Prasad Eye Institute, Hyderabad, among others. Aravind Eye Hospital conducts the largest number of cataract surgeries in the world. Costs of comparable treatment in India are on average one-eighth to one-fifth of those in the West. For instance, a cardiac procedure costs anywhere between US$ 40,000-60,000 in the United States, US$ 30,000 in Singapore, US$ 12,000-15,000 in Thailand and only US$ 3,000 -6,000 in India. Likewise, the associated costs of surgery are also low. Not only are skilled Indian surgeons available for less, they are also less susceptible to costly litigation. The cost of malpractice insurance in New York is around US$ 100,000 but only US$ 4000 in India. This brings down the overall cost of treatment.

With diagnostic tests in India being inexpensive, India also has the potential to emerge as a hub for preventive health screening. At a private clinic in London a health check-up for men that includes blood tests, electro-cardiogram tests, chest X-Rays, lung tests and abdominal ultrasound costs around £350. In comparison, a comparable check-up at a clinic operated by Delhi-based health care company Max Health Care costs US$ 84. A Magnetic Resonance Imaging (MRI) scan costs US$ 60 at Escorts Hospital in Delhi, compared with roughly US$ 700 in New York.

The overall cost of travel and treatment in India is still far less than the expense of just the medical treatment in many western countries. A study by the India Brand Equity Foundation (IBEF) in 2004 shows how competitive India is in comparison with Thailand, another leading medical tourism destination. Thailand has a cost advantage over India in only two categories: plastic surgery and breast augmentation. India is cheaper than Thailand across a whole range of other—and more serious—surgery categories.

Cutting edge technology

The gamma knife treatment for brain tumors costs US$ 10,000 (for a two-day package) in Thailand while the same costs US$ 45,000 in the US and Euro 25,000 in Europe. However, India still has a cost advantage here with the same treatment costing roughly about US$ 6,000. India's value proposition goes far beyond cost; quality second to none. Cost is not the only factor weighing in India's favour. Escorts Hospital, for instance, is one of the only handful treatment facilities worldwide that specialize in robotic surgery. The death rate of coronary bypass patients at Escorts is 0.8 per cent. By contrast, the 1999 death rate for the same procedure at New York-Presbyterian Hospital, was 2.35 per cent, according to a 2002 study by the New York State Health Department. The overall success rate of cardiac bypasses is 98.7 per cent in India, as opposed to only 97.5 per cent in the United States. India's health care industry is thus both competitive on cost and quality. US-based private health insurers Blue Cross and Blue Shield and British health insurer Bupa now insure clients treated at a number of private hospitals in India.

Further, hospital chains are offering special packages, which include airport pickups, visa assistance and boarding and lodging. Apollo Group of hospitals for instance has a full fledged international patients department, which offers assistance to patients from the time they land in India to the time they depart. Apollo has about 14 health care facilitators, besides tie ups with two travel agents. Similarly, Escorts Hospital (now a part of the Fortis Group) has an in-house hospitality department that provides all pre and post-treatment assistance, including receiving patients at the airport, arranging accommodation and travel packages to various tourist destinations in the country. Wockhardt group has also been taken over by the fortis group, which is now coming up as the largest conglomerate of health care in the country. Tie-ups and alliances are taking interesting forms. Manipal hospital has tie-ups with the governments of Tanzania and Mauritius. The health expenses of Tanzanians and Mauritians in Manipal Hospital are covered by the respective governments. Further, the hospital's agreements with foreign travel insurance providers give it significant international exposure.

Medical devices

The medical devices market in India is highly promising. The market size for medical devices in India is expected to touch US$ 1.7 billion by 2010, against US$ 1.2 billion presently. The demand for hi-tech products constitutes close to 80 per cent of the overall market in India. Since domestic production comprises primarily of low-tech devices; there is a higher involvement of foreign companies in sourcing hi-tech devices, which alone account for US$ 770 million of market value. Presently, nearly 90 per cent of the demand is being met by imports from countries like USA, Japan and Germany.

The Israel-based US$ 2 billion Europe-Israel Group of companies has evinced interest to set-up an US$ 222.2 million medical equipment factory in the state of West Bengal. Steris, a US$ 1.1 billion health care equipment company, plans to set-up a wholly-owned arm in India to sell its devices and products in the country's booming medical device market. Steris plans to make an initial investment of US$ 1,00,000 to set-up the wholly-owned subsidiary. The Indian arm will also be involved in servicing of medical, surgical and other sterilization products. The German medical device company BSN Medical GmbH—a joint venture of Beiersdorf and Smith and Nephew—plans to set-up a new joint venture in India with 61 per cent foreign equity. The joint venture will be involved in manufacturing and importing products, as well as in distributing, marketing and sales.

Siemens' success story in India

German electrical engineering major Siemens plans to source medical equipment from the Goa facility in India for the regulated markets. The Goa facility earlier used to work as a component manufacturing unit and the products were integrated in Germany from where they were exported. The company has recently completed 40 per cent capacity expansion at its Goa unit and is in the process of receiving regulatory approval from the US FDA and European authorities.

While the global orders will be placed through Siemens, it will be serviced out of India once the regulatory approvals are in place. The Goa plant will now operate as a global production hub. The facility will export products to about 30 countries and is targeting export growth of about 45-50 per cent. Siemens currently exports four models from India and will increase the product portfolio to 8-10 models by the end of next fiscal. The main focus will be on X-ray systems and it will also undertake all global R&D activities for this product segment in this unit. The company's medical solutions division currently generates sales of about US$ 111.1 million for it in India.

Pathology Services

The US$ 500 million domestic pathology industry has been growing over the last five years at an estimated Compound Annual Growth Rate (CAGR) of 20 per cent per annum. It currently comprises almost 2.5 per cent of the overall health care delivery market. With 40,000 independent pathology laboratories in the country, the industry is highly competitive and price-driven.

Labs form an essential and prominent component of health cities

Presently, the lab testing market is largely serviced by small unorganised players and hospitals. Believing that diagnostics is a high-margin and asset-intensive business, many focused players are in the process of developing national networks—such as Dr. Lal's Pathlabs, Metropolis, SRL Ranbaxy, Thyrocare, and Nicholas Piramal. Most renowned path labs are expanding regionally and foraying into the international markets as well. For instance, SRL Ranbaxy Ltd. has signed outsourcing contracts with several UK hospitals to provide pathological services. The Group with 17 labs, 550 collection centres distributed in 350 towns across the country and seven franchisee labs is looking for both franchisees and acquisitions in all the major cities of the country. Metropolis Health Services too plans to increase its collection centres and franchisee systems. It currently has 13 laboratories in India and plan to open at least another 9 labs by the end of next year. Some national players have been successful in attracting the interest of foreign investors. For instance, WestBridge Capital Partners picked up a 26 per cent stake in Dr. Lal's Pathlabs for US$ 9.7 million. Dr. Lal's PathLabs plans to build South Asia's biggest laboratory in Delhi besides expanding in the country. The chain currently has 13 laboratories in the country and plans another 50 labs in the next five years. It plans to double its sample collection centres from 250 at present, in the next five years. These collection centres would be in addition to the 500 pick-up points like major hospitals, nursing homes, other pathology laboratories, doctor's Molecular diagnostics and pharmacogenomic testing to be future growth Molecular diagnostics is the fastest growing segment of the *in-vitro* diagnostics (IVD) market with a projected growth of 25 per cent per annum. Viral diagnostics, immune system disease diagnostics, bacterial, parasitic and fungal identification, cancer diagnosis and monitoring are the segments where molecular technologies enjoy significant cost-benefit advantage. Similarly, pharmacogenomic testing too is believed to usher in an era of personalised medicine where diagnostic tests that will help in selecting the best of the several therapies will be a prerequisite for prescribing a therapy. With the Government expected to bring in a relaxation on customs duty and service tax, molecular diagnostics and pharmacogenomic testing too are touted as the future drivers of the diagnostic industry. By 2010, two million patients are expected for clinical trials in India; translating into 20 million tests.

Preventive aspects of health care and health cities

Increasing health consciousness among common people has created avenues for preventive health care. Hospitals have started witnessing a number of patients who visit for health check-ups as a preventive measure. The various health check-up packages offered include a combination of CBC, blood sugar, cholesterol, urine, stool, digital chest X-Ray, ECG, general examination, blood group, blood sugar, liver profile, proteins, lipid profile, cholesterol, and renal profile. Around 70 per cent of treatment decisions in the country are based on lab results. This trend has further led to newer avenues for companies involved in carrying out diagnostic tests. The entry of foreign health insurance companies in India is proving to be an important driver of the domestic diagnostic industry as coverage of pathology services is inevitable in the policy.

Outsourcing opportunity for hospitals in the west

Outsourcing of pathology and laboratory tests by foreign hospital chains is becoming is a huge opportunity because of the high cost differential in India. A thyroid profile blood test costs anywhere from US$ 30-50 in the US, the same can be analysed by Indian companies for less than US$ 5 per patient. The outsourcing opportunity from UK alone is about 450 million pounds or US$ 800 million. Chennai-based Metropolis Labs has inked a partnership with a US-based consortium to bid for outsourced pathology work from the National Health Services (NHS) of the UK. The consortium, which bagged US$ 600 million of outsourced work last year, is aiming for US$ 1 billion this year. Metropolis would be investing approximately US$ 1 million on technology up-gradation in its Mumbai lab for handling outsourcing jobs. SRL Ranbaxy has tied up with a large UK-based private hospital to outsource work to India.

International players beginning to eye Indian diagnostics pie Apollo Hospitals Enterprise Ltd. has entered into a joint venture with Amcare Labs, an affiliate of Johns Hopkins International of the US, to set-up a diagnostic laboratory in Hyderabad. An initial amount of US$ 2.2 million is to be invested and the laboratory is likely to be operational by mid-2006. General and high-end tests such as tests based on genetic mutation and tests to assess the effect of particular drug on a patient would be done in the lab.

Development of Tele-medicine and health cities

In India, only about 27 per cent of the population lives in urban areas, while a sizeable 73 per cent of the population is rural. While 72 per cent specialist doctors practice in urban areas, only 25 per cent reside in semi-urban areas and a mere 3 per cent in rural areas. The outcome of this lop-sided distribution is that 80 per cent of the medical facilities are concentrated in urban areas and a mere 20 per cent in rural areas, which continue to remain deprived of proper health care facilities. The answer to patient treatment in inaccessible areas in India with fewer medical facilities, is tele-medicine.

The exponential growth in the ICT (Information and Communication Technologies) sector and the plummeting telecom costs are making India highly competitive in tele-medicine. The early successes of pioneers such as Apollo Hospitals, Narayana Hridulaya, AIMS Kochi, SGPGI Lucknow, and SRMC Chennai has resulted in increased acceptance and proliferation of tele-medicine. At present, there are around 120 tele-medicine centres spread. Government and public sector initiatives lend credence to tele-medicine. Though India is yet to pass legislation on tele-medicine-related issues, a beginning has been made. 'Guidelines and Standards for Practice of Tele-medicine in India' has already been recommended by the Ministry of Information Technology, Government of India, to standardise digital communication in tele-medicine. The Medical Council of India has also constituted committees to look into this and other legal aspects of The role played by the Indian Space Research Organisation (ISRO) in not only providing VSATs but also tele-medicine hardware and software has also contributed immensely to the growth. ISRO has taken the initiative to establish tele-medicine centres across India. It plans to set-up 100 tele-medicine centres across the country. ISRO plans to have a minimum number of 650 district hospitals across the country to be networked through tele-medicine by 2008.

Leading corporate hospitals take the lead in tele-medicine. Among private players, the Apollo Hospitals Group established India's first formal tele-medicine centre in a village in Andhra Pradesh, linking it to its hospital in Chennai. The Group has further established a tele-medicine link between Indraprastha Apollo Hospitals at Delhi and Apollo Information.

Asian Heart Institute (AHI) is planning to establish 60 tele-medicine satellite-centres across the interiors of Maharashtra. The company plans to expand its tele-medicine operations across the country. Africa and Middle East are next on the company's radar. Escorts Hospital (now part of the Fortis Group), Wockhardt Hospital and Heart Institute and Max Health Care are other private players providing tele-medicine services.

Tele-radiology emerging as a major niche

The global demand for radiology services in is growing rapidly while the supply of radiologists is not growing enough to match the requirements. Such professionals are is short supply world-over. For instance, reports claim that one in every seven radiology positions in the UK is vacant. On the other hand, in India, there is a relative abundance. By outsourcing tele-radiology to India, overseas hospitals can be assured of competent and trained professionals, time zone advantages, skill set availability, HIPAA mandates adhered to and year-round, round-the-clock services. Patients can be diagnosed and effectively treated at any time of the day or night, with a diagnosis provided from across the globe within 30 minutes. It is cost-effective to the overseas hospital, as the need to recruit night shift personnel is minimized.

According to an estimate, approximately 50 per cent of the 6,000-odd hospitals in the US still do not have the technology for tele-radiology, and this represents a huge potential market to be tapped. Indian health care providers have recognized the opportunity to deliver quality radiology services arising out of this shortage of radiologists internationally. Manipal Education and Medical Group (MEMG) has a global radiology centre jointly operated with Wipro that employs five Indian radiologists and four technologists to read CT scans and MRIs for US patients. Metropolis Clinical Laboratories, which is already in the pathology space is looking to enter tele-radiology. The Indian health imaging market is expected to double from the existing US$ 350 million by 2010. X-ray, ultrasound, CT, and MRI are expected to collectively account for 68.6 per cent of the health imaging market.

Tele-radiology Solutions

Tele-radiology Solutions, started in 2002, was the first company in India to provide US hospitals with tele-radiological services and is today a leader in the imaging markets field. The company today serves 50 hospitals in the US and boasts of an accuracy rate of 99.8 per cent—above the accepted US standard of 96-97 per cent—Tele-radiology Solutions has recently become the first Indian. health care company to be fully accredited by the Joint Commission of Accreditation of Health Care Organisations (JCAHO). The company provides tele-radiology-based services such as diagnostic interpretation of all emergently and non-emergently performed non-invasive imaging studies, including computed tomography, MRI, ultrasound, X-ray, nuclear medicine studies and conventional plain films (digital format). These services are provided with a turnaround time of less than 30 minutes in the emergency setting.

The 75 people-strong company counts among its employees eight US and 14 Indian radiologists, apart from support staff like IT people, transcriptionists, data entry professionals and call centre staff. The company transmits digital images over a distance using standard telephone lines, satellite connections, or wide area networks (WANs). Further, the company is in constant communication with the client hospitals and is readily accessible to all the referring physicians/hospitals at all times. The company is currently expanding its operations to Europe. Spiraling health care costs, unbearable squeeze on margins, process inefficiencies, acute talent shortage and an aging population are compelling health care establishments in the US and Europe to look at Indian health care BPOs. Outsourcing health care business processes to Indian service providers can result in cost savings to the tune of 20-30 per cent. The global market for outsourced services from the health care industry was estimated to be worth US$ 3.6 billion in 2004 and is projected at US$ 24 billion in 2008. The estimated opportunity for India is US$ 4.5 billion by 2008, employing about 200,000 people.

India is capable of offering a wide spectrum of outsourced Health Care Services

The types of services being offered by Health Care BPOs in India include:

- *Data capture*—include reporting of diagnostic tests and radiology.
- *Documentation*—data coding, medical transcription, billing and data
- *Commercial*—invoicing, disbursal, expense reporting, procurement, cash management, general ledger and receivables management.
- *Administration*—claims processing, adjudication, mailroom services and records management.
- *Human resources*—employee assistance, training and payroll
- *Customer care*—dispatch and activation services, technical support.

Companies are further involved in various functions such as

converting existing data to HIPPA format (Health Insurance Portability and Accountability Act), USA, administrative functions, billing and coding tasks, processing forms, including scanning written documents, converting them into an electronic format, and sending them back. BPOs are further involved in claims forms processing for health insurance companies. Number of Indian health care BPOs eyeing the US opportunity The Apollo Group was one of the early entrants in the health care BPO business. Its IT and BPO division—Apollo Health Street (AHS) is set to expand to other countries. Having invested about US$ 3 million in its BPO operations, Apollo is now planning to expand its US operations and is actively looking at a Greenfield venture in the UK. The company is currently doing about US$ 100 million worth of transactions. At present, it has a workforce of 20 people in the US and about 600 in the Hyderabad facility. The company is planning to double its workforce in India in the next few months. The company was also reported to be planning investments close to US$ 10 million for its medical BPO expansion. Among others, AHS has a US$ 6.7 million multiple year contract from a 600 bed hospital in New York. Apollo Health Street's back office work for the provider is primarily revenue cycle management, which includes billing and coding services. The company is also doing billing and coding work for three more providers in the US. Manipal Education and Medical Group (MEMG) provides medical billing and coding services to US hospitals. Here, trained US-approved coders in India work with hospitals to prepare patient bills formatted in a manner required by US insurance companies. Other firms such as Hinduja TMT work with insurance companies on the other side of the chain doing medical claims verification.

Foreign health care BPOs scaling up Indian presence

Integreo Inc., an Atlanta-based health care BPO, is in the process of ramping up its operations in India. Integreo India was formed with the acquisition of Symphony Data in February 2005. The company plans to invest US$ 10 million in its facility at Hyderabad. Integreo is establishing a 60,000 sq. feet facility in Hyderabad and it expects to increase its headcount from 600 employees currently, to 3,000 people by January 2008. It is further planning to set-up a second centre in India, which is expected to be in Pune.

BPO HealthScribe

Bangalore-based health care BPO HealthScribe, which is today a fully owned subsidiary of the Spheris, a US-based medical transcription company, has opened its facility at the STPI IT Park in the Kumaraguru College of Technology campus at Coimbatore under its new name—Spheris India Pvt. Ltd. The Coimbatore-arm is the second location for Spheris in India. The company has invested about US$ 2.2 million on this facility, which covers an area of 35,000 sq feet. The company is planning to add another 15,000 sq feet. It has commenced operations with a workforce of

300, but by the end of 2006, it intends to ramp up its headcount to 3,000 from the existing 2,000 in India. The company expects to see a 30-50 per cent growth over the next two years, consequent to expanding its operations. Health insurance premium is set to touch US$ 533.3 million by the end of 2005-06 as against US$ 385 million in 2004-05, primarily due to growing awareness. Industry analysts believe the figure could even go upto US$ 777.8 million by 2007, in case the insurers decide to increase the premium rate while tapping virgin markets. With escalating medical costs, companies are already looking at the option of increasing the premium by about 15 per cent to 20 per cent for health insurance.

In order to spur the private health insurance sector, the Insurance Regulatory and Development Authority (IRDA) has increased the FDI limit from 26 per cent to 51 per cent. It has further reduced the minimum capital requirement to US$ 11.1 million. The government is mulling over a proposal to further lower the minimum threshold limit for standalone health insurance companies to US$ 5.6 million.

Health insurance is a rapidly growing market in India. The number of lives covered under health plans has improved from 4-5 million about six years back to over 12 million today. With benefits being offered to private players in the health insurance market, a number of international insurers are making their presence felt in India. Along with offering general insurance, Iffco Tokio has made an entry into the health insurance market. Chubb is another entrant into India. It has formed an alliance with HDFC for offering health insurance. Miliman is the latest multinational to make a foray into the Indian health insurance sector. A large number of companies are also waiting in the wings to make a foray into the market, including leading global players such as Aetna, Brooke Shield, and Blue Cross, among others.

Accreditation of health cities and other hospitals

The Government of India has formed a task force consisting of experts from the Ministries of Health and Family Welfare, Tourism, Railways, External Affairs, Civil Aviation, and the Director-General of Health Services. This task force has been set-up with the objective to suggest policy measures and norms for the National Accreditation Board to provide accreditation to all public and private hospitals to ensure quality and timely health services. The draft on standards of health care accreditation, prepared by the technical committee of National Accreditation Board of Hospitals and Health Care Providers (NABH), is ready. The draft would ensure uniform access, assessment, care of patients and protect patient's The Government is further expected to release a Clinical Establishment Act by 2006 to make sure that fair and quality health services are provided to The Ministry of Health and Ministry of External Affairs have reached a policy decision so that 'medical visas', which are issued to overseas patients seeking medical care in India, are granted within a month or in even lesser time to all incoming patients.

Allowing 100 per cent FDI subject to approval by the Foreign Investment Promotion Board under the Department of Industrial Policy and Promotion in the Ministry of Industry and Commerce has assisted in opening up the Indian health care market for international investors. Health Ministry has finalized a notification amending the Drugs and Cosmetics Rules to include medical devices. It has further finalized regulations related to medical devices wherein companies manufacturing or importing stents, pacemakers, valves, catheters, and other such implants would have to seek prior approval from the regulator. Implants for hips and knee replacements will also be brought under the ambit of licensing. While *in-vivo* devices will be regulated initially, it is planned that *in-vitro* implants would later be added. The Drug Controller General of India (DCGI), which gives clearances to medicines before they are introduced in the market, will be the nodal agency.

5

Medical and Health Cities can Boost Biotechnology

Health and disease is the subject for scientific scrutiny and the development of biotechnological aids. It has implications on life and death, suffering and well-being. This makes it important to analyze how knowledge concerning health and sickness is being created, is being maintained and is changing. Biotechnology, in its broadest sense, is the use of biological systems to carry out technical processes. Red biotechnology involves medical processes such as getting organisms to produce new drugs, or using stem cells to regenerate damaged human tissues and perhaps re-grow entire organs. From a spit test for cancer to a shot that helps your body re-grow nerves along your spinal cord, these new advances in the world of medicine blur the line between biology and technology to help restore, improve and extend our lives.

Research, medical education and patient care

Health and medical cities can boost biotechnology as a part of research and futuristic development in addition to clinical care of the patients and enhancement of skill and training. Thus Health city is not the clinical and investigative aspects of patients alone, it entails many other aspects viz. health and fitness, preventive medicine, development of new devices and innovation of new equipment, molecular biology and nanotechnology, development of new drugs and molecules, disposal of bio-waste, production of more nutritive food and vaccines, study of stem cells and their application in chronic ailments and much more. Setting up of such a institute as a part of a health city augurs well for overall improvement of quality of life of humans. Examples of this kind of set-up can be seen in several countries. Recently a new drug-development institute was set-up in collaboration of Hamner Institutes for Health Sciences U.S.

and China Medical City. The new institute, called the Hamner-China Medical City Institute for International Drug Development, will receive $5 million from Chinese-American CRO New-summit Biopharma, and will attempt to leverage each partner's strengths in translational research, business development, and education to produce new biomedical technologies. During the first phase of the agreement, the partners will establish the new institute at Hamner's campus in Research Triangle Park, NC, where scientists will focus on preclinical drug development and compliance with US Food and Drug Administration regulatory standards. After the partners validate research capabilities and new technologies at the Hamner campus, they will transfer them to China Medical City, a life-science park located in the Yangtze River Delta north of Shanghai. As part of the agreement, Hamner will work with the North Carolina Department of Commerce and North Carolina Biotechnology Center to create a North Carolina-China partner network to support Chinese business and educational initiatives.

China Medical City takes a lead

The Hamner institute began in 1974 as The Chemical Industry Institute of Toxicology, an independent research institute formed by leaders from 11 major chemical companies to address growing concerns about the effects of small-molecule chemicals on the environment and human health. Since then, the institute, named for North Carolina and RTP biotech pioneer Charles Hamner, has broadened its mission to include translational research in biopharmaceutical safety, metabolic disorders, respiratory disease, oncology, and nanosafety. Last year, the institute signed an agreement with the University of North Carolina-Chapel Hill to create an integrated Center for Drug Safety Sciences to study the safety of biotechnology and pharmaceutical products. The institute has also established research and business-development agreements with Duke, North Carolina State University, and Wake Forest University.

BIOTECHNOLOGY IN MEDICINE

Biotechnology entails any technique that is used to make or modify the products of living organisms in order to improve plants or animals, or to develop useful microorganisms. In modern terms, biotechnology has come to mean the use of cell and tissue culture, cell fusion, molecular biology, and in particular, recombinant deoxyribonucleic acid (DNA) technology to generate unique organisms with new traits or organisms that have the potential to produce specific useful products. Biotechnology also holds great promise in the production of vaccines for use in maintaining the health of animals. Interferons are also being tested for their use in the management of specific diseases.

Animals may be transformed to carry genes from other species including humans and are being used to produce valuable drugs. For example, goats are being used to produce tissue plasminogen activator, which has been effective in dissolving blood clots. Genetic engineering has enabled the large-scale production of proteins which have great potential for treatment of heart attacks. Many human gene products, produced with genetic engineering technology, are being investigated for their potential use as commercial drugs. Recombinant technology has been employed to produce vaccines from subunits of viruses, so that the use of either live or inactivated viruses as immunizing agents is avoided. Cloned genes and specific, defined nucleic acid sequences can be used as a means of diagnosing infectious diseases or in identifying individuals with the potential for genetic disease. The specific nucleic acids used as probes are normally tagged with radioisotopes, and the DNAs of candidate individuals are tested by hybridization to the labeled probe. The technique has been used to detect latent viruses such as herpes, bacteria, mycoplasmas, and plasmodia, and to identify Huntington's disease, cystic fibrosis, and Duchenne muscular dystrophy. It is now also possible to put foreign genes into cells and to target them to specific regions of the recipient genome. This presents the possibility of developing specific therapies for hereditary diseases, exemplified by sickle-cell anemia.

Modified micro-organisms are being developed with abilities to degrade hazardous wastes. Genes have been identified that are involved in the pathway known to degrade polychlorinated biphenyls, and some have been cloned and inserted into selected bacteria to degrade this compound in contaminated soil and water. Other organisms are being sought to degrade phenols, petroleum products, and other chlorinated compounds.

However, in the future, the most significant breakthroughs in human medicine will result from mapping and understanding the human genome—in elucidating the exact sequence of the billions of nucleotides that constitute the estimated 30,000-40,000 genes that are the collective blueprint for human beings and are responsible for some 10,000 genetic disorders. The Human Genome Project was launched in 1990 as a 15-year, $3 billion international effort to map and sequence all human genes. Innovations in sequencing technology have ensured that the project moved ahead of schedule. With less than 5% of all human genes identified at the start of the project, it has become increasingly clear that each new gene discovery proffers new drugs for the diagnosis, treatment, and prevention of human disease. These drugs include therapeutic proteins, diagnostics, gene therapy reagents, and small molecules. A significant proportion of the human genome has been sequenced and many new human disease genes are being characterized. These advances will enable biotechnologists not only to measure disease potential and expand the applications for genomic diagnostics but also to devise fundamental new therapeutic approaches.

Biotechnology revolution in health care and medicine

Biotechnology is facilitating the development of new medicines, producing them faster, cheaper, safe and more efficient. Instead of just studying the new drugs in clinical trials, scientists are identifying the generic cause of diseases. By stimulation, they are able to design and study the action of new products. An estimated 400 pharmaceutical companies worldwide are conducting research and development into genetically engineered products and industry predicts that in few years several hundred genetically engineered products will be on the market. Many scientists believe that the impact of genetics in medicine will revolutionize the concept of human health and the scientific revolution in medical genetics is happening at a very fast pace. By year 2010 genetic tests will be available for 25 commonly encountered genetic disorders and by year 2020, drugs based on pharmogenomics will be routine part of common diseases such as diabetes and high blood pressure and by year 2040, individualized medicines will be produced.

Biotechnology revolution in health care

Biotechnology revolution in health care and medicine started with the recombinant DNA technology (often referred as genetic engineering) revolution that began around 1970's. It allowed scientists to transfer genes from one organism to another, circumventing the sexual process. Several enzymes (such as restriction enzymes that cut DNA molecule at specific sites; DNA ligase that join DNA fragments end to end; DNA polymerase that synthesize DNA on a complementary template and DNA modification enzymes that are used to control ligation bacteria manipulate DNA as a part of their normal cellular process enabled the recombinant DNA (rDNA) technology to flourish. In any exercise, the final objective of genetic engineering or rDNA technology is the stable and inheritable expression of a new trait in different organisms and certain basic steps are common to all rDNA experiments. To construct an rDNA molecule, DNA is isolated from a donor cell (animal or plant) and a plasmid is cut with the same restriction enzyme and mixed. "Sticky ends" of donor DNA form hydrogen bonds with the sticky ends of plasmid DNA fragment and recombinant molecule is sealed with another specific enzyme (ligases). Modified plasmid (rDNA) is introduced into a bacterium, which reproduces and clones the gene from donor cell that was spliced into the plasmid. The initial advances made in rDNA technology have increased our fundamental knowledge of the molecular basis of human diseases and this has resulted into the development of new field of medicine, known as molecular medicine. Stanley Cohen and Herbert Boyer in 1973 and their work are the basis of much of the current work in biotechnology.

Biotechnology will shape the future research as this field is being driven forward both by private biotechnology companies and also by academicians who are introducing new technologies required for the parallel identification of individual proteins. Economic impacts of biotechnology will surpass the information technology and there will be a greater demand for qualified biotechnologists. As such the developing countries need to focus on the production of highly trained manpower in the field of biotechnology not only for local market but also for export purposes.

Benefits of biotechnology

(i) disease prevention,
(ii) disease detection,
(iii) therapeutic agents,
(iv) new smart gadgets,
(v) correction of genetic diseases,
(vi) fertility control, and
(vii) forensic medicine.

It is aimed to highlight the major developments under each of these categories by citing appropriate examples.

Glamorous illustrations of biotechnology in health care

Decay-Fighting Microbes; Swab SMaRT

Bacteria living on teeth convert sugar into lactic acid, which erodes enamel and causes tooth decay. BioPharma US has engineered a new bacterial strain, called SMaRT, that cannot produce lactic acid-plus, it releases an antibiotic that kills the natural decay-causing strain. Dentists will only need to swab SMaRT, onto teeth once to keep them healthy for a lifetime.

Artificial Lymph Nodes

Scientists from Japan's RIKEN Institute have developed artificial versions of lymph nodes, organs that produce immune cells for fighting infections. The artificial nodes may initially be used as customized immune boosters. Doctors could fill the nodes with cells specifically geared to treat certain conditions, such as cancer or HIV.

Asthma Sensor

Asthma accounts for a quarter of all emergency room visits round the world, but a sensor developed at the University of Pittsburgh, USA, may finally cause that number to decline. Inside the handheld device, a polymer-coated carbon nanotube—100,000 times thinner than a human hair—analyzes breath for minute amounts of nitric oxide, a gas that lungs produce prior to asthma attacks.

Cancer Spit Test

Forget biopsies—a device designed by researchers at the University of California—Los Angeles detects oral cancer from a single drop of saliva. Proteins that are associated with cancer cells react with dyes on the sensor, emitting fluorescent light that can be detected with a microscope. The same principle could be applied to make saliva-based diagnostic tests for many diseases.

Biological Pacemaker

Electronic pacemakers save lives, but the hardware used eventually wears out. Now, researchers at several universities are developing a battery-less alternative: pacemaker genes expressed in stem cells that are injected into damaged regions of the heart. Better suited for physical exertion, biological pacemakers have been shown to bring slow canine hearts back upto speed without complications.

Prosthetic Feedback

One challenge of prosthetic limbs is that they're difficult to monitor. Skin is sensitive to being stretched-it can detect even small changes in direction and intensity—so Bark is developing a device that stretches an amputee's skin near the prosthesis in ways that provide feedback about the limb's position and movement.

Contact Lens to monitor glaucoma

Glaucoma, the second-leading cause of blindness, develops when pressure builds inside the eye and damages retinal cells. Contact lenses developed at the University of California-Davis contain conductive wires that continuously monitor pressure and fluid flow within the eyes of at-risk people. The lenses then relay information to a small device worn by the patient; the device wirelessly transmits it to a computer. This constant data flow will help doctors better understand the causes of the disease. Future lenses may also automatically dispense drugs in response to pressure changes.

Speech Restorer

For people who have lost the ability to talk, a new "phonetic speech engine" from Illinois-based Ambient Corporation provides an audible voice. Developed in conjunction with Texas Instruments, the Audeo uses electrodes to detect neuronal signals traveling from the brain to the vocal cords. Patients imagine slowly sounding out words; then the quarter-size device (located in a neck brace) wirelessly transmits those impulses to a computer or cell phone, which produces speech.

Absorbable Heart Stent

Stents open arteries that have become narrowed or blocked because of coronary artery disease. Drug-eluting stents release medication that keeps the artery from narrowing again. The bio-absorbable version made by Abbott Laboratories in Illinois goes one step further: Unlike metal stents, it does its job and disappears. After six months the stent begins to dissolve, and after two years it's completely gone, leaving behind a healthy artery.

Muscle Stimulator

In the time it takes for broken bones to heal, nearby muscles often atrophy from lack of use. Israeli company StimuHeal solves that problem with the MyoSpare, a battery-operated device that uses electrical stimulators-small enough to be worn underneath casts—to exercise muscles and keep them strong during recovery.

Nerve Regenerator

Nerve fibers can't grow along injured spinal cords because scar tissue gets in the way. A nanogel developed at Northwestern University eliminates that impediment. Injected as a liquid, the nanogel self-assembles into a scaffold of nanofibers. Peptides expressed in the fibers instruct stem cells that would normally form scar tissue to produce cells that encourage nerve development. The scaffold, meanwhile, supports the growth of new axons up and down the spinal cord.

Stabilizing Insoles

When Erez Lieberman's grandmother suffered a dangerous fall, he wanted to ensure it never happened again. "But it wasn't till a few years later at NASA that I found a way to channel that into something tangible". Using technology developed to monitor the balance of astronauts who have just returned from space, Lieberman's iShoe analyzes the pressure distribution of the feet. Doctors can use the insole to diagnose balance problems in elderly patients before falls occur.

Smart Pill

California-based Proteus Biomedical has engineered sensors that track medication use by recording the exact time drugs are ingested. "To really improve pharmaceuticals, we need to do what is now common in every other industry-embed digital technology into existing products and network them," says David O'Reilly, senior vice-president of corporate development.

Autonomous Wheelchair

MIT researchers have developed an autonomous wheelchair that can take people where they ask to go. The chair learns about its environment by listening as a patient identifies locations—such as "this is my room" or "we're in the kitchen"—and builds maps using Wi-Fi, which works well indoors (unlike GPS). The current model, which is now being tested, may one day be equipped with cameras, laser rangefinders and a collision-avoidance system.

Gastrointestinal Liner

Obesity is associated with type II diabetes, which over time wears out the pancreas. A gastrointestinal liner developed by Massachusetts—based GI Dynamics may restore the obese to a healthy weight by preventing food from contacting the intestinal wall. Unlike a gastric bypass, no surgery is necessary—and lines the first 2 ft of the small intestine, where the most calories are absorbed (nutrients are still absorbed farther down the intestine).

Liver Scanner

How healthy is your liver? Until recently, answering that question often required a painful biopsy. French company EchoSens has developed a machine that scans the organ for damage in just 5 minutes. Studies have shown that damaged livers become stiffer and less elastic, so the scanner, called the Fibroscan, measures the organ's elasticity using ultrasound.

Nanoscale Adhesive

Gecko feet are covered with nano-size hairs that exploit intermolecular forces, allowing the lizards to stick firmly to surfaces. By replicating this nanoscale topography, MIT scientists have developed an adhesive that can seal wounds or patch a hole caused by a stomach ulcer. The adhesive is elastic, waterproof and made of material that breaks down as the injury heals.

Portable Dialysis

Standard dialysis involves three long sessions at a hospital per week. But an artificial kidney developed by Los Angeles-based Xcorporeal can clean blood around the clock. The machine is fully automated, battery-operated, waterproof and, at less than 5 pounds, portable.

Walking Simulator

Stroke victims are being tricked into recovering more quickly with a virtual-reality rehabilitation program developed at the University of Portsmouth in Britain. As patients walk on a treadmill, they see moving images that fool their brains into thinking they are walking slower than they are. As a result, patients not only walk faster and farther, but experience less pain while doing so.

Rocket-Powered Arm

Adding strength to prosthetic limbs has typically required bulky battery packs. Vanderbilt University scientist Michael Goldfarb came up with an alternative power source: rocket propellant. Goldfarb's prosthetic arm can lift 20 pounds—three to four times more than current prosthetics—thanks to a pencil-size version of the mono-propellant rocket-motor system used to maneuver the space shuttle in orbit. Hydrogen peroxide powers the arm for 18 hours of normal activity.

Biotechnology in Indian medicine

Biotechnology in India has made great progress in the development of infrastructure, manpower, research and development and manufacturing of biological reagents, bio-diagnostics, bio-therapeutics, therapeutic and, prophylactic vaccines and bio-devices. Many of these indigenous biological reagents, bio-diagnostics, therapeutic and prophylactic vaccines and bio-devices have been commercialized. With the liberalization of Indian economy, more and more imported biotechnology products will enter into the Indian market. The conditions of internal development of biotechnology are not likely to improve in the near future and it is destined to grow only very slowly. Even today biotechnology in India may be called to be in its infancy.

Sports Medicine; technological revolution in diagnostic, clinical and rehabilitation areas

With different sports finally gaining the desired recognition in India and people getting increasingly concerned about their health and fitness quotient, the sports medicine specialty also seem to have dropped the veil of anonymity. This segment has witnessed a technological revolution in diagnostic, clinical and rehabilitation areas which has taken the treatment in sports medicine to the next level.

Gait and Motion Analysis, Multi-joint Dynamometer with Sports Simulator, balance assessment and training system, EMG biofeedback, Human performance evaluation, Muscular strength testing, advanced arthroscopic interventions are just few of the many examples of latest advancements in sports medicine technology and techniques, which has opened up a plethora of options for the advanced treatments in sports injuries, performance enhancement and fitness. Says Dr Chandra Siddaiah, HOD and Consultant, Department of Sports and Exercise Medicine

Manipal Hospital, Bangaluru, "There are plenty of options for the sports doctors to diagnose, treat and rehabilitate athletes with injuries. Now almost all parameters of sports performance can be scientifically assessed like VO2 Max, Lactate threshold tests, Gait analysis, Resting Metabolic Rate

Musculoskeletal strength power, and endurance. Since a long time, biomechanical assessment of sports specific movements like running, throwing, swimming, etc. has been done using highly advanced motion analysis systems.

Revolution in Diagnostic and Rehabilitation

Gait and Motion Analysis

An athlete needs efficient movement of flexible joints, strong muscles and balance between different muscle groups. If this is not there, the athlete is prone to many injuries. This is seen in many conditions of the foot and ankle, which maybe bony (leg length difference), muscular imbalances or tendon disorders. Gait and motion analysis has helped the doctors in finding the cause of many of these lower limb problems. Gait and motion analysis is an assessment of the way a sportsman walk and run. This analysis gives in-depth insight about the technology is available in India in various centers (approximately at 6-7 centers in India), but skilled biomechanist who can analyse the data are not available. Further, database of Indian athletes is not available for comparison. "These systems are essential to improve skill and performance. This technology is also being presently used to treat patients with gait abnormalities," states Dr Parag Sancheti, Chairman, SIOR, Pune.

Multi-joint Dynamometer with Sports Simulator

As the name suggests, the system serves two separate functions. The multi-joint dynamometer can measure muscle strength of any major muscle group in three different modes; isokinetic, isotonic and isometric. This assessment helps in making rehabilitation programme and strength training schedule for patients with sports or other injuries, targeting isolated weaker muscle groups specifically. The training can be initiated on the machine using isokinetic mode in the early stage after injury reducing the impact on the joint. Sports simulator can simulate many activities/actions in sports like throwing, bowling, driving, etc. This gives objective evidence in performing functional capacity evaluation and disability assessment.

The Primus Rehabilitation System

Primus is a highly advanced musculoskeletal evaluation and rehabilitation machine. This machine is designed for assessment of muscle strength, power and endurance of any group of muscles and also rehabilitates any musculoskeletal injuries. This can perform muscle training in various modes such as isometric, isotonic, isokinetic and also improves range of movements of a joint in a controlled graded manner. Sportsmen for example, cricket bowlers can get their shoulder strength, power, and endurance assessed before and after a training regime to know their prognosis. "It allows testing and exercise of patients across an extensive range of conditions. It is According to Dr Sancheti, this is good equipment for functional training and testing. It can be used from the sub-acute stage of the injury upto end stage rehabilitation and return to play. Again, the only drawback is the equipment is expensive.

Balance Assessment and Training System (BATS)

This system helps in assessing the balance capabilities of a sportsman and evaluates the underlying cause of impaired balance in patients with sports injuries. "Balance Master is one of its kinds as it helps in both balance assessment as well as training. Balance and proprioception are a key component of sports performance and sometimes all that separates top level sportsmen is their somatosensory, visual, or proprioceptive capability," shares Dr Pardiwala. Balance can be impaired because of somatosensory, visual or vestibular dysfunction.

EMG Btoftedback

EMG stands for electromyography, measures the electrical response of the muscles when contracting. The electrical response is measured with pads placed muscular tension. EMG biofeedback produces more rapid and significantly greater development of strength when combined with more traditional form of strength training.

Diagnostic

- *MRI scan*: State-of-the-art machines to diagnose soft tissue injuries.
- *Diagnostic ultrasound*: Cheap, non-invasive to detect muscle/soft tissue injuries.
- *Diagnostic arthroscopy*: Minimally invasive for accurate diagnosis and treatment.

Rehabilitation

- Electrotherapy modalities.

Combination therapy units

Gives multiple treatment options for acute/ sub-acute and chronic injuries. Easy to carry when travelling with a team.

Shockwave Therapy

Latest in treatment of tendon injuries.

Laser, longwave therapy, traction systems (Eg. DTS)

Gait analysis

Biomechanical gait analysis can be used extensively to prevent injuries and injury recurrence. Strength testing and training.

Use of Isotonic/Isokinetic machines having a dynamometer can be used to find inherent weakness in muscles and muscle imbalance.

Helpful in injury prevention and preventing injury recurrence.

Training Equipment

Swiss balls, therabands, balance boards.

Essentially used during the sub-acute and final stages of rehab to improve strength and proprioception which is essential for return to play.

Balance trainer

Sophisticated equipment (eg. Core Balance) available to train proprioception, balance and co-ordination which is commonly affected after an injury.

Rehab Gym Equipment

Sophisticated gym equipment (eg. Proxomed) which gives visual feedback to the athlete during rehab, speed/poundage, range of motion power can be controlled during exercise with the help of this equipment.

Human Performance Evaluation (VO2 max)

Maximal oxygen uptake (VO2 max) is the maximum capacity of an individual's body to transport and utilise oxygen during graded exercise, which reflects the physical fitness of the individual. It is an important determinant of endurance performance which represents a true parametric measure of cardio-res-piratory capacity of an individual at a given degree of fitness and oxygen availability.

It involves a graded exercise test (either on treadmill or cycle ergo meter) in which exercise intensity is progressively increased while measuring ventilation and oxygen and carbon dioxide concentration of the inhaled and exhaled air. VO2 max is reached when oxygen consumption reaches a peak and remains at steady state despite achieving maximal or sub-maximal heart rate of the individual. "Use of sophisticated equipment such as VO2 analysers can definitely help in performance enhancement, to improve the cardio-respiratory endurance depending on the nature of the sport," states Dr Sancheti.

Experts consider this technology extremely important in India since it reflects the physical fitness and athletic capability of the sportsman, and is also utilized in planning cardiopulmonary and sports rehabilitation programmes. However, this equipment too is expensive and few centers in India have this facility. Also there is very limited Indian database available for comparison.

3 Tesla MRI is used for more accurate imaging studies of joint injuries, especially useful for cartilage injuries and 3 dimensional mapping of articular cartilage defects.

Surge in Surgical techniques

Advanced arthroscopic intervention of not just the knee, but all major joints (hip, ankle, shoulder, elbow, wrist) has been possible because of better endoscopic instrumentation and advances in visualization systems. This has resulted in all operations on joints (except replacement surgery and major fractures) now being performed arthroscopically (as against open surgery), enabling minimal surgical morbidity and early return to full function and sports.

Better Arthroscopic Fixation Systems

Better arthroscopic fixation systems (for example in knee ligament surgery and shoulder surgery) including bioabsorbable screws and anchors ensure early rehabilitation with no need for subsequent implant removal.

Computer Navigated Knee Ligament Surgery and Osteotomy

This surgical technique is available worldwide since the past few months. This ensures precision surgery especially in complex and revision knee arthroscopy cases and ACL/PCL ligament reconstruction.

Platelet Rich Plasma (PRP) Therapy

A number of orthopedic and sports conditions remain a major therapeutic challenge to orthopaedic surgeons. Some of these difficult conditions include plantar fasciitis (chronic pain in the sole of the foot), tennis elbow (chronic pain in the elbow), ligament and muscle injuries (around the knee and other joints) and tendo-achelles (heel) injuries. Persistent symptoms, due to these conditions, in young sporty individuals have lead to premature ending of their competitive careers. PRP therapy is now being effectively used to mend ligaments and repair tendon injuries.

Whole blood (about 30 ml) is drawn from the patient, prior to the injection, in the blood bank. The blood is then centrifuged. to separate the plasma (buffy coat) from the blood. This concentrate, which contains platelets and growth factors (multiplied several fold), is then mixed with activating agents and is injected back into the patient's own damaged tissue where it begins to initiate the process of repair. The repair response in the injured tissue is kick-started by the formation of a blood clot. This is then followed by the implanted platelets being dissolved, triggering the release of growth factors which in turn leads to the formation of a fibrous scar.

ESWL

Non-invasive modalities such as ESWL; Extracorporeal Shock Lithotripsy are now available for muscle and tendon problems (tennis elbow, elbow, heel pain, calcific tendonitis of shoulder, Achilles tendinitis) in athlete modality has ensured that many sportsmen will severe tendonitis problem avoid surgery as a means of return to sport.

Even though the technology is available worldwide, in India the conditions doesn't seem very promising. Moreover, the sports medicine personnel have limited exposure to above equipment.

CT coronary Angiography

Heart disease is the single largest cause of mortality and morbidity amongst all diseases. As India's economy is flourishing, there appears to be a rise in Coronary Artery Diseases (CAD) especially in the affluent class. In fact, India has become the heart disease capital of the world. An increasingly sedentary lifestyle, changing food habits and an ever increasing stressful and competitive work culture have just multiplied the risk factors for coronary artery disease. The need of the hour is a non-invasive, out-patient investigation that accurately diagnoses coronary artery disease early. CT Coronary angiography plays this role to perfection.

Multi-Slice CT (MSCT) has gained clinical acceptance for cardiac imaging, owing to improved temporal and spatial resolution with the latest multi-detector technology which allows amazingly accurate 3-D imaging from a beating heart. With this advanced machine, every routine CT scan is a 3-D image. It takes only five seconds and one breath hold for the whole heart scan.

What is GT Coronary Angiography?

CT coronary angiography is a simple non-invasive method that uses X-rays to visualize blood flow in coronary arteries which supply blood to the heart. The size of the heart and the thickness of the wall of the heart chambers are evaluated and even the surrounding area of the heart, including the lungs are visualized.

The Procedure

- This is a simple, non-invasive OPD test just like a routine CT scan test. There is no need for admission.
- The person is placed on a comfortable CT scanner table.
- Deposits of calcium in the heart are first calculated.

A CT angiogram is obtained following contrast injection:

- The entire procedure hardly takes 10 to 15 minutes after which the person is ready to continue his/her routine.

Information Obtained

Firstly, detection and quantification of calcium within the coronary vessels is obtained. Calcification in the vessel wall is an indicator of degree of damage that has occurred to the vessels. A high calcium score is consistent with a moderate to high risk of CAD. A negative calcium score is predictive of a comparatively very low incidence of CAD. The coronary arteries, their lumen, wall and plaques are seen and assessment of luminal obstruction is done. The adjacent lungs are also visualized.

What Else?

The 64-slice in a single rotation, high quality imaging allows triple heart 'rule out', i.e. the three critical causes of serious heart condition namely, CAD, pulmonary embolism and aortic dissection are evaluated in one scan.

Working on the Same Day?

Can the patient go back to work on the same day? Yes, since it is a non-invasive OPD procedure, the work can be resumed on the same day after the test.

Eligibility

Who should undergo CT coronary angiography?

- Asymptomatic patient with family history of coronary artery disease.
- Patient with high risk factors.
- Prior to non-coronary surgery in the adult population, e.g. pre-ASD repair, pre-valvular repair and pre-tumour surgery.
- Follow-up for post-CABG.
- Atypical chest pain with doubtful coronary origin.

- Evaluation of coronary anomalies.
- Assessment of cardiac neoplasm.
- Diagnosis of pericardial disease.
- Non-conclusive stress tests.
- 64 Slice MDCT is an excellent, fast, non-invasive modality for pre-operative as well post-operative assessment of pulmonary arteries and its associated anomalies and complications in pediatric patients.

Who Does Not Qualify CT Coronary Angiography

Patient with hypersensitivity to iodinated contrast, renal insufficiency with serum Creatinine > 1.5 mg/dl, congestive heart failure, atrial fibrillation and inability to hold breath for five seconds should not be referred for CT coronary angiography.

Who are at Risk?

Patients with strong family history, heavy smokers, diabetics, patients with high blood pressure, obese patients, patients with high cholesterol and triglycerides, people with high stress and high tension jobs, alcoholics, etc.

What are Asymptomatic Patients?

People may be suffering from Coronary Artery Disease without being aware of it, because many of them may not have any typical clinical symptoms like chest pain or may have atypical symptoms like chest tightness or breathlessness or gaseous discomfort. These are cases which can go undetected for a long time. For many of these cases, heart attack may be first sign of Coronary Artery Disease and many of such patients never reach the hospital.

Difference with Catheter Angiography

- Unlike catheter angiography, CT coronary angiography does not require admission in the hospital. In contrast, with the conventional catheter angiogram, where a dye is injected into the lumen of the coronary artery, the CT angiogram is able to demonstrate the wall of the artery as well as heart itself.
- At times, though there: large cholesterol plaque deposit on the wall of artery, the artery remodels its lumen and become wider. This is called positive remodeling. These plaques may not be picked up on catheter angiogram, as there is no reduction in the vessel caliber. However, CT scanner is able demonstrate these plaques with ease.
- Abnormal courses of coronary arteries and cogenital anomalies are demonstrated by the model of the heart on 64-slice CT. It may be tedious and difficult to demonstrate such abnormalities in arteries by catheter angiogram.

- CT coronary angiogram is an excellent test for coronary artery bypass grafts.

PET/CT

Hailed as the investigation of this century, Positron Emission Tomography—Computed Tomography (better known by its acronym PET-CT) is a medical imaging device which combines in a single gantry system both a Positron Emission Tomography (PET) and an X-Ray Computed Tomography, so that images acquired from both devices can be taken sequentially, in the same session from the patient and combined into a single superposed (co-registered) image. Thus, functional imaging obtained by PET, which depicts the spatial distribution of metabolic or biochemical activity in the body can be more precisely aligned or correlated with anatomic imaging obtained by CT scanning. Two- and three-dimensional image reconstruction may be rendered as a function of a common software and control system.

PET-CT has revolutionized many fields of medical diagnosis, by adding precision of anatomic localization to functional imaging, which was previously lacking from pure PET imaging. For example, in oncology, surgical planning, radiation therapy and cancer staging have been changing rapidly under the influence of PET-CT availability, to the extent that many diagnostic imaging procedures and centers have been gradually abandoning conventional PET devices and substituting them by PET-CTs. Although the combined device is considerably more expensive, it has the advantage of providing both functions as stand-alone examinations, being, in fact, two devices in one.

The Story of PET/CT

Doctors, especially cancer surgeons, were often frustrated in trying to match PET images with CT images to determine the precise location of a tumor in relation to an organ or the spinal column. They had little choice other than to 'eyeball' the two separate images and make an educated guess as to the tumor's exact location until 1992, when engineer Ron Nutt and combined PET and CT concept for three years, Nutt and Townsend installed a prototype machine at the university of Pittsburgh medical centre in 1998. Time Magazine honored PET/CT as the 'Medical Science Investigation of the year' in 2000, noting that the PET/CT scanner has 'provided medicine with a powerful new diagnostic tool'.

How Does PET/CT WORK?

The PET/CT systems now in wide clinical use combine a multi-detector PET system with a multi-detector (currently 4-16 slice) Computed Tomography (CT) scanner in a single unit with a patient couch which traverses the bore of both imaging components. Approximately 30 to 60 minutes after intravenous FDG administration the patient is placed on the examination couch. The CT data is acquired first (lasting around 30 seconds) followed by a repeat slower transit of the patient through the bore for PET data acquisition (lasting around 30-45 minutes).

The CT and PET data sets are fused or 'co-registered' electronically by the scanner's computer system and presented to the interpreter on a work station. The data can then be simultaneously and interactively viewed as CT data, PET data, and superimposed CT and PET data in any percentage combination of these data sets desired (e.g. 100 per cent PET data, 100 per cent CT data, 50 per cent CT/50 per cent PET data).

PET/CT Indications

PET/CT is particularly effective in identifying whether cancer is present or not, if it has spread, if it is responding to treatment, and if a person is cancer free after treatment.

Cancers for which PET/CT is considered particularly effective include lung, head and neck, colorectal, esophageal, lymphoma, melanoma, and breast, as well as a variety of other tumors.

Early Detection

Conversely, because a PET/CT scan images the entire body, conformation of distant metastases can alter treatment plans, in certain cases, from surgical intervention to chemotherapy. PET/CT is extremely sensitive in determining the full extent of disease, especially in lymphoma, malignant melanoma, breast, lung and colon cancers. Conformation of the presence or absence of metastatic disease allows the physician to more effectively decide how to proceed with the patient's management.

Checking for Recurrences

PET/CT is currently considered to be the most accurate diagnostic procedure to differentiate tumor recurrences from radiation necrosis or post-surgical changes in many types of cancer. Such an approach allows for the development of a more rational treatment plan for the patient.

Assessing the Effectiveness of Chemotherapy

The level of tumor metabolism is compared on PET/CT scans taken before and after a chemotherapy cycle. PET/CT can provide important about the effectiveness of a chemotherapy treatment plan. Treatment regime can be altered or modified according to the PET/CT scan evidence of treatment response.

Neurology

PET/CT's ability to measure metabolism has significant implications in localizing the site or origin of epilepsy, because it can vividly illustrate areas where brain actively differs from the normal. PET/CT can also be used to differentiate Alzheimer's disease, Pick's disease from other causes of dementia in cases where the clinical picture is atypical. The device can also evaluate extent of stroke and recovery following therapy as well as image malignant brain tumors.

PET/CT has become the standard of for oncology imaging:

A whole body scan, which usually is made from mid-thighs to the top of the head, takes from five minutes to 40 minutes depending on the acquisition protocol and technology of the equipment used. FDG imaging protocols acquires slices with a thickness of two to three mm. Hyper metabolic lesions are shown as false color-coded pixels or voxels onto the gray-value coded CT images. Standardized uptake values are calculated by the software for each hyper metabolic region detected in the image. It provides a quantification of size of the lesion, since functional imaging does not provide a precise anatomical estimate of its extent. The CT can be used for that, when the lesion is also visualized in its images (this is not always the case when hyper metabolic lesions are not accompanied by anatomical changes).

In PET/CT, both the multi-detector CT apparatus and the PET detectors are mounted in the same gantry, one immediately behind the other. Both PET and CT scanning are performed with the patient lying in the same position on the imaging table resulting in optimal correlation of anatomic and metabolic information. For interpretation, the PET data is actually superimposed upon the CT data (co-registration) resulting in improved anatomic localization of normal and abnormal FDG activity. This fusion process has proven beneficial in more exactly localizing tissues involved by tumor. Better co-registration is especially significant in regions of complex anatomy, such as in the abdomen and in the head and neck. More exact localization of the involved tissues results in more accurate staging and more appropriate treatment planning including surgical therapy, radiotherapy, and medical therapy.

3D techniques have better sensitivity (because more coincidences are detected and used) and therefore less noise, but are more sensitive to the effects of scatter and random coincidences, as well as requiring correspondingly greater computer resources. The advent of sub-nanosecond timing resolution detectors affords better random coincidence rejection, thus favouring 3D image reconstruction

Safety

PET scanning is non-invasive, but it does involve exposure to ionising radiation. The total dose of radiation is not insignificant, usually around 11 mSv. This can also be compared to 2.2 mSv average annual background radiation, 0.02 mSv for a chest X-ray and 6.5-8 mSv for a CT scan of the chest, according to the Chest Journal and ICRP.

Benefits

The benefits of a combined PET/CT scanner include:

- Greater detail with a higher level of accuracy; because both scans are performed at one time without the patient having to change positions, ferent times.

Risks

- Because the doses of radio-tracer administered are small, diagnostic nuclear medicine procedures result in low radiation exposure, acceptable for diagnostic exams. Thus, the radiation risk is very low compared with the potential benefits.
- Nuclear medicine diagnostic procedures have been used for more than five decades, and there are no known long-term adverse effects from such low-dose exposure.
- Allergic reactions to radio-pharmaceuticals may occur but are extremely rare and are usually mild. Nevertheless, you should inform the nuclear medicine personnel of any allergies you may have or other problems that may have occurred during a previous nuclear medicine exam.
- Injection of the radiotracer may cause slight pain and redness which should rapidly resolve.
- Women should always inform their physician or radiology technologist if there is any possibility that they are pregnant or if they are breastfeeding their baby.

Limitations

Limitations to the widespread use of PET arise from high cost of cyclotrons needed to produce the short-lived radionuclide for PET scanning and the need for specially adapted on-site chemical synthesis apparatus to produce radiopharmaceuticals. Because half life of F-18 is about two hours, the prepared dose of a radiopharmaceutical bearing this nuclide will undergo multiple half lives of decay during the working day. This necessitates frequent recalibration of the remaining dose and careful planning with respect to patient scheduling.

3D techniques have better coincidences, as well as requiring correspondingly greater computer resources. The advent of sub-nanosecond timing resolution detectors affords better random coincidence rejection, thus favouring 3D image reconstruction hours to days for the radiotracer to accumulate in the part of the body under study and imaging may take upto several hours to perform, though in some cases, newer equipment is available that can substantially shorten the procedure time.

The resolution of structures of the body with nuclear medicine may not be as clear as with other imaging techniques, such as CT or MRI. However, nuclear medicine scans are more sensitive than other techniques for a variety of indications, and the functional information gained from nuclear medicine exams is often unobtainable by any other imaging techniques.

PET scanning can give false results if chemical balances within the body are not normal. Specifically, test results of diabetic patients or patients who have eaten within a few hours prior to the examination can be adversely affected because of altered blood sugar or blood insulin levels.

Medical Diagnosis

Medical conditions and diseases are now being detected more accurately and quickly due to the advancement of biotechnology-based tools, an example of the benefits biotechnology has brought us, and one which most people will be able to relate to, is the home pregnancy testing kit. The new generation of home testing kits are able to provide results which are more accurate and are able to be used much earlier than the ones a few years ago. Illnesses such as strep throat and other infectious diseases are now diagnosed within minutes enabling treatment to begin at a much earlier time where previous tests could take a few days.

Without biotechnology, a new simpler blood test couldn't have been developed which allows us to measure the amount of "bad" cholesterol in the blood, before this conventional methods required separate blood tests which took longer to obtain the results and were much more costly.

Certain types of cancer such as ovarian and prostrate cancer now rely on biotechnology-based tests by taking a simple blood test and thus eliminating the need for expensive and invasive surgery.

We benefit because not only are the tests cheaper but they are a lot more accurate and quicker than any previous tests prior to the use of biotechnology, this allows Doctors to make a diagnosis earlier in the diseases progress and begin treatment of the disease quicker, which greatly increases the patients prognosis. Prior to the use of biotechnology-based tests diagnosis could only be made when the disease had progressed far enough to provide measurable indicators. Researchers studying Proteomics have discovered that molecular markers can indicate the signs of disease even before visible changes to the cells or symptoms have appeared; soon in the very near future physicians will have access to tests which are able to detect biomarkers even before the disease begins. This information of course is invaluable in treating and diagnosing hereditary diseases such as diabetes, cystic fibrosis and the early onset of Parkinson's and Alzheimer's disease. Previously all of these diseases were only diagnosed after the symptoms began to show, genetic tests would also be able to reveal and identify those people who could be prone to diseases such as cancers, asthma, osteoporosis, emphysema and type II diabetes.

Biotechnology-based diagnostic tests are not only altering how quickly and easily we can detect disease but is also making improvements in the way health care is provided. As many of the tests are now portable, with equipment being smaller, Doctors can literally conduct the tests, get the results and prescribe the appropriate treatment without even leaving the patients bedside. Technically trained staff and expensive equipment are no longer needed to read the results from tests as now most rely on a simple colour change system, which is seen in the home pregnancy test.

Indian biotechnology industry dominated by the health care sector

The results have shown that the evolution/growth of health care biotechnology firms has its roots in the pharmaceuticals industry, which reflects the phenomenon taking place globally. Key pharmaceutical firms established in pre-80s in the country like Wockhardt Ltd., Hindustan Antibiotics Ltd., Lupin Ltd., Glen Pharma Ltd., etc. have ventured or adopted at a later stage the biotechnology in manufacturing, marketing and also research. Majority of the biotechnology companies were established after 1980s and this period incidentally coincides with the initiatives started by the government during the Sixth Five Year Plan (1980-85) to set-up a dedicated Department of Bio-technology and to nurture and promote biotechnology. The growth of health care biotechnology companies gained momentum in post-1990s, with phenomenal growth being observed in the post-WTO period, i.e. 1995 onwards.

large pharmaceutical firms adopting BT, spin-offs from the established pharma majors like Dabur, Ranbaxy, Reddy, Cadila, etc. as well as biotechnology majors like Biocon and Shantha Biotechnics. The first successfully established spin-off company from the Indian Institute of Science (IISc), Strand Genomics, also emerged in this period. Majority of the health care biotechnology companies established in post-1990s are private limited companies. Interestingly, MNC subsidiaries like Eli Lilly, GlaxoSmith-Kline, Pfizer, etc. also gained entry during this period. The reasons for the active participation by MNCs during this period could possibly be the signing of the WTO treaty by India, coupled with the comparative advantages the country offers like cost, skilled manpower, etc. in the health care domain. The growth of health care biotechnology firms has largely taken place in clusters. The results showed a large concentration of companies in four states, namely, Andhra Pradesh, Maharashtra, Karnataka and Delhi. The state governments are giving a special thrust for the promotion of biotechnology cluster development by evolving liberal/favourable policies, including tax and excise concessions as well as the much needed venture capital support. This has resulted in an upsurge of new biotechnology firms, especially in states like AP and Karnataka. 'Baddi' in Himachal Pradesh is a recent witness of this phenomena. Perhaps this could be one of the reasons that Gujarat, despite being recognized as a traditional pharma hub along with Maharashtra is yet to catch up with other states in adopting biotechnology.

The firms that are active in the health care sector mainly comprised of medium sized and newly dedicated biotechnology firms. The activity profile of these firms though quite diverse, is mainly concentrated in the domain of recombinant therapeutics, vaccines, diagnostics and anti-bodies. Biotechnology is a knowledge or research-intensive industry; the results portend that biotechnology firms, irrespective of their size, are engaged in multi-disciplinary R&D activities. Thus, there is a realization by the firms to carry out innovative research for achieving growth by bringing out new products in the post-WTO era.

Globally, the growth of biotechnology has been characterized by large alliances or networks of learning. Indian BT firms have exhibited alliances both with national and international organizations. A study on Indian biopharmaceuticals also supports this assertion. Foreign collaboration dominated among the firms, thereby reflecting their tendency to catch up with the new or cutting-edge technology or align with the global research network for higher growth.

The R&D efforts of Indian biotechnology firms are substantially lower than those of global counterparts. One of the prime reasons for this is the lack of research infrastructure compared to that of other developing countries like Brazil, Taiwan, China and Israel. In India, the government has played a key role in building capacities and capabilities in terms of research infrastructure, human resources, fiscal support and R&D incentives, apart from synergizing the various actors through new initiatives and programmes such as PRDSF (DST), NIMTLI (CSIR), etc. aimed at utilizing the results of the public research institutions for commercialization. The National Biotechnology Policy (National Biotechnology Development Strategy, Draft, 2005) announced recently by the government is a step forward in encouraging innovative enterprises and addresses appropriately issues such as quality of manpower, regulatory environment, effect of WTO, etc. for the growth of biotechnology in India. Though there has been a slow transition to product model by Indian biotechnology companies, India is still a generic market. To achieve global presence, Indian firms need to have product focus and should come up with blockbuster drugs. There exist boundless opportunities for pharma and biotech firms to find innovative ways of working together by leveraging the committed government support. According to Padmanaban, 'India has just crossed the lag phase of the biotechnology growth and is at the beginning of the log phase of growth'. India's advantages lie in vaccine development, traditional herbal medicine as the cheapest mode of protecting health as well as bioinformatics, because of strong capabilities in software, and for these areas India should aim for global leadership.

Promising applications

- pharmacogenomics;
- gene therapy;
- genetic testing; and
- drug production;

Pharmacogenomics

Pharmacogenomics is the study of how the genetic inheritance of an individual affects his/her body's response to drugs. It is a coined word derived from the words "pharmacology" and "genomics". It is hence the study of the relationship between pharmaceuticals and genetics. The vision of pharmacogenomics is to be able to design and produce drugs that are adapted to each person's genetic makeup.

Pharmacogenomics results in the following benefits:

1. Development of tailor-made medicines. Using pharmacogenomics, pharmaceutical companies can create drugs based on the proteins, enzymes and RNA molecules that are associated with specific genes and diseases. These tailor-made drugs promise not only to maximize therapeutic effects but also to decrease damage to nearby healthy cells.
2. More accurate methods of determining appropriate drug dosages. Knowing a patient's genetics will enable doctors to determine how well his/her body can process and metabolize a medicine. This will maximize the value of the medicine and decrease the likelihood of overdose.
3. Improvements in the drug discovery and approval process. The discovery of potential therapies will be made easier using genome targets. Genes have been associated with numerous diseases and disorders. With modern biotechnology, these genes can be used as targets for the development of effective new therapies, which could significantly shorten the drug discovery process.
4. Better vaccines. Safer vaccines can be designed and produced by organisms transformed by means of genetic engineering. These vaccines will elicit the immune response without the attendant risks of infection. They will be inexpensive, stable, easy to store, and capable of being engineered to carry several strains of pathogen at once.

Pharmaceutical products

Most traditional pharmaceutical drugs are relatively simple molecules that have been found primarily through trial and error to treat the symptoms of a disease or illness. Biopharmaceuticals are large biological molecules known as proteins and these usually target the underlying mechanisms and pathways of a malady (but not always, as is the case with using insulin to treat type 1 diabetes mellitus, as that treatment merely addresses the symptoms of the disease, not the underlying cause which is autoimmunity); it is a relatively young industry. They can deal with targets in humans that may not be accessible with traditional medicines. A patient typically is dosed with a small molecule via a tablet while a large molecule is typically injected.

Small molecules are manufactured by chemistry but larger molecules are created by living cells such as those found in the human body: for example, bacteria cells, yeast cells, animal or plant cells. Modern biotechnology is often associated with the use of genetically altered microorganisms such as E. coli or yeast for the production of substances like synthetic insulin or antibiotics. It can also refer to transgenic animals or transgenic plants, such as Bt corn. Genetically altered mammalian cells, such as Chinese Hamster Ovary (CHO) cells, are also used to manufacture certain pharmaceuticals. Another promising new biotechnology application is the development of plant-made pharmaceuticals.

Biotechnology is also commonly associated with landmark breakthroughs in new medical therapies to treat hepatitis B, hepatitis C, cancers, arthritis, hemophilia, bone fractures, multiple sclerosis, and cardiovascular disorders. The biotechnology industry has also been instrumental in developing molecular diagnostic devices that can be used to define the target patient population for a given biopharmaceutical.

Modern biotechnology can be used to manufacture existing medicines relatively easily and cheaply. The first genetically engineered products were medicines designed to treat human diseases. To cite one example, in 1978 Genentech developed synthetic humanized insulin by joining its gene with a plasmid vector inserted into the bacterium Escherichia coli. Insulin, widely used for the treatment of diabetes, was previously extracted from the pancreas of abattoir animals (cattle and/or pigs). The resulting genetically engineered bacterium enabled the production of vast quantities of synthetic human insulin at relatively low cost. According to a 2003 study undertaken by the International Diabetes Federation (IDF) on the access to and availability of insulin in its member-countries, synthetic 'human' insulin is considerably more expensive in most countries where both synthetic 'human' and animal insulin are commercially available: e.g. within European countries the average price of synthetic 'human' insulin was twice as high as the price of pork insulin. Yet in its position statement, the IDF writes that "there is no overwhelming evidence to prefer one species of insulin over another" and "[modern, highly-purified] animal insulins remain a perfectly acceptable alternative.

Modern biotechnology has evolved, making it possible to produce more easily and relatively cheaply human growth hormone, clotting factors for hemophiliacs, fertility drugs, erythropoietin and other drugs. Most drugs today are based on about 500 molecular targets. Genomic knowledge of the genes involved in diseases, disease pathways, and drug-response sites are expected to lead to the discovery of thousands more new targets.

Genetic testing

There are two major types of gene tests. In the first type, a researcher may design short pieces of DNA ("probes") whose sequences are complementary to the mutated sequences. These probes will seek their complement among the base pairs of an individual's genome. If the mutated sequence is present in the patient's genome, the probe will bind to it and flag the mutation. In the second type, a researcher may conduct the gene test by comparing the sequence of DNA bases in a patient's gene to disease in healthy individuals or their progeny.

Genetic testing is now used for:

- Carrier screening, or the identification of unaffected individuals

who carry one copy of a gene for a disease that requires two copies for the disease to manifest;
- Confirmational diagnosis of symptomatic individuals;
- Determining sex;
- Forensic/identity testing;
- Newborn screening;
- Prenatal diagnostic screening;
- Presymptomatic testing for estimating the risk of developing adult-onset cancers; and
- Presymptomatic testing for predicting adult-onset disorders.

Some genetic tests are already available, although most of them are used in developed countries. The tests currently available can detect mutations associated with rare genetic disorders like cystic fibrosis, sickle cell anemia, and Huntington's disease. Recently, tests have been developed to detect mutation for a handful of more complex conditions such as breast, ovarian, and colon cancers. However, gene tests may not detect every mutation

Gene therapy

Gene therapy may be used for treating, or even curing, genetic and acquired diseases like cancer and AIDS by using normal genes to supplement or replace defective genes or to bolster a normal function such as immunity. It can be used to target somatic (i.e., body) or gametes (i.e., egg and sperm) cells. In somatic gene therapy, the genome of the recipient is changed, but this change is not passed along to the next generation. In contrast, in germline gene therapy, the egg and sperm cells of the parents are changed for the purpose of passing on the changes to their offspring.

There are basically two ways of implementing a gene therapy treatment:

1. *Ex vivo,* which means "outside the body"—Cells from the patient's blood or bone marrow are removed and grown in the laboratory. They are then exposed to a virus carrying the desired gene. The virus enters the cells, and the desired gene becomes part of the DNA of the cells. The cells are allowed to grow in the laboratory before being returned to the patient by injection into a vein.
2. *In vivo,* which means "inside the body"—No cells are removed from the patient's body. Instead, vectors are used to deliver the desired gene to cells in the patient's body.

As of June 2001, more than 500 clinical gene-therapy trials involving about 3,500 patients were identified worldwide. Around 78% of these are in the United States, with Europe having 18%. These trials focus on various types of cancer. Recently, two children born with severe combined immunodeficiency disorder ("SCID") were reported to have been cured after being given genetically engineered cells.

The obstacles

1. *Gene delivery tools.* Genes are inserted into the body using gene carriers called vectors. The most common vectors now are viruses, which have evolved a way of encapsulating and delivering their genes to human cells in a pathogenic manner. Scientists manipulate the genome of the virus by removing the disease-causing genes and inserting the therapeutic genes. However, while viruses are effective, they can introduce problems like toxicity, immune and inflammatory responses, and gene control and targeting issues. In addition, in order for gene therapy to provide permanent therapeutic effects, the introduced gene needs to be integrated within the host cell's genome. Some viral vectors affect this in a random fashion, which can introduce other problems such as disruption of an endogenous host gene.
2. *High costs.* Since gene therapy is relatively new and at an experimental stage, it is an expensive treatment to undertake. This explains why current studies are focused on illnesses commonly found in developed countries, where more people can afford to pay for treatment. It may take decades before developing countries can take advantage of this technology.
3. *Limited knowledge of the functions of genes.* Scientists currently know the functions of only a few genes. Hence, gene therapy can address only some genes that cause a particular disease. Worse, it is not known exactly whether genes have more than one function, which creates uncertainty as to whether replacing such genes is indeed desirable.
4. *Multigene disorders and effect of environment.* Most genetic disorders involve more than one gene. Moreover, most diseases involve the interaction of several genes and the environment. For example, many people with cancer not only inherit the disease gene for the disorder, but may have also failed to inherit specific tumor suppressor genes. Diet, exercise, smoking and other environmental factors may have also contributed to their disease.

Human Genome Project

The Human Genome Project is an initiative of the U.S. Department of Energy ("DOE") that aims to generate a high-quality reference sequence for the entire human genome and identify all the human genes. The DOE and its predecessor agencies were assigned by the U.S. Congress to develop new energy resources and technologies and to pursue a deeper understanding of potential health and environmental risks posed by their production and use. In 1986, the DOE announced its Human Genome Initiative. Shortly thereafter, the DOE and National Institutes of Health developed a plan for a joint Human Genome Project ("HGP"), which officially began in 1990. The HGP was originally planned to last 15 years. However, rapid technological advances and worldwide participation accelerated the completion date to 2003 (making it a 13 year project). Already it has enabled gene hunters to pinpoint genes associated with more than 30 disorders.

Cloning

Cloning involves the removal of the nucleus from one cell and its placement in an unfertilized egg cell whose nucleus has either been deactivated or removed.

There are two types of cloning:

1. *Reproductive cloning*. After a few divisions, the egg cell is placed into a uterus where it is allowed to develop into a fetus that is genetically identical to the donor of the original nucleus.
2. *Therapeutic cloning*. The egg is placed into a Petri dish where it develops into embryonic stem cells, which have shown potentials for treating several ailments.

Genomics and Public Policy

The Executive Courses on Genomics and Public Health Policy that took place between 2002 and 2004 in five regions of the developing world had three goals:

1. To familiarize the participants with the current status and implications of health genomics and biotechnology, and to provide information relevant to public policy-making in these fields.
2. To provide frameworks for analyzing and debating the policy issues and related ethical questions in health genomics and biotechnology, and to help people to understand, anticipate and influence the legal and regulatory frameworks under which health biotechnology industries will operate, both nationally and internationally.
3. To begin developing a leaders' network reaching across different sectors (including industry, academic, government and NGOs) by sharing perspectives and building relationships.

Science does not have borders

Although the recommendations from the five courses display nuances linked to regional differences in biotechnology capacity and development, financial conditions, political frameworks, and population needs, fundamental lessons emerge from their insights. These lessons highlighted the key forces: science; finance; ethics, society, culture; and politics. An Indian participant invited to speak at the EMRO Course explained that although the Course occurred amidst Indian-Pakistani tensions, his presentation received a "warm response" from Pakistani delegates that led not only to the bulk transfer of the hepatitis B vaccines from India to Pakistan, but also the technology transfer that facilitated their manufacture in Pakistan. "Every small cooperation matters," he said.

Miracles of biotechnology; from killing bacteria to cancer cell destruction

Biotechnology has been in existence for thousands of years, originating in food production, but when was the first biotechnological application in medicine? The revolution began with the advent of biologically-produced antibiotics and the discovery of penicillin by Alexander Fleming in 1929. Fleming observed that cultures of Staphylococcus aureus were killed when accidentally contaminated with the fungus Penicillium notatum. Similarly, new technology will help to assess the aggressiveness of tumors and their susceptibility to chemotherapy may become easier to predict based on a mathematical model developed at The University of Texas Health Science Center at Houston. In spite of extensive experimental and clinical studies, the process of cancer growth is not well understood. Tumors are complex systems, with changes at the molecular and cellular levels influencing shape and behaviour in sometimes unpredictable ways. New research by a scientist in mathematical oncology at the Health Science Center at Houston suggests that mathematical modeling based on data from the molecular and cellular levels could shed light on tumor development and lead to better treatments.

Solution to these chronic diseases could come through genetic medicine and that modern biotechnology will play a major role.

It must be recognized that many chronic diseases will most probably not have a single, identifiable genetic cause but rather arise from a complex, cascading series of biological events interacting with environmental factors. The impact of pharmaceuticals on human health care is an area where biotechnology innovations are likely to have the earlier commercial realization. New medical treatments based on biotechnology are appearing almost daily in the market place. These include: therapeutic products (hormones, regulatory proteins and antibiotics) prenatal diagnosis of genetic diseases vaccines immunodiagnostics and DNA probes for disease identification and genetic therapy (This is the largest commercially developed area of new biotechnology, with massive present and future markets and can only be selectively examined here).

Biotechnology coupled with genomics can act both as a catalyst to foster overall development of science and technology as well as the development of practical solutions to local health needs. However, the benefits of biotechnology, driven by market incentives of the developed world, have accrued primarily to rich countries, with billions in the developing world largely excluded from these advances. Developing nations are also taking steps to build long-term plans to benefit from biotechnology innovation. To assess the potential of genomics to address health needs in the developing world, the McLaughlin-Rotman Centre for Global Health, organized five courses in the developing world. The overall objective of the courses was to collectively explore how to best harness genomics to improve health in each region viz. Nairobi, Kenya with the African Centre for Technology Studies for the African continent; Kerala, India with Indian Council of Medical Research for the Indian subcontinent; Muscat, Oman with the World Health Organization's Regional Office for the Eastern Mediterranean region (EMRO); Caracas, Venezuela with the United Nations University's Biotechnology for Latin America and the Caribbean (BIOLAC) and the Pan American Health Organization for Latin America and the Caribbean; and Hong Kong SAR China with the University of Hong Kong for the Western Pacific and Southeast Asia region.

Drug delivery and gene therapy in medicine; Nanotechnology

Nanotechnology as applied to drug delivery systems will undoubtedly dramatically improve the therapeutic potential of many water-insoluble and unstable drugs. Microsensors interfaced to a nanoscale drug delivery system could dispense precise amounts of drugs for optimum functionality and minimum toxicity. However, significant challenges still remain in synthesis and processing of drug-carrier nanoparticles at the industrial scale. Nanotechnology may also help reach the hitherto elusive goal of active drug targeting to selected cells within the body. Nanotechnology that can further reduce the size and reproducibly attach targeting ligands to the drug-loaded nano-particles may help localize the drug to the desired tissues in the body. These nano-particles may also be valuable tools for molecular and cell biologists to study fundamental cellular processes such as receptor-mediated endocytosis and intracellular trafficking.

The nanoscale chemical and topographical details of the implanted materials determine the reaction of the body. If we can gain sufficient understanding and control of these biological reactions to surface nanostructure, we may be able to control the rejection of artificial implants. Similarly, it may be possible to surround implanted tissue with a nano-fabricated barrier that would thwart the rejection mechanisms of the host, allowing wider utilization of donated organs. Ultimately, better materials and understanding of their interaction with the body may lead to implants that the body will not only accept, but that will actually become integrated into the body. Nanofabrication and nano-synthesis give us powerful new tools to address these important medical issues for which a great deal of research is still necessary.

Nanotechnology and its relevance to health care

"Nanotechnology has the potential to generate enormous health benefits for the more than five billion people living in the developing world," said Dr. Peter A. Singer, senior scientist at the McLaughlin-Rotman Centre for Global Health and professor of medicine at the University of Toronto. Dr. Singer joined the Wilson Center's Andrew Maynard; the National Cancer Institute's Piotr Grodzinski; and moderator, Jeff Spieler, from the U.S. Agency for International Development (USAID) at an event on February 27, 2007, to discuss the use of nanotechnology to improve health in developing countries. Dr. Singer continued by discussing a number of possible advances in nanotechnology which could potentially have a huge impact on public health, such as tools for diagnosing and treating diseases in less-industrialized countries as well as being able to increase the availability of clean water.

Comparatively speaking, the size differential between a one meter child and a nanometer is roughly the same as the size differential between the moon and the head of a pin. Working with particles at this size is enabling scientists to "move into an area that they've never really been able to work with before and never really been able to take advantage of before." In practice, consumer nanotechnology products include better stain-resistant products, more effective sun-screens, and thermal insulating shoe insoles. Scientists, however, have only scratched the technological surface when it comes to health products.

Dr. Piotr Grodzinski, described nanotechnology as an opportunity for early diagnosis and novel therapy as well as a means for prevention and quality of life enhancement among cancer patients. However, the technology is not without its risks, and there is still quite a bit of work to be done in order to help different scientific fields work together in developing this technology as well as making sure that the products are safe. Improved energy storage, production and conversion would help to improve environmental sustainability. Better food processing and storage would help in eradicating extreme hunger. While some technology transfer from the industrialized nations could be used to jump-start programs in the developing world, these countries should not rely on such programs in the long-run.

Why Nanotechnology came to the fore only recently

Emerging tools, including scanning probe microscopy, quantum mechanical computer simulation and soft X-ray lithography, have combined with new synthesis methods, such as chemical vapour deposition, leading to a significantly greater, ever accelerating understanding of scientific endeavour at the nano-scale. Nanotechnology aims to produce devices commencing with the self-assembly of individual atoms into precise configurations, as has been the case with combinational chemistry for many years. Thirdly, the recognition of nanotechnology as an emerging field demands and creates new levels of multi-disciplinary collaboration and cross-fertilisation amongst the sciences. Whilst nanotechnology is projected by the U.S. National Science Foundation (NSF) to have a global market value of $1 trillion by 2011, early signs in the information and communications technology (ICT) and textile industries are that nanotechnology is more complementary than displacing.

Applications in Health Care

Representatives from the U.N. Conference on Trade and Development and Commission on Science and Technology for Development have suggested that nanotechnology can help "reduce the cost and increase the likelihood of attaining the Millennium Development Goals". In a recent study that ranked nanotechnology applications according to their potential benefit for developing countries, water treatment, disease diagnosis/screening and drug delivery systems respectively rated 3rd, 4th and 5th, behind energy storage, production, and conversion (1st) and agricultural productivity enhancement (2nd). Salvarezza believes nanotechnology offers an area such as developing country health care, "safer drug delivery, new methods for prevention, diagnosis and treatment of diseases". In rural areas, Harper argues that pulmonary or epidermal drug delivery applications utilizing nanotechnology, "have the potential to free up the large numbers of trained medical personnel who are currently engaged in administering drugs via hypodermic needles". In a joint project between groups in the U.S., India and Mexico, inexpensive, maintenance free solar panels, aimed at powering rural clinics and refrigerating medicines, are currently being developed. Could nanotechnology empower local health care auxiliaries, in rural settings worldwide, to address diagnostic and therapeutic concerns by reducing reliance on trained specialists or technical assistance?

Diagnosis and Treatment of Tuberculosis

Many believe nanotechnology offers new ways to address residual scientific concerns for Mycobacterium tuberculosis (TB). Treatments with improved sustained release profiles and bioavailability can increase compliance through reduced drug requirements and therein minimize MDR-TB. Additionally, improved diagnostic tools are required to meet the needs of the WHO's expansion of the Directly Observed Treatment, Short-course, MDR and co-infection with HIV. A nanotechnology-based TB diagnostic kit, designed by the Central Scientific Instruments Organization of India and currently in the clinical trials phase, does not require skilled technicians for use and offers efficiency, portability, user-friendliness and availability for as little as 30 rupees (less than US$1). In the Medical Sciences division of the U.S. Department of Energy, researchers are investigating an optical biosensor for rapid TB detection. Furthermore, a group at RMIT University, in Australia, is conducting research into the application of novel tethered nano-particles as low-cost, color-based assays for TB diagnosis. So far, all groups have registered high levels of drug encapsulation efficiency, whilst both the Indian and South African groups have demonstrated sustained release profiles. Furthermore, the Indian group have reported increased bioavailability and "undetectable bacterial counts in the lungs and spleens of Mycobacterium tuberculosis-infected mice" 21 days post-inoculation.

Prevention of HIV/AIDS

An Australian company, Starpharma, is developing a preventative, clear, HIV microbicidal, based on nanotechnology, that would remain effective when applied by women upto four hours in advance of sexual intercourse. Also in Australia, the Austin Research Institute has conducted successful trials into nano-vaccines for malaria. Researchers at the State University of Campinas, Brazil, are investigating drug and vaccine delivery for leishmaniasis. At the Chidicon Medical Center in Nigeria, researchers are studying nano-scale copolymer assemblies for diagnostic imaging and therapeutic management of infectious diseases. Furthermore, in a joint project between the Rensselaer Polytechnic Institute (U.S.) and Banaras Hindu University (India), scientists are investigating easy-to-manufacture, carbon nano-tube filters that remove nano-scale germs, such as the polio viruses, E. coli and Staphylococcus aureus bacteria, from water.

Risk *versus* Benefits of Nanotechnology

The debate surrounding Genetically Modified foods, that focuses upon issues of risk, threatens to divert attention from identifying and applying nanotechnology to the developing world. An engagement with 'risk' and the consideration of nanotechnology's application to the developing world need not be mutually exclusive. In fact, although technological 'risk' affects countries indifferent ways depending on the nature of their engagement with change, it remains a universal consideration and a crucial factor in ensuring the appropriateness of new technology, to any setting. It is clear that a number of issues remain unresolved and require greater consideration that incorporates truly global perspectives.

China, India and South Korea have established national activities in nanotechnology; Thailand, The Philippines, South Africa, Brazil and Chile had some form of government support and national funding programs were being developed; whilst Mexico and Argentina had some form of organized nanotechnology activity but no specific government funding.

Assessing Global Engagement with Nanotechnology

In 2003, White noted that bio-nanotechnology patenting was occurring in three main areas: cosmetics and consumer health; instrumentation, focussed on general diagnostic processes; and drug delivery. Furthermore, with relatively little research directed towards some of the health problems affecting the majority of the world's population, they chose to analyse every title and abstract for references to diseases in order to assess one aspect of early orientation within health-related

Global Distribution of Nanotechnology Activity Based on Countries' Human Development Groupings

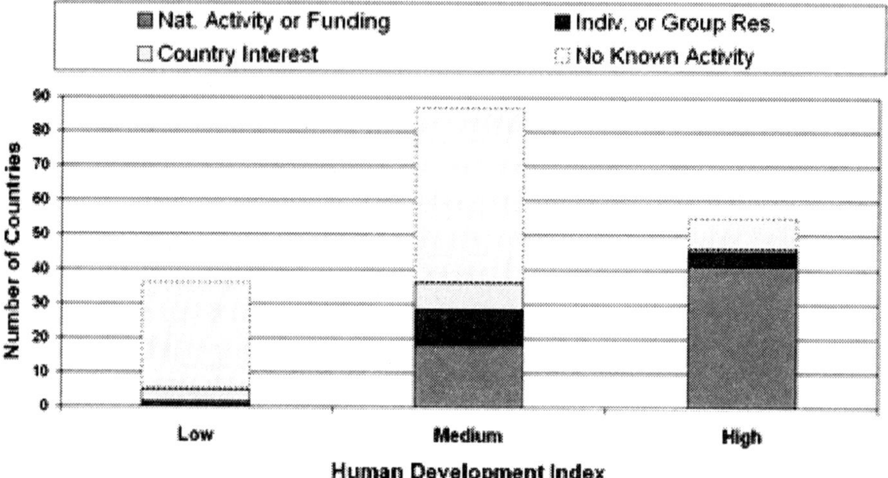

nanotechnology research. China, India and Brazil lead developing country investment in nanotechnology, ahead of many developing countries with a higher HDI rank.

The correlation between lower average incomes and lower government spending on R&D and health care, presents an initial challenge for nanotechnology to even be considered in less-developed countries. Infrastructure; human and policy capacity; cost; intellectual property rights; education relating to academics and the public; brain drain; trade barriers and the political context, constitute further barriers, although these are not unique to nanotechnology.

The cost of establishing nanotechnology institutes has been claimed at approximately $5 million in both Vietnam and Mexico, whereas the new national nanotechnology facility in Costa Rica, including a 'clean room', was reportedly built for "about $50,000", and will be equipped for an extra several hundred-thousand dollars.

Health-Related Patent Activity

35 countries have a share in the global distribution. The three leading countries are the U.S. (32.8%), China (20.3%) and Germany (12.9%), with the top 7 countries holding 88% of the overall patent share.

Health-Related Nanotechnology Development in India

With India touted as "likely to become a leader in nanotechnology within the next ten years" (Pillai), the country remains behind the rest of the world by about 6 years in nanotech patenting. Yet these results come at a time of great transition for developing country patent regimes in light

Distribution of Health-related Nanotechnology Patent Activity (1975-2004), by Country

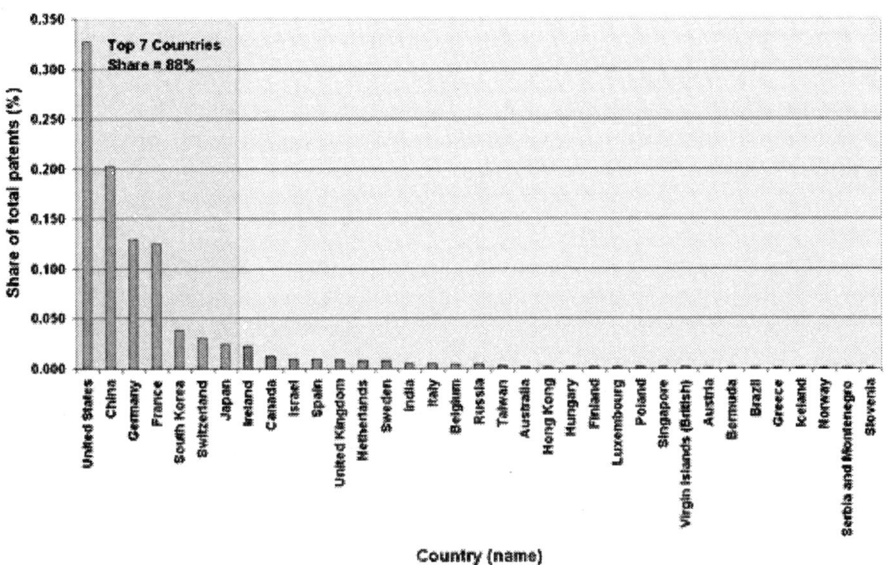

of required accession to the Trade Related Aspects of Intellectual Property Rights Agreement. Furthermore, Indian research has been strengthened by a number of domestically-based, international nanotechnology health care conferences. In both 2003 and 2005, an international workshop on 'Nanotechnology and Health Care' saw a wide range of researchers and industry professionals, including Nobel laureates, gather in India to discuss

Global Distribution of Nanotechnology Health-related Patent Share, by Region

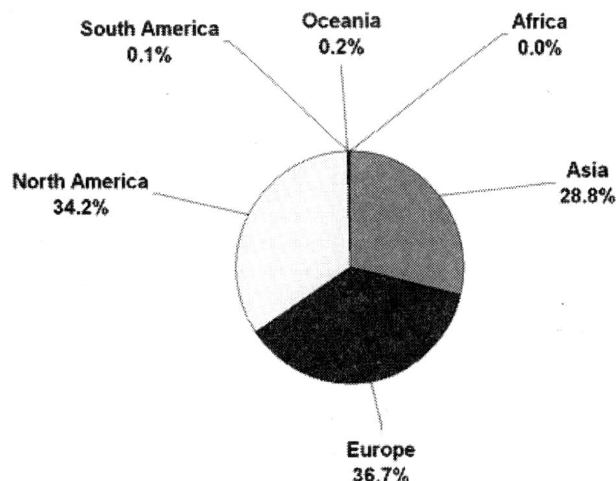

applications of nanotechnology in frontier areas. These conferences flanked 'The First World Congress on Nano-biotechnology' in 2004, and "Nanobiotechnology: Implications on Food, Health and Nutrition Security", in 2005.

Of the top 10 pharmaceutical companies on the U.S. market, Sanofi-Aventis, GlaxoSmithKline, AstraZeneca and Merck have all engaged in nanotechnology patenting. Two further drug giants: Elan Pharma International and Novartis, hold strong patent positions in health-related nanotechnology.

Patents Classified by Disease

Patenting is strongest for non-communicable diseases. By citation, cancer is receiving the greatest focus, propelled by funding such as the $144 million committed to nanotechnology cancer research in the U.S. Yet cancer's burden, in terms of overall numbers, is greatest in the developing world. Hepatitis is the second most cited disease, yet the majority of patents relate to Hepatitis B which is most prevalent in the developing world. Non-communicable diseases include osteoporosis, beri-beri, stroke and diabetes mellitus. Yet, much of the projected doubling of diabetes mellitus cases by 2025 will stem from increases in developing countries. Influenza, acne, AIDS and vaginitis represent the remaining communicable diseases and are conditions prevalent in both the developed and developing world. Numerous references to various waterborne diseases, staph infections and

The 10 Most Cited Diseases in Health-related Nanotechnology Patent Abstracts

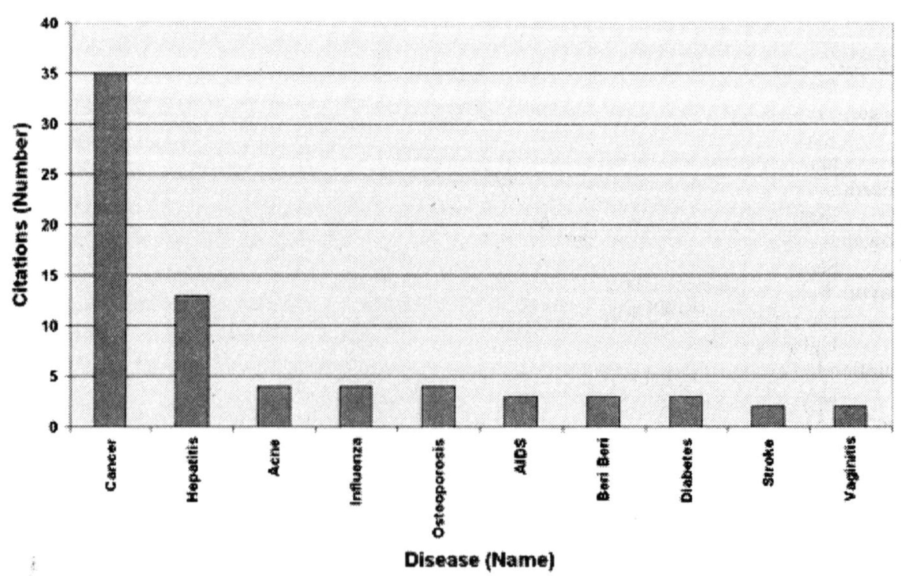

viruses such as HIV were not included in this research but would have shown HIV/AIDS receiving a greater focus than represented in our disease citation data.

Two of the worlds greatest killers, malaria and tuberculosis, are noticeably absent from any significant level of nanotechnology patenting. In one respect, this could mean that little research being undertaken in these areas has been transferred to the commercial setting. However, what is more likely is its signifying that these diseases are receiving attention disproportionate to their global impact. Viewing the overall picture of health-related nanotechnology patents, we see that control lies firmly with the industrialised countries of the North, although China is ensuring strong representation from the developing world, relative to its general patent input. The U.S. holds a strong lead in health-related nanotechnology patenting.

Sources

Acharya, T., Abdur Rab, M., Singer, P.A., Daar, A.S., Harnessing genomics to improve health in the Eastern Mediterranean Region—an executive course in genomics policy. BioMed Central. 2005; 3:1. http://www.health-policy-systems.com/content/3/1/1.

Acharya, T., Kumar, N.K., Muthuswamy, V., Daar, A.S., Singer, P.A., Harnessing genomics to improve health in India—an executive course to support genomics policy. Bio-Med Central. 2004; 2:1. http://www.health-policy-systems.com/content/2/1/1

Albano, I., Padma, T.V., Learn from Brazil and Thai drug licenses, say MSF. Sci Dev Net. 25 July 2007.

Asia Pacific Nanotechnology Forum, "Executive Summary First Workshop on 'Human Resources Development in Nanotechnology' in Asia", Asian Institute of Technology, Bangkok, 2003.

Bachmann, G., "IPTS-ESTO Techno-Economic Analysis Report 1999-2000", Joint Research Centre, European Commission, Spain, 2000.

Bai, C., "Progress of Nanoscience and Nanotechnology in China", *Journal of Nanoparticle Research*, 3 (4), pp. 251-56, 2001.

Barker, T. *et al.*, 2005, "Nanotechnology and the Poor: Opportunities and Risks". Accessed on: January 26, 2005. http://nanotech.dialoguebydesign.net/rp/NanoandPoor2.pdf

Biosante Pharmaceuticals, 2002, "Biosante Pharmaceuticals Announces Positive Trial Results for Tuberculosis Vaccine". Accessed on: April 7, 2004.

Biowatch South Africa, 2002, "The Cape Town Declaration". Accessed on: September29, 2004.http://www.biowatch.org.za/ctdecform.htm.

Brown, M.M., Foreword in Human DevelopmentReport: Making new technologies work for human development, United Nations Development Programme (Ed.), Oxford University Press, New York 2001.

Bruntland, G. (Ed.), Our common future: The WorldCommission on Environment and Development, Oxford, Oxford University Press, Oxford, 1987.

Byerlee, D., Fischer, K. Accessing modern science: policy and institutional options for agricultural biotechnology in developing countries. World Bank Report, Washington, DC. 2001.

Changsorn, P., "Firms See Lower Costs, More Profit in Nanotech", *The Nation*, November 22, p. unknown, 2004.

Choi, K., "Ethical Issues Of Nanotechnology Development in the Asia-Pacific Region", Regional Meeting on Ethics of Science and Technology, UNESCO Regional Unit for Social andHuman Sciences in Asia and Pacific, Bangkok, pp. 327-76, 2003.

Choi, K., Ethical Issues Of Nanotechnology Development in the Asia-Pacific Region in Ethics in Asia-Pacific, Bergstrom, P. (Ed.), Regional Unit for Social and Human Sciences in Asia and the Pacific, Asia and the Pacific Regional Bureau for Education, UNESCO, Bangkok pp. 327-76, 2003.

Chrispeels, M.J., "Biotechnology and the Poor", Plant Physiology, 124 (1), pp. 3-6, 2000.

Chrispeels, M.J., Biotechnology and the poor. Plant Physiology. 2000; 124:3-6. doi: 10.1104/pp. 124.1.3. [PubMed]

Cientifica Ltd., 2004, "Nanowater: Technology Helping the Environment". Accessedon: September 1, 2004.http://www.nanowater.org.

Cohen, J.I., Harnessing Biotechnology for the Poor: challenges ahead for capacity, safety and public investment. Journal of Human Development. 2: 239-263. doi: 10.1080/14649880120067275. 2001 Jul 1.

Compañó, R. and Hullman, A., "Forecasting the development of nanotechnology with the help of science and technology indicators", Nanotechnology, 13, pp. 243-47, 2002.

CORDIS News, 2003, "Nanotechnology: Opportunities or Threat?" Accessed on: December 9, 2003. http://dbs.cordis.lu/cgi-bin/srchidadb?CALLER=NHP_EN_NEWS&ACTION=D&SESSION=&RCN=EN_RCN_ID:20401.

CORDIS, 2004, "Nanotechnology". Accessed on: September 15, 2004. http://www.cordis.lu/nanotechnology/src/sitemap.htm.

Council for Scientific and Industrial Research South Africa, 2005, "New nanodrugcarriers to target TB sufferers". Accessed on.

Court, E., Daar, A.S., Martin, E., Acharya, T. and Singer, P.A., 2004, "Will Prince Charles Et Al Diminish the Opportunities of Developing Countries in Nanotechnology?" Accessed on: February 23, 2004. http://www.nanotechweb.org/articles/society/3/1/1/1.

Daar, A.S., Martin, D.K., Nast, S., Smith, A.C., Singer, P.A., Thorsteinsdóttir, H. Top 10 Biotechnologies for Improving Health in Developing Countries. Toronto: University of Toronto Joint Centre for Bioethics; 2002.

Dayrit, F.M. and Enriquez E.P., Nanotechnology Issues for Developing Economies (revised) (essay), Philippines, 2001.

deAlmeida, A.O., 2003, "Responses to questionnaire on nanotechnology; Brazil". Accessed on: September 22, 2004.

Drexler, K.E., Engines of Creation: The Coming Era of Nanotechnology, Doubleday, New York 1986.

Dwivedi, K.K., 2004, "Questionnaire Response for the International Dialogue on Responsible Research and Development of Nanotechnology". Accessed on: December 12, 2004.http://www.nanodialogues.org/international.php.

ETC Group, "Nanotech Un-gooed! Is the Grey/Green Goo Brouhaha the Industry's Second Blunder?" Communiqué, (80) 2003.

ETC Group, "The Big Down: From Genomes To Atoms", ETC Group, Winnipeg, 2003.

ETC Group, 2002, "Patenting Elements of Nature". Accessed on: August 1, 2004.

ETC Group, 2004, "26 Governments Tiptoe toward Global Nano Governance: Grey Governance". Accessed on: September 27, 2004. http://www.etcgroup.org/article.asp?newsid=466.

ETC Group, 2004, "Itty-bitty Ethics: Bioethicists see Quantum Plots in Nanotech Concern.and Quantum Bucks in Buckyball Brouhaha?" Accessed on: October 7, 2004. http://www.etcgroup.org/article.asp?newsid=436.

European Commission, 2004, "Opening to the World: International Co-operation". Accessed on: January 16, 2004. http://www.cordis.lu/nanotechnology/src/intlcoop.htm.

European Patent Office, 2005, "European Classification (ECLA)". Accessed on: April 20, 2005.http://ep.espacenet.com/ep/en/helpv3/ecla.html.

Fawcett, A., "Where the Bright Sparks Are", Sydney Morning Herald, February 8, p. 12, 2005.

Fifis, T. *et al.*, "Size-DependentImmunogenicity: Therapeutic and Protective Properties of Nano-Vaccines Against Tumors", *The Journal of Immunology*, 173 (5), pp. 3148-54, 2004.

Genomics and World Health. Report of the Advisory Committee on Health Research Geneva. 2002.

Global Forum: Building Science, Technology, and Innovation Capacity for Sustainable Growth and Poverty Reduction. Washington DC. 2007 February 13

Hamdan, H., 2003, "Nanotech Initiative in Malaysia (Part 1)". Accessed on: May 30, 2004.

Hamdan, H., 2005, "Nanotechnology in Malaysia". Accessed on: March 13, 2005.http://www.ics.trieste.it/Documents/Downloads/df2676.pdf.

Harper, T., "What is Nanotechnology?" Nanotechnology, 14(1), p. introduction, 2003.

Harper, T., 2003, "Nanotechnology in Kabul? Taking the First Steps". Accessedon: October 10, 2003.

Hassan, M.A., Nanotechnology. Small Things and Big Changes in the Developing World. Science. 309:65. doi: 10.1126/science.1111138. 2005 Jul 1. [PubMed]

Haum, R., Petschow, U. and Steinfeldt, M., "Nanotechnology and Regulation within theframework of the Precautionary Principle. Final Report for ITRE Committeee ofthe European Parliament", Institut für ökologische Wirtschaftsforschung (IÖW)gGmbH, Berlin, 2004.

Heines, H., 2003, "Patent Trends in Nanotechnology". Accessed on: December 3, 2003.http://library.findlaw.com/2003/Nov/4/133136.html

Henderson, R., 2002, "The Next Technological Revolution: Predicting the Technical Future and its Impacts on Firms, Organisations and Ourselves". Accessedon.mitsloan.mit.edu/50th/tech.pdf.

Hoet, P.H.M., Nemmar, A. and Nemery, B., "Health Impact of Nanomaterials?"Nature Biotechnology, 22 (1), p. 19, 2004.

Huaizhi, Z. and Yuantao, N., "China's ancient gold drugs", Gold Bulletin, 34(1), pp. 24-29, 2001.

Huang, Z., Chen, H., Chen, Z.-K. and Roco, M.C., "International nanotechnology development in 2003: Country, institution, and technology field analysis based on USPTO patent database", *Journal of Nanoparticle Research*, 6, pp. 325-54, 2004.

India, Pakistan establish closer cooperation in Biotechnology. Pakistan Times, Business and Commerce Desk. 2004 Feb 29.

Institute of Nanotechnology, "Nanotechnology in China", Institute of Nanotechnology, London, 2004.

Inter-Academy Council, "Strong Science and Technology Capacity a Necessity for Every Nation", Inter-Academy Council, New York, 2004.

International Association of Nanotechnology, 2004, "International Association of Nanotechnology". Accessed on: November 20, 2004. http://www.ianano.org/aboutus.htm.

International Council on Nanotechnology, 2004, "International Council on Nanotechnology: About Us". Accessed on: March 12, 2005. http://icon.rice.edu/about.cfm.

International Nanotechnology and Society Network, 2005, "International Nanotechnology and Society Network". Accessed on: June 17, 2005. http://www.nanoandsociety.com/index.htm.

Invernizzi, N. and Foladori, G., 2005, "Nanotechnology as a solution to the problems of developing countries?" Accessed on: June 17, 2005.

Juma C.and Yee-Chong L., 2005, "Innovation: Applying Knowledge in Development". Accessed on: January 27, 2005.

Juma, C. and Yee-Chong, L., "Innovation: Applying Knowledge in Development", UN Millennium Project Task Force on Science, Technology and Innovation, London, 2005.

Kalam, A.A.P.J., 2004, "Our Future Lies in Nanotechnology". Accessed on: September 1, 2004.Our Future Lies in Nanotechnology.

Kalaugher, L., 2004, "Nanoparticles Clean Up Arsenic". Accessed on: December 23, 2004.http://www.nanotechweb.org/articles/news/3/5/15/1.

Karim, S.S.A., 2003, "Creating Equal Access to Scientific Information". Accessed on: September 1, 2004. http://www.scidev.net/Opinions/index.cfm?fuseaction=readOpinions&itemid=122&language=1.

Khuller, G.K. and Pandey, R., "Sustained Release Drug Delivery Systems inManagement of Tuberculosis", *Indian J Chest Dis Allied Sci*, 45, pp. 229-30, 2003.

Khuller, G.K., "Subcutaneous nanoparticle-based antitubercular chemotherapy inexperimental model", *Journal of Antimicrobial Chemotherapy*, 54 (1), pp. 266-68, 2004.

Kumar, N.K., Quach, U., Thorsteinsdóttir, H., Somsekhar, H., Daar, A.S., Singer, P.A.., Indian biotechnology—rapidly evolving and industry led. Nat Biotechnol. 22 Suppl: DC31-DC36. [PubMed]

LaVan, D.A. and Langer, R., Implications of Nanotechnology in the Pharmaceutics and Medical Fields in Societal Implications of Nanoscience and Nanotechnology: NSET Workshop Report, edited workshop report,, Roco, M.C. and Bainbridge, W.S. (Eds), National Science Foundation, Arlington, Virginia. pp. 79-83, 2001.

Leahy, S., 2004, "'Nano Divide' No Small Matter". Accessed on: February 27, 2004.

Lee, K., "The Global Dimensions of Health: Background paper for the Global Health, a Local Issue Seminar", London School of Hygiene and Tropical Medicine, London, 1999.

Lee-Chua, Q.N., 2003, "Nanotechnology". Accessed on: September 23, 2003.http://www.inq7.net/inf/2003/jun/25/inf_24-1.htm.

Leite, J.R., 2004, "Questionnaire Response for the International Dialogue on Responsible Research and Development of Nanotechnology". Accessed on: January 15, 2005.http://www.nanodialogues.org/international.php.

Liu, L., "Societal Impact of Nanotechnology in the Asia Pacific Region", Asia Nanotechnology Forum, Beijing, 2004.

Liu, Y., Tsapis, N. and Edwards, D.A., "Investigating Sustained-release Nanoparticles for Pulmonary Drug Delivery", Harvard University, Cambridge, Massachusetts, 2003.

Lux Research, 2005, "Why Big Pharma is Missing the Nanotech Opportunity". Accessed on: March 20, 2005. http://www.azonano.com/news.asp?newsID=525.

Maclurcan, D.C., Ford, M.J., Cortie, M.B. and Ghosh, D., "Medical Nanotechnology and Developing Nations", Proceedings of the Asia Pacific Nanotechnology Forum, World Scientific Publishing Co., Singapore, pp. 165-72, 2004.

Mahajan, R., 2005, "North South Dialogue on Nanotechnology: Challenges and Opportunities". Accessed on: April 1, 2005.

Mantell, K., 2003, "Developing nations 'must wise upto nanotechnology'". Accessed on: September 25, 2003. http://www.scidevnet/News/index.cfm?fuseaction=readNews&itemid=992&language.

Marinova, D. and McAleer, M., "Nanotechnology Strength Indicators: International Rankings Based on US Patents", Nanotechnology, 14, pp. R1-R7, 2003.

Maruping, P., 2005, "South African Nanotechnology Strategy". Accessed on: March 12, 2005.

Maugh II, T.H., 1996, "Worldwide Study Finds Big Shift in Causes of Death". Accessed on: November 25, 2004. http://www.aegis.com/news/lt/1996/LT960902.html.

McArthur, J.W. and Sachs, J.D., "The Growth Competitiveness Index: MeasuringTechnological Advancement and the Stages of Development", 2001.

Merkle, R., "It's a small, small, small, small world", MIT Technology Review,100 (Feb/March), pp. 25-32, 1997.

Ministério Das Relaçõs Exteriores, 2003, "Titulo: Nanotechnology R&D: Sweating the Small Stuff". Accessed on: October 22, 2004.http://www.mre.gov.br/portugues/noticiario/internacional/selecao_detalhe.asp?ID_RESENHA=4139.

Mnyusiwalla, A., Daar, A.S. and Singer, P.A., "'Mind the gap': science and ethics innanotechnology", Nanotechnology, 14, pp. R9-R13, 2003.

Mooney, P., "The ETC Century Erosion, Technological Transformation and Corporate Concentration in the 21st Century", Development Dialogue, 1999 (1-2), pp. 1-128, 1999.

Moore, R., 2004, "Medical nanotechnology: a new challenge forstandardization?" Accessed on: March 23, 2005.

Morris, M.L., Hoisington, D., Bringing the benefits of biotechnology to the poor:the role of the CGIAR centers. In: Qaim M, Krattiger AF, von Braun J, editor. Agricultural Biotechnology in Developing Countries: Towards Optimizing the Benefits for the Poor. Boston, Kluwer Academic Publishers; 2000. pp. 327-356.

Morrison, S., (date unknown), "The Emerging Nanotech Industry; Lessons from Biotech Experience". Accessed on: December 9, 2003.

Munroe, P., 2003, "Nano, Nanotechnology (Or Nanoscience, or Nanomaterials) at UNSW". Accessed on: November 11, 2004.

Nanoscale Science and Engineering Subcommittee, 2000, "Nanotechnology Definition". Accessed on: September 5, 2003.

National Cancer Institute, U.S. National Institutes of Health, 2004, "National Cancer Institute Announces Major Commitment to Nanotechnology for Cancer Research". Accessed on: December 15, 2004. http://www.nci.nih.gov/newscenter/pressreleases/nanotechPressRelease.

National Science Foundation, "International Dialogue on Responsible Research and Development of Nanotechnology", National Science Foundation, Arlington, Virginia, 2004.

National Science Foundation, Sri Lanka, "Cutting-edge technology and developing countries", *Techwatch Lanka*, Vol. 2, no. 2, p. 1, 2002.

New Partnership for Africa's Development. http://www.nepad.org/[cited 7 Mar 2007]

Njemanze, P.C., Receptor mediated nanoscale copolymerassemblies for diagnostic imaging and therapeutic management of hyperlipidemia and infectious diseases In esp@cenet, European Patent Office, 2005.

Nordan, M.M. *et al.*, "The Nanotech Report 2004™", Lux Research Inc., New York 2004.

Office of Science and Technology Policy, Executive Office of the President, 2005, "National Nanotechnology Inititiative: Research and Development Funding in the President's 2005 Budget". Accessed on.http://www.ostp.gov/html/budget/2005/FY05NNI1-pager.pdf.

Pan-Asian Biotech Federation Formed. Sci Dev net. 2005 Feb 23 [cited 2007 Feb 28]

Patil, R., 2005, "If Tomorrow Comes". Accessed on: February 3, 2005. http://www.indianexpress.com/full_story.php?content_id=62323.

Peters, S. and Page, P., 2003, "Building Bonds across the Ocean". Accessed on: December 13, 2004. http://www.princeton.edu/~seasweb/eqnews/spring03/feature1.html.

Poullier, J.-P., Hernandez, P., Kawabata, K. and Savedoff, W.D., "Patterns of Global Health Expenditures: Results for 191 Countries", World Health Organisation, Geneva, 2002.

Powell, K., "Green Groups Baulk At Joining Nanotechnology Talks", Nature, 432 (7013), p. 5, 2004.

Pratap, R., 2005, "Engaging Private Enterprise in Nanotech Research in India". Accessed on: April 3, 2005.http://www.ics.trieste.it/Documents/Downloads/df2684.pdf.

President's Council of Advisors on Science and Technology, "The National Nanotechnology Initiative at Five Years: Assessment and Recommendations of the National Nanotechnology Advisory Panel", Office of Science and Technology Policy, Washington, D.C., 2005.

Proceedings of the Biotechnology and Rural Livelihood - Enhancing the Benefits Conference. The Hague, the Netherlands. International Service for National Agricultural Research Consultation; 2001 June 25-28.

Proceedings of the Way Forward to Strengthen National Plant Breeding and Biotechnology Capacity. Food and Agriculture Organization of the UN. Headquarters, Agriculture Department, Plant Production and Protection Division, Crop and Grassland Service; 2005 Feb 9-11.

Public Intellectual Property Resource for Agriculture, Date unknown, "Public Sector Collaboration". Accessed on: March 30, 2005. http://www.pipra.org/main/background.htm.

Rader, R.A., 1990, "Trends in Biotechnology Patenting". Accessed on: February 8, 2005.http://www.bioinfo.com/patrev.html.

Railey, C.J., 2004, "Fourth Asan-HMI symposium highlights nanotechnology". Accessed on: September 9, 2004.

Rensselaer Polytechnic Institute, 2004, "Efficient Filters Produced fromCarbon Nanotubes". Accessed on: April 10, 2005.

Roco, M.C. and Murday, J., "Nanotechnology—A Revolution in the Making—Vision for R&D in the Next Decade", Interagency Working Group on Nano Science, Engineering and Technology, Washington, D.C., 1999.

Roco, M.C., "International Strategy for Nanotechnology Research and Development", *Journal of Nanoparticle Research*, 3 (5-6), pp. 353-60, 2001.

Roco, M.C., "National Nanotechnology Initiative and a Global Perspective", "Small Wonders", Exploring the Vast Potential of Nanoscience, (ed.) National Science Foundation, Washington D.C., 2002.

Runge, C.F. and Ryan, B., "The Global Diffusion of Plant Biotechnology: International Adoption and Research in 2004", University of Minnesota, Minnesota, 2004.

Salamanca-Buentello, F. *et al.*, "Nanotechnology andthe Developing World", PLoS Medicine, 2 (4), pp. 300-03, 2005.

Salvarezza, R.C., "Why Is Nanotechnology Important For Developing Countries?"Third Session of the World Commission on the Ethics of Scientific Knowledge and Technology, UNESCO, Rio De Janeiro, pp. 133-36, 2003.

Schubert, M., 2005, "Global Nanotechnology Network". Accessed on: March 30, 2005. http://www.cc-nanochem.de/gnn2005/GNN2005-Flyer3.pdf.

Scott, A., 2003, "Nanotechnology and Nanoscience". Accessed on: February 17,2004.http://www.nanotec.org.uk/evidence/77aAndrewScott.htm.

Scott, J., 2002, "New Technologies 'Central to Sustainable Development'". Accessed on: September 1, 2004.

Service, R.F., "Nanotech Forum Aims To Head Off Replay of Past Blunders", Science, 306 (5698), p. 955, 2004.

Shanahan, M., 2004, "Nanotech 'threatens markets for poor nations' goods'".Accessed on: February 2, 2005.

Singer, P.A., Berndtson, K., Tracy, C.S., Cohen, E.R.M., Masum, H., Daar, A.S., A Tough Transition. Nature. 449:160-163. doi: 10.1038/449160a. [PubMed]

Singer, P.A., Daar, A.S. Harnessing Genomics and Biotechnology to Improve Global Health Equity. Science. 294:87. doi: 10.1126/science.1062633. 2001 Oct 5.

Smith, A.C., Mugabe, J., Singer, P.A., Daar, A.S., Harnessing genomics to improve health in Africa—an executive course to support genomics policy. Bio-Med Central. 2005; 3:2. http://www.health-policy-systems.com/content/3/1/2

South African Nanotechnology Initiative, "National Nanotechnology Strategy: Nanowonders—Endless Possibilities, Volume 1, Draft 1.5", South African Nanotechnology Initiative and the Department of Science and Technology, Pretoria, 2003.

South African Nanotechnology Initiative, "South African Nanotechnology Strategy, Volume 1, Draft 1.4", South African Nanotechnology Initiative, Pretoria, 2003.

South Asian Peasants' Assembly, 2003, "Dhaka Declaration". Accessed on: March 22, 2005. http://www.nadir.org/nadir/initiativ/agp/en/index.html.

Starpharma Ltd., 2004, "Product Focus: Vivagel... Applying Dendrimer Nanotechnology to Prevent HIV and Other STDs". Accessed on: September 20, 2004.

Taniguchi, N., "On the Basic Concept of NanoTechnology", International Conference of Production Engineering Part II, Japan Society of Precision Engineering, Tokyo, pp. 18-23, 1974.

Tegart, G., "Nanotechnology The Technology for the 21st Century", APEC Center for Technology Foresight, Bangkok, 2001.

Thao, T., 2004, "Ho Chi Minh City Thinks Nano Labs". Accessed on: October 1, 2004.http://english.vietnamnet.vn/tech/2004/09/261046/.

The Coalition Against Biopiracy, 2004, "Ahoy and Welcome to The 2004 Captain Hook Awards: Nominations for Outstanding Achievements in Biopiracy". Accessed on: March 25, 2005. http://www.captainhookawards.org/history.html.

The Ecologist, "Promising the World, or Costing the Earth?" *The Ecologist*, Vol. 33, no. 4, pp. 28-39, 2003.

The Hindu, 2005, "India becoming a Pioneer in Nano Technology". Accessed on: May 3, 2005. http://www.hindu.com/2005/03/25/stories/2005032518320300.htm.

The Press Trust of India, 2003, "In The News—TB News". Accessed on: March 10, 2004.

The Royal Society and Royal Academy of Engineering, "Nanoscience and Nanotechnologies: Opportunities and Uncertainties", The Royal Society and Royal Academy of Engineering, London, 2004.

The Special Programme for Research and Training in Tropical Diseases, "Executive Summary of Meeting Report "Diagnosis of Tuberculosis: Countdown to New Tools" Geneva, Switzerland, 29-30 June 2000", UNDP/WORLD BANK/WHO, Geneva, 2000.

The Times of India, 2004, "CSIO Develops Nanotechnology for TB Diagnostic Kit". Accessed on: February 21, 2004.

Thorsteinsdóttir, H., Quach, U., Daar, A.S., Singer, P.A.S., Promoting Biotechnology Innovation in Developing Countries. Nature Biotechnology. 2004; 22:DC48-DC52. doi: 10.1038/nbt1204supp-DC48. [PubMed]

U.S. Department of Energy, Office of Science, 2003, "Faster Test forTuberculosis". Accessed on: December 20, 2003.

UNCTAD, 2004, "Interactive Dialogue on Harnessing Emerging Technologies to Meetthe Millennium Development Goals". Accessed on: September 3, 2004. http://stdev.unctad.org/unsystem/emerging.htm.

UNIDO, 2004, "2004 Technology Fair of the Future". Accessed on: September 30, 2004. http://www.unido.org/en/doc/20219.

Unisearch, "Final Report: Survey for Current Situation of Nanotechnology Researchers and R&D in Thailand", Chulalongkorn University, Bangkok, 2004.

United Nations Development Program, Human Development Report 2003, Oxford University Press, New York 2003.

Vargas, M., 2004, "Costa Rica Opens Region's First Lab for Nanotechnology". Accessed on: October 22, 2004.

Viet Nam News Agency, 2004, "Viet Nam Initially Penetrates into Nanotechnology". Accessed on: October 28, 2003.http://nanotechwire.com/news.asp?nid=655&ntid=116&pg=18.

Waga, M., 2002, "Emerging Nanotechnology Research in Vietnam". Accessed on: October 28, 2003. http://www.glocom.org/tech_reviews/geti/20021028_geti_s29/.

Walsh, M., 2004, "Nanoscale Particle Systems Suitable for New Microdevices andBio-Diagnostics". Accessed on: November 16, 2004.

Watanabe, M., "Small World, Big Hopes", Nature, 426 (6965), pp. 478-79, 2003.

White, E., 2003, "Nano-Robots Not Yet On The Patenting Horizon". Accessed on: January 5, 2005.http://scientific.thomson.com/knowtrend/ipmatters/nanotech/8238656/.

Whittingham, J. and Bateman, A., 2003 "???" Accessed on: May 25, 2004.

WHO, Global Tuberculosis Program, "Anti-tuberculosis drug resistance in the world:third global report", World Health Organisation, Geneva, 2004.

Wilsdon, J. and Willis, R., 2004, "Will nanotechnology go the GM way?" Accessedon: September 15, 2004.

World Health Organisation, "Hepatitis B", Department of Communicable Disease Surveillance and Response, World Health Organisation, Geneva, 2002.

World Health Organisation, "The World Health Report, 1997: Conquering Suffering, Enriching Humanity", World Health Organisation, Geneva, 1997.

World Health Organisation, 2005, "Diabetes Mellitus". Accessed on: June 13, 2005. http://www.who.int/mediacentre/factsheets/fs138/en/index.html.

World Health Organisation, 2005, "Global tuberculosis control: surveillance, planning, financing". Accessed on: May 20, 2005.

Xinhua News Agency, 2003, "China's Nanotechnology Patent Applications Rank Third in the World". Accessed on: January 27, 2004. http://www.chinadaily.com.cn/en/doc/2003-10/03/content_269182.htm.

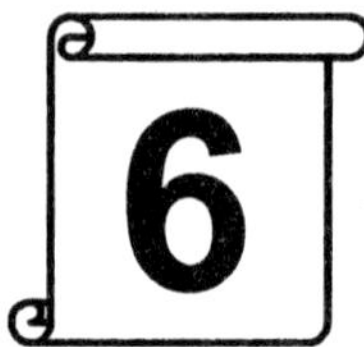

Foreign Collaboration in Health and Medical Cities

Public health expenditure accounts for less than 1 percent of GDP compared to 3 percent of GDP for developing countries and 5 percent for high income countries. The private health care sector in India accounts for over 75 percent of total health care expenditure. India's health care sector, however, falls well below international benchmarks for physical infrastructure and manpower, and even falls below the standards existing in comparable developing countries. It is estimated that over a million beds have to be added, which translates into a total investment of $78 billion (Rs. 350,830 crores) in health infrastructure. An additional 800,000 physicians are required over the next 10 years, which translates into huge investments in training facilities and equipment. In order to reach even 50-75 percent of the present levels of other developing countries, the sector will require an estimated investment of $20-30 billion. Thus, India's health care sector needs to scale up considerably in terms of the availability and quality of its physical infrastructure as well as human resources. Given the growing demand, the emergence of reputed private players, and the huge investment needs in the health care sector, in recent years, there has been growing interest among foreign players and non resident Indians to enter the Indian health care market. There is also growing interest among domestic and international financial institutions, private equity funds, venture capitalists, and banks to explore investment opportunities across a wide range of segments. (Rupa Chanda, IIMB).

Private health *vs.* Public health

Studies by the Central Bureau of Health Intelligence have shown that a majority of Indians trust private health care despite a higher average cost of US$ 4.3 compared to US$ 2.7 in government-owned health care agencies.

Only 23.5 percent of urban residents and 30.6 percent of rural residents choose government facilities, reflecting the widespread lack of confidence in the public health care system. The private sector's role is expected to grow in the future. Government spending on health care infrastructure (excluding land) is projected to rise only marginally, by 0.12 percent of GDP and is expected to meet only 12 percent of the huge investment required in the health care sector, with the private sector providing some 88 percent of investment requirements. There has been growing interest among foreign players and non-resident Indians to enter the Indian health care market.

Government policy is liberal

The foreign investment policy is very liberal for hospitals. Since January 2000, FDI is permitted upto 100 percent under the automatic route in hospitals in India. Controlling stake is also permitted in hospitals for foreign investors. In addition, FIIs and private equity funds can individually purchase upto 10 percent and collectively upto 24 percent of the paid-up share capital of the company, through open offers or private placement, or through the stock exchange. Proprietary funds, foreign individuals and foreign corporates can register as a sub-account and invest through the FII, subject to limits of 10 percent and 5 percent, respectively for these sub-accounts. Foreign venture capital investments (FVCIs) are also permitted, though subject to certain restrictions. No major regulatory hurdles seem to exist with regard to the setting up of hospitals. Although various forms of financing may be classified as FDI, industry experts distinguish between these various modes as they have different implications for the absorption of costs, benefits to patients, expectations of returns, and improved capacity in health care delivery.

Thus no government approval is required as long as the Indian company files with the regional office of the RBI within 30 days of receipt of inward remittances and file the required documents along with form FC-GPR with that Office within 30 days of issue of shares to the non-resident investors.

The hurdles are felt mostly at the operational level rather than in the regulatory framework *per se*.

Constraints to foreign investment in hospitals in India

There are certainly many factors that could drive foreign funding into hospitals in India. The most important driving factor is the demand-supply mismatch and the huge amount of private sector investment that is required in this sector to raise its infrastructure even marginally to meet international metrics. With the growing economy, rising incomes, increased willingness among Indian consumers to pay for quality health care and to go to institutional providers, the comparably lower costs of establishment in India, and the health care packages offered by companies which are increasing affordability of health care for consumers, this is a potentially attractive sector for both foreign and domestic investors.

The main factors that make India unattractive is the uncertainty of its regulatory environment, issues of income flow, license and red tape, difficulties in developing business, and corruption. Investing in service industries is different from that in production industries...There are two reasons why investors are waiting and watching. One is the lack of infrastructure and the second is the bureaucracy for setting up."

One senior doctor noted that an estimated that about one crore is required per bed, which works out to Rs. 200 crores for a 200-bed hospital. If this cost could be reduced then the break-even period could be quicker. Thus, investment in hospitals is characterized by low returns, high capital intensity, and long-term commitment. This is not the most attractive combination for foreign investors.

The following discussion examines four issues. These are: (1) set-up costs and in particular costs of procuring land; (2) required investments in and depreciation of medical equipment and devices; (3) medical manpower constraints; and (4) regulations in related areas and the overall regulatory environment and policy direction affecting investment in hospitals. one respondent noted that land accounts for 10-15 percent of a hospital's existing fixed assets, and buildings, IT, and engineering services account for a sizeable 30 percent or so of fixed assets. Thus land and buildings together remain an important part of the hospital's total stock of assets and clearly for its initial establishment costs. Respondents also noted that given the hard infrastructure requirements and long repayment periods, scale is essential to make hospital projects viable. For example, if there is infrastructure of around 5,000 beds, then costs can be lowered significantly, and margins can be improved. Such investments are only possible with inflows from international agencies. However, the cost of land is a major deterrent to setting up such large-scale establishments and the viability of hospital projects. Many noted that there needs to be land allocated within SEZs for hospitals as this would lower the cost of establishment and enable the setting up of large hospitals. Many also pointed out that if land is subsidized, then this should not come with conditions to serve below poverty line patients as such conditions are not enforceable and create perennial obligations on hospitals rather than making the procurement of land a one-time transaction.

In addition to the procurement of land, there are also issues concerning the supporting infrastructure (such as getting water supply and electricity) and the process of obtaining clearances for buildings (getting legal documents, environmental and fire clearances) which are not always transparent, may involve corruption, varying levels of efficiency and interest on the part of state governments, and vested interests, which may delay establishment and drive up initial costs.

Equipment constitutes around 30 percent of all fixed assets; depending on the kind of technology acquired and some 40 percent of revenues are spent on drugs and supplies. However, 70 percent or more of medical devices are imported, often at high cost notwithstanding recent reductions in import duties. It is felt that these duties could be rationalized further and flat uniform rates introduced for a wide range of medical devices, without conditions. According to industry experts, unless companies establish Indian subsidiaries or enter into tie-ups with local companies, hospitals will need to continue importing and these input costs will not come down.

Organized equipment manufacturers often engage in opportunistic pricing and make big margins when selling to hospitals. The prices paid generally exceed their true manufacturing cost. A catheter may be procured at ten times its actual manufacturing cost. Partnerships between hospitals and medical equipment manufacturers to develop indigenous technologies and greater involvement of medical faculty in research and product development at such companies could help lower input costs for hospitals. It was also pointed out that if there were larger hospitals, then economies of scale would enable the hospitals to bring down the share of medical equipment costs from the current level of 40 percent to around 20 percent.

Strategy for multilateral liberalization in hospital services

Should India further liberalize its offer on hospital services to 100 percent with no prior approval requirement, i.e., bind in its existing FDI regulations in this area? The concern in policy circles is that such a binding would lead to entry by foreign players and increased FDI in this segment, with possible negative effects on equity and on the public sector. A binding commitment would be irreversible and thus caution may be required in taking such a step towards further multilateral liberalization. The findings of this study, however, suggest that India could bind in its existing FDI policy in hospitals and permit 100 percent on automatic route. The justifications for such a strategy relate to two facts:

First, as investors see a lack of clarity and roadmap for the health sector, a binding commitment would signal that the liberal foreign investment policy for hospitals is there to stay and that the government is committed to facilitating investments in India's hospital segment.

Second, to the extent that additional FDI does flow into hospitals, there are several likely benefits that could accrue while the negatives that could arise will not really be a direct result of foreign investment but of existing structural distortions and inadequacies in India's health care sector.

The study also suggests possible conditions that could be inscribed in India's commitments to ensure that certain objectives are realized. The existing revised offer puts a technology transfer-related condition. Another possible condition could pertain to corporate social responsibility measures, such as outreach and extension services and reinvestment of part of profits in medical research and education or in tele-medicine to serve a wider population base if any subsidies or concessions have been granted in related areas. While other conditions could be inscribed, such as requiring tie ups with local players in terms of referral services, education and training of personnel, transfer of older equipment, and pooling of resources, it may not be advisable to impose too many conditions as these could adversely affect incentives for investors and their bottom lines. As investors would adopt different investment models (hub and spoke, local franchises, medicity, etc.), depending on their profile, the location of the investment, and the pattern of financing, among other factors, attaching too many conditions on the commitment may reduce the flexibility of investors to enter into what is a very location specific business.

While external factors influence foreign investors in their decision to invest in this segment, the main factors that influence overall profitability of hospitals pertain to domestic factors, in particular:

- High upfront costs due to physical infrastructure (land) constraints;
- High input costs for medical devices and technology resulting from reliance on imports, the structure of this industry, and lack of local manufacturing capacity;
- Manpower constraints in terms of quantity and quality arising from inappropriate regulations on medical education suppliers and inadequacies in medical education;
- The low level of insurance penetration resulting from limited opening up of the insurance sector and lack of a universal health insurance scheme to make health care affordable to a larger number of people;
- Other regulatory inadequacies affecting standards and practices in health care establishment; and
- Lack of policy clarity and thrust on health care as a priority area.

The study also throws up several policy measures required by government and initiatives required by private players to make the hospital segment more attractive to both domestic and foreign investors if the ultimate aim is to expand capacity, improve standards, and make health care affordable and accessible to a wider segment. Some of these measures include:

- Facilitating land acquisition—some subsidization of initial project costs or PPP arrangements with possible cost discounting or cross subsidization arrangements built into the valuation of land;
- Consider other forms of obtaining land—through leasing arrangements, joint development with real estate developers and arrangements with public sector units owning land and hospital facilities and government facilitation of such arrangements;

to enter into medical education and training to expand the supply of medical personnel at all levels;

- Incentivising domestic manufacturing of medical devices and technologies through increased investment in this sector and tie-ups with foreign companies and efforts to standardize output;
- Opening up the health insurance sector to enable greater scrutiny of processes and standards of hospitals, which would also help attract foreign funds, as well as introduction of a national or community-based health insurance scheme to increase affordability of health care and mitigate potential adverse effects of corporatization on equity;
- Improving the regulatory framework for health insurance by standardizing norms for payouts, coverage, reduce malpractice;
- Facilitating public private partnerships in hospitals, with private sector hospitals entering into limited period management contracts with public hospitals, under well-defined revenue sharing arrangement, along with CSR responsibilities through cross subsidization mechanisms;
- Greater sharing of resources (equipment, knowledge, research facilities) between public and private hospitals and between larger private hospitals and smaller local players;
- Establishing a regulatory framework and an independent regulator in the health care sector to address issues of standardization, classification, information disclosure, etc.; and
- Improved regulation and monitoring of mid and small size establishments to improve standards and quality, weed out substandard establishments, and enable consolidation in health care delivery.

It needs to be pointed out that there have been repeated demands to grant infrastructure status to the health care sector so as to facilitate access to viability gap financing and improve cash flows for private players; the study finds that there are practical difficulties in implementing this proposal. In order to get infrastructure status, the existence of a regulatory body is required. The feasibility of setting up such a body may be questioned given there are incumbents such as the Medical Council of India and there are likely to be conflicts of interest with regard to regulatory jurisdiction. The real issue as highlighted by this study is not whether the industry gets infrastructure status but the availability of cheaper domestic financing and tax benefits in view of the long gestation of hospital projects, both of which are possible on a case-to-case basis, even without infrastructure status.

Some illustrative examples of foreign collaboration in Indian hospitals

- Singapore's Pacific Health Care has made its first foray into the Indian market, opening an international medical centre, which is a joint venture with India's Vitae Health Care, in the Indian city of Hyderabad.

- The Singapore based Parkway Group Health Care Pte. Ltd. penetrated into the Indian health care market in 2003 through a joint venture with the Apollo group to build the Apollo Gleneagles hospital Kolkata, a 325-bed multi-specialty hospital at a cost of US$ 29 million.
- Columbia Asia Group, a Seattle-based hospital services company, a worldwide developer and operator of community hospitals, has started its first American- style medical centre in Hebbal, Bangalore. Columbia Asia is the first hospital to enter the Indian health care market through the Foreign Direct Investment route.
- Wockhardt, the international arm of the Harvard Medical School, which also has a strategic association with Harvard Medical International, has set-up a new hospital (a tertiary service provider) in Bangalore at a cost of around Rs. 200 crores.
- The Parkway group has also entered into a joint venture with a Mumbai-based Asian Heart institute and research centre to set-up specialized centers of medical excellence in Mumbai.
- Max Health Care and Singapore General Hospital (SGH) have entered into collaboration for medical practice, research, training and education in health care services.
- Steris, a US$ 1.1 billion health care equipment company, plans to set-up a wholly owned arm in India to sell its devices and products in the country's booming medical device market. Steris plans to make an initial investment of US$ 1,00,000 to set-up the wholly owned subsidiary.
- Apollo Hospitals Enterprise Ltd has entered into a joint venture with AmcareLabs, an affiliate of Johns Hopkins International of the US, to set-up a diagnostic laboratory in Hyderabad. An initial amount of US$ 2.2 million is to be invested and the laboratory is likely to be operational by mid-2006.
- India's first geriatric hospital, the Heritage Hospital of Hyderabad has formed a joint venture with US-based United Church Homes to recruit, train and provide placement to registered Indian nurses in USA.
- The US-based health care products major, Proton Health Care has made an entry into India with its range of digital health monitoring devices and has a strategic tie-up with the Delhi-based SM Logistics for distributing its products in the Indian market.
- The American Association of Physicians of Indian Origin (AAPI), a Non-Resident Indian group launched two pilot projects in Bihar and Andhra Pradesh to help improve India's health care in rural areas. The AAPI has committed itself to the

improvement of primary health care under a MOU during the Pravasi Bharatiya Divas, the annual conclave of the Indian diaspora, with the government.

According to one estimate, foreign investors have tapped only 10 percent of the Indian health care market and thus the scope for FDI remains large.

The main source countries for foreign investment are seen to be the US, UK, Australia, and Singapore.

Visible players

The Singapore-based Parkway Group Health Care Pte. Ltd. is aggressively penetrating the Indian health care market. The group came up with its first Indian project in 2003 through a joint venture with the Apollo Group to build the Apollo Gleneagles Hospital, a 325-bed multi-specialty hospital at a cost of US$ 29 million. The partnership will further explore collaboration in oncology and orthopedics. The Parkway Group has also entered into a JV with the Mumbai-based Asian Heart Institute and Research Centre (AHIRC) to set-up specialized centres of medical excellence in Mumbai with Parkway holding a majority stake. These superspecialty centers will be set-up in AHIRC's facility and will be co-branded by both the partners. The Group is also looking for hospital projects in Chennai and other cities.

The Parkway Health, controlled by the US-based private equity firm Texas Pacific Group (TPG) announced that it has plans to set-up several multi-specialty hospitals in India. The group is also tying up with some of the leading health care providers in India apart from its plans to build hospitals on its own. Currently, it has agreement with Apollo Hospitals Group and has bought a 50 per cent stake in the Khubchandani Hospital in Mumbai which is jointly owned by the Mauritius-based Koncentric Investments. It plans to initially invest approximately US$ 83 million (Rs. 350-400 crore) in the Mumbai-based Khubchandani Hospital.

Location—Parkway Health plans to set-up the multispeciality hospitals all over India.

Budget—The hospital firm plans to invest US$ 125 thousand (Rs. 50-60 lakh) per bed in the project.

Features—Starting with 5-6 hospitals in metros, Parkway Health has plans to set-up 300-400-bed multispeciality hospitals all over the country.

The Khubchandani Hospital, which will be a 1,000-bed facility, is expected to be operational by 2011. The agreement with Apollo Group is intended to help Parkway develop hospitals across West Bengal. This JV currently runs Apollo Gleneagles Hospital, a 325-bed multispeciality hospital in Kolkota. This hospital will cater to Eastern India and neighbouring countries like Bangladesh, Myanmar, Nepal and Bhutan

Pacific Health Care Holdings

One of Singapore's leading health care service providers, is coming up with Pacific Medical Centre, an international medical centre at Hyderabad in a joint venture with Vitae Health Care Pvt Ltd. In the pipeline are two more medical facilities. The Pacific Women's and Children's Hospital will be a 150-bed state of the art hospital specializing in fetal-maternal medicine, reproductive medicine, gynecological oncology, neonatology and pediatrics. The Pacific Stem Cell Bank will provide both private and public cord blood stem cell storage facilities, which has clinical applications in the treatment of blood cancers and disorders. The other cities that the group is trying to foray into are Chennai and Mumbai.

Columbia Asia

Malaysia-based Columbia Asia has set-up its first 75-bed hospital in Hebbal, Bangalore through the FDI route. The company has chosen India to expand as private health care is recognised here by consumers and the government as a necessary supplement to the public health care system and also because there is a presence of a large and growing middle and upper income groups, options for quality health care are relatively limited or under served, growing number of third party payors and increasing health-insurance penetration. In the pipeline, the group has two more hospitals in Bangalore: a 150-bed tertiary care facility and another 75-100 bed. The group is also exploring markets in the southern and northern parts of the country.

MoU with Malaysia

The Malaysian government is expected to sign an agreement with the Indian government for the development of a medical city in Kerala within the next two months, Malaysian Works Minister said. Under the government-to-government cooperation, the Construction Industry Development Board Malaysia (CIDB) is given the mandate to select Malaysian companies to participate in the project with a gross development value (GDV) of over 1.5 billion ringgit (441.2 million U.S. dollars) spanning eight years. A Memorandum of Understanding (MoU) had been signed two months ago with the Indian Kerala state government, Works Minister Samy Vellu said after presenting certificates to contractors who had obtained the ISO 9001:2000 certification under CIDB's scheme. Proposals on developing the designated 500-hectare site in phases according to zones have been submitted, he said.

"The medical city will be complemented with industrial and township precincts," the national news agency Bernama quoted the minister as saying.

CIDB chief executive Hamzah Hasan, who returned from Kerala early this morning, said companies have not been short listed but those selected must have the capability and capacity to handle big projects, such as Grade G7 contractors. Grade G7 contractors are the highest in the registration hierarchy of contractors of Malaysia's construction industry, and are involved in projects with value of more than 10 million ringgit (2.9 million U.S. dollars).

Besides Kerala, he had also talked with the chief ministers of Gujarat and Delhi recently on the possibility of Malaysian contractors undertaking projects in their states, Samy Vellu said. The minister also called on Grade G7 contractors to obtain the ISO 9001:2000 certification as soon as possible as it would be a requirement for them from next year. "According to CIDB statistics, only about 400 or 10 percent of Grade G-7 contractors have the certification as opposed to the total number of 4,000 at present," he said.

Behrain interest

A leading Bahraini businessman has proposed to set-up a medical city in Bangalore with the help of investors from Gulf countries. Abdulnabi Al Sho'ala, Chairman of the Bahrain-India Society has proposed to the Federation of GCC Chambers of Commerce and Industry to establish a committee to examine the proposal and arrange a feasibility study. The former Labour and Social Development minister, who led a delegation from Bahrain to a meeting organized by the Federation of Indian Chambers of Commerce and Industry also made a presentation on the proposed project at a conclave in New Delhi last week, said a report.

India should be preferred as the natural destination as it has many advantages. GCC nationals feel at home and feel familiar with the culture, food habits, environment in India, he said. "While GCC nationals are currently not utilizing the potential of India as a medical care destination for various reasons, India, however, is perceived as the preferred choice for medical treatment by Western nationals," Al Sho'ala said. "Europe and the US are the destinations of some members of the affluent segment of GCC citizens. However, the majority of GCC citizens cannot afford the expensive treatment in US and Europe to such segments the only alternative is Asian destinations." The proposed project would not only cater to the needs of GCC market, but also to the Indian market as a whole, he said, adding that Gulf Finance House has already taken a similar initiative by establishing the new Energy City in Mumbai. A Medical and health care city is even more viable and very attractive to the investors of both the countries, he added.

IIM study

A study was carried out by IIMB under supervision of Prof. Rupa chandra. It covered 19 hospitals in 6 cities around the country. All the hospitals were of a minimum size of 100 beds, multi-specialty, and included a mix of for profit private hospitals with and without foreign financing and not for profit private hospitals categorized as charitable/trust hospitals. The study indicates that FDI presence in Indian hospitals is very limited at present. There are only three or hospitals, which qualify as FDI hospitals in India. However, it is perceived that there will be increased inflow of foreign funds into India's hospital segment in the near future given major expansion plans by existing and prospective corporate players. These include huge Medicities with large superspecialty and multi-specialty hospitals and integrated health care services as well as scaling up of existing operations and setting up of new hospitals around the country. The constraints to FDI include the fact that the number of such foreign players are limited, there are competing investment destinations, there are difficulties for foreign players in entering independently and in maintaining joint ventures that the gestation period in hospital projects is long and that investors may not be willing to make such a long-term commitment. domestic factors that adversely affect the returns to investment include high initial establishment costs and in particular the prohibitive cost of procuring land, low health insurance penetration in the country, which reduces the consumer base for corporate hospitals, restrictions on medical education and training providers, which create a supply bottleneck and adversely affects the quality of medical personnel at all levels, the high cost of importing medical devices and the limited domestic manufacturing capacity in this area, other regulatory deficiencies, which result in lack of standardization, proper governance, and quality assurance in the health care sector, and lack of policy clarity and priority to the health care sector.

The likely colour and contour of FDI hospitals in India

- Such hospitals are likely to focus on advanced procedures and specialty areas.
- They are more likely to focus on curative and intervention-oriented treatment than on preventive and long-term kind of treatment.
- They are likely to employ a higher ratio of technology to personnel in their health care delivery and thus involve a substitution of human resources with technology and equipment.
- They are likely to invest much more in medical equipment and devices and also in specialized and experienced medical personnel, thus involving a focus on high-end human resources and high-end technology.
- Such hospitals tend to have better systems and processes and usage of IT, which creates a more efficient and professional work environment.
- Foreign funded hospitals pay higher rates to staff at all levels and particularly to senior medical personnel.
- They are likely to attract overseas doctors and specialists than other hospitals.
- They are more likely to be accredited domestically and/or internationally.
- Their costs are likely to be higher than those of non foreign funded hospitals

- Their costs will tend to be higher than for small and medium size nursing homes but this is mainly due to greater capital intensity and focus on quality systems and processes and focus on hygiene.
- There could be positive externalities in other areas, some of which could further drive foreign investment in hospitals.
- Foreign funded hospitals could draw away medical personnel at all levels from other hospitals (both large non-foreign-funded and medium and small size hospitals/nursing homes, and public sector hospitals) and could adversely impact the quality of medical manpower available to competing institutions.
- There is likely to be closure of substandard institutions, some consolidation of the hospital segment, and new kinds of arrangements could emerge between larger and smaller players as the health care sector evolves.
- There could be greater segmentation between the public and private sector.

Foreign investment and greater corporate presence in hospitals could aggravate structural problems. The solution lies in strengthening the public health care system, in amending certain regulations that affect all players, and in introducing schemes, which provide affordable access to health care for all and not in restricting foreign investment. The benefits of foreign investment in hospitals are likely to outweigh these adverse effects.

IIMB recommendations to promote and develop FDI hospitals

- *Facilitating land acquisition*—some subsidization of initial project costs or PPP arrangements with possible cost discounting or cross subsidization arrangements built into the valuation of land.
- *Consider other forms of obtaining land*—Through leasing arrangements, joint development with real estate developers and arrangements with public sector units owning land and hospital facilities and government facilitation of such arrangements.
- Freeing up medical education and encouraging private hospitals to enter into medical education and training to expand the supply of medical personnel at all levels.
- Incentivizing domestic manufacturing of medical devices and technologies through increased investment in this sector and tie ups with foreign companies and efforts to standardize output.
- Opening up the health insurance sector to enable greater scrutiny of processes and standards of hospitals, which would also help attract foreign funds, as well as introduction of a national or community-based health insurance scheme to

increase affordability of health care and mitigate potential adverse effects of corporatization on equity.

- Improving the regulatory framework for health insurance by standardizing norms for payouts, coverage, reduce malpractice;
- Facilitating public private partnerships in hospitals, with private sector hospitals entering into limited period management contracts with public hospitals, under well-defined revenue sharing arrangement, along with CSR responsibilities through cross subsidization mechanisms.
- Greater sharing of resources (equipment, knowledge, research facilities) between public and private hospitals and between larger private hospitals and smaller local players.
- Establishing a regulatory framework and an independent regulator in the health care sector to address issues of standardization, classification, information disclosure, etc.
- Improved regulation and monitoring of mid and small size establishments to improve standards and quality, weed out substandard establishments, and enable consolidation in health care delivery.

Foreign investment can yield many benefits but if structural and regulatory deficiencies are not addressed, these benefits may not materialize and existing structural distortions may be aggravated. Hence, government needs to take a proactive role by initiating domestic reforms and creating an enabling environment so that the benefits of liberalization do ensue and any adverse effects are mitigated.

Hospitals covered by the survey:

1. Indraprastha Apollo, New Delhi
2. Max Health Care, New Delhi
3. Fortis a/New Delhi
4. Escorts Health Care a/New Delhi
5. Woodlands, Kolkata
6. Anandlok Hospital, Kolkata
7. Jitendra Narayan Ray Sishu Seva Bhavan and General Hospital, Kolkata
8. Apollo Gleneagles a/Kolkata
9. Sarvodaya Hospital, Bangalore
10. Suguna Ramaiah Hospital Pvt. Ltd., Bangalore
11. Chinmaya Mission Hospital, Bangalore
12. Columbia Asia Hospital Pvt. Ltd., Bangalore
13. Wockhardt Hospitals a/Bangalore
14. Manipal Hospitals a/Bangalore
15. Narayana Hrudayalaya, Bangalore
16. CSI Kalyani General Hospital, Chennai
17. KHM Hospitals, Chennai

18. Kumaran Hospitals (P) Ltd., Chennai
19. Apollo Hospitals a/Chennai
20. P.D. Hinduja National Hospital and Medical Research Centre, Mumbai
21. Joy Hospital, Mumbai
22. Sir H.N. Hospital and Research Centre, Mumbai
23. Sowmya Hospital, Hyderabad
24. Pacific Medical Centre, Hyderabad
25. St. Theresa's Hospital, Hyderabad

Proposed/Newly Established Medical City Projects

- **Medicity, Gurgaon**
  Dr. Naresh Trehan's Medicity, a Rs. 1,200 crores project in Gurgaon, spread over 43 acres will consist of a 1,600 bed hospital. The project is modeled along the lines of the Mayo Clinic.
- **Fortis Medicity, Gurgaon**
  It is worth an investment of over Rs. 1,200 crores. It will have two campuses. The hospital campus will contain a high-end, multi and superspecialty hospital and research centre.
- **Fortis Medicity, Lucknow**
  This project is worth an investment of between Rs. 500 crores to Rs. 800 crores and is spread over 52 acres. It will include an 800-bed hospital, a medical college offering undergraduate, postgraduate, and postdoctoral courses, a dental college, nursing college, a college of physical medicine and rehabilitation, and a college of allied medical science.
- **Narayan Health City, Bangalore**
  This 5,000-bed health city will be spread over 35 acres with a project cost of Rs. 2,000 crores. It will consist of 10 hospitals, which will come up over several phases.

Other sources of foreign investment in hospitals

There are various other forms of foreign funding, which are being used by hospitals in India to either expand their operations or to set-up new operations.

Pattern of financing in major corporate hospitals

It is clear that there is scope for expansion in FDI as well as private equity funding, especially in larger hospitals. However, if one looks at the current pattern of financing, both domestic and foreign, for some of the major corporate hospitals in India, one finds that these constitute a relatively small share. It is domestic financing that predominates, in particular domestic long-term bank borrowings.

Over half of the finances are obtained through long-term bank loans.

From the other categories of financing the share of foreign sources is not readily apparent, but roughly less than 20 percent could be funded through external sources. This corroborates the earlier discussion that although the sector has a lot of potential, to date, the role of foreign investment remains limited.

Human resources; availability and quality issues

Another major operating challenge is human resources at all levels-doctors, nurses, paramedics, front and back end support staff, managers, and administrators. This gap is both in terms of quantity and quality. As a result, the cost of talent is rising by some 20 percent per year and is even higher at around 50 to 60 percent at the junior and middle levels. Poaching and attrition problems are rampant. There is a dearth of qualified and trained technicians who can operate sophisticated health care equipments. One reason, why FDI in health care may not be happening is because of the dearth of qualified manpower in the country, both for doctors and paramedics. Ironically, as experts commented, while the Medical Council has not permitted corporate hospitals to set-up training facilities, which would benefit them and the health care sector at large, it has permitted a plethora of substandard private medical colleges, which have political patronage and make money through huge capitation fees. Many of these private institutes lack basic faculty, equipment, and infrastructure and are unable to provide relevant and quality training. It was also suggested that the constraints on the supply of trainers and faculty could be alleviated if more flexibility were provided to professionals in this sector. It is also noted that opening up the higher education sector to FDI would alleviate the manpower constraint in the health care sector as much of the resulting investment is expected to flow into medical education.

Some private hospitals are tying up with overseas institutions like medical schools in the UAE for training their staff e.g. Narayana Hrudalaya has a tie up with Hyatt College of Technology and with Queen Mary's Medical School for training. It has also tied up with the University of Ohio to train nurses and with University of Minnesota for temporary registration of its doctors to train there.

There are several ways in which liberalization of health insurance and the entry of foreign as well as domestic health insurance companies could help. First is by increasing accountability, transparency, and efficiency in health care delivery e.g. accreditation. The second is by increasing the paying consumer-base and thus making health care affordable to a larger percentage of the population. It was felt that without a critical mass of insured patients, at around 10-20% of the population, foreign players would not enter the Indian hospital market in a big way. The low share of insured patients is seen as one of the main reasons that health care services have not grown as much as they could in India. Health care is expensive and needs to be made more affordable. Health insurance can provide a reliable payer source.

Health has never been seen as a core sector so far. The government has given little emphasis on organized health care. It has not been seen as a priority from the privatization perspective and so its influence remains peripheral.

What would be required for foreign investors to show more interest is a roadmap of where the government sees health care from a domestic and international perspective, clarity on the government's position on urban, rural, and semi-urban health care, what is desired from foreign participation, and how the government will support the sector. Greater transparency and predictability in the policy environment is required if the existing liberal FDI regulations are to elicit greater foreign participation in this sector.

Impact of foreign investment in hospitals

Some 800,000 beds are required over the next five years to raise our infrastructure status in health care to an acceptable level and for this Greenfield investments are essential. The latter is not possible with domestic resources alone. There is an estimated gap of $10-15 billion, which foreign investment can provide to double existing infrastructure. Investments are also needed beyond the metros to expand access to health care. There are many positive implications of foreign investment in hospitals. In addition to helping increase physical capacity in the health care sector, such as increasing the number of hospital beds, diagnostic facilities, and increasing the supply of specialty and superspecialty centers, foreign investment can also help in raising the standards and quality of health care, in upgrading technology, and in creating employment opportunities, with potential benefits to the health sector and the economy at large.

The presence of foreign investors in the health care sector could also provide a boost to medical tourism and help India in achieving its goal of establishing itself as a medical tourism hub in the region. There are also spill over benefits in other areas, such as the growth of the health insurance sector, clinical trials and other health services outsourcing, and the pharmaceutical market.

The survey results indicate resource pull effects from the non-foreign-funded to the foreign funded segment. If one were to take this analysis further and also consider public sector hospitals, then one can make the argument that internal brain drain is likely from the public sector to the private sector in general, and especially towards the foreign funded and large corporate hospitals, given the much lower wages and poor working conditions in the public sector. Overall it appears that foreign funded hospitals may be better placed at retaining and attracting good quality medical personnel. Discussions also made it clear that the these hospitals also rely on their investments in state of the art equipment and the good work environment and infrastructure as an important means of attracting and retaining good personnel. Several of the respondents from such hospitals noted that they have efficient computerized systems for maintaining patients' records, for pay rolls, billings, and inventory management, which make the work environment much more professional and streamlined. It appears that the foreign funded hospitals tend to be more expensive than the non-foreign-funded hospitals. While the cost for EMG in foreign funded hospitals is around Rs. 1,500, for non-foreign-funded hospitals the cost is half this amount at around Rs. 750. In the case of endoscopy, the cost in foreign funded hospitals varies from Rs. 4,000 to over Rs. 9,000 while that in non foreign funded institutions it ranges from less than Rs. 1,000 in several of the responding hospitals to as much as Rs. 7,000 and Rs. 9,000 in others. If one removes the very low cost hospitals the average cost in the non foreign funded category is around Rs. 5,000, still lower than that in foreign funded hospitals at around Rs.7,000. For dialysis, the cost in foreign funded hospitals is around Rs. 2,500 compared to an average cost of around Rs. 1,000 for the reporting non-foreign-funded hospitals.

The picture is different, however, if one examines costs for cardio-thoracic surgery. Here, foreign funded hospitals reported a cost of around Rs. 1.1 lakh to Rs. 1.25 lakhs compared to a range of Rs. 1.2 lakhs to over Rs. 1.6 lakhs in the case of non-foreign funded hospitals.

However, when compared to small and medium size establishments, the general view is that most medical procedures and services are likely to be 15-30 percent costlier in the larger corporate hospitals, with some variability within this range depending on the procedure concerned and the kind of equipment involved.

Public-private partnership

Another way in which the growth of the private hospitals could benefit society is through public-private partnership. Seven of the hospitals, mainly the ones with foreign funding, covered in this sample noted that they have some form of PPP.

One form of PPP is the reserving of beds and procedures for below poverty line patients. One major corporate hospital noted that it provides 15 percent of its beds and procedures free to the state government for BPL patients. It also provides a 15 percent discount on the total bill for all state government employees. A second area of PPP is in medical education and training. A few of the major corporate hospitals noted that they provide training to students of a state medical college in particular programmes such as cardiology. But this is seen as an untapped area for collaboration. A third form of PPP was between private and state run hospitals, wherein the former is allowed to operate a public hospital under contract and take care of poor people. This was seen as one of the most promising areas for partnership as many state governments are interested in collaborating with reputed private sector hospitals. The government hospitals are too focused on quantity with no regard to quality and this is why even the poor do not go to these hospitals.

Some of the large hospitals covered in this study indicated that they have partnerships with state Governments e g Wockhardt Gujarat. There is a subsidized rate for the beneficiaries while private patients pay at their capacity, thus providing a mechanism for cross subsidization. In terms of helping the poor, cross subsidy mechanisms rather than quantitative targets were considered a better model for such partnerships.

It was stated that the supply chain needs to be sorted out and the entire experience made more attractive, to create a positive image and to further develop the infrastructure for medical tourism. Employment and foreign exchange can be generated from medical value travel, which is of course beneficial to any country. But medical value travel will never constitute a significant percentage of all customers in Indian hospitals. Greater foreign investor presence in hospitals, however much limited, is expected to help expand medical value travel to India by enabling tie ups with foreign health insurance providers to develop customized insurance products for target groups overseas to undertake elective surgeries in India and follow ups abroad, by facilitating tie ups with medical schools, and through greater investment in tele-diagnostic and other tele-health facilities. When questioned about the likely impact on availability of beds for domestic patients, most respondents noted that there is unlikely to be any major squeezing out of lower paying segments as the number of medical value travelers is never expected to be large, though some respondents did note that such an impact could arise. It was argued that medical value travel could be used to generate resources for investments in the health care system as hospitals today are charging medical value travelers at higher rates. Higher fees can be used to cross subsidize domestic consumers.

Apollo Gleneagles has a relationship with Johns Hopkins for research and training and for second opinions but there is no collaboration in terms of investment in any facilities. Joint venture type of approach could potentially yield more benefits.

Positive implications

Some of the areas of positive impact that were highlighted are:

- Infrastructure development,
- Upgrading and investment in technology,
- Increased availability of high end and niche procedures,
- Improved systems and processes,
- Integration of information technology in health care delivery,
- Improved standards and focus on accreditation,
- Improved work environment,
- Increased employment opportunities at all levels,
- Greater emphasis on medical research and training,
- Greater opportunities for knowledge transfer due to tie ups with overseas hospitals and collaborative ventures,
- Spillover in related areas such as diagnostics, labs, and medical

equipment supply and manufacturing, outsourcing (clinical trials, billings, insurance processing), medical value travel, and
- Increased insurance penetration

Infrastructure, technology, and standards were the most commonly cited areas of impact. Several respondents noted that foreign investment would augment resources available for investing in new technologies and that foreign direct investment, joint ventures, and tie ups in particular would bring in new technologies. The latter would include more effective and new ways of management, better governance, increased accountability through audits of medical practices, better methods of health care delivery, which would improve efficiency. More hospitals would turn towards international accreditation. It was also noted that the process of accreditation would reduce violations in medical ethics, such as reducing unnecessary tests and procedures, as there would be greater accountability. The offshoot of such improvements in standards and practices would be shorter hospital stay, lower infection rates, benefiting both patients and doctors. There would also be a demonstration effect on other hospitals with many more getting accredited and registering for NABH/NABL certification.

Some points were also made about the likely evolution of the health care delivery system. Several respondents noted that greater corporatization and inflow of FDI in the hospitals segment would also enable more healthy competition among the big corporate players and could encourage consolidation and economies of scale in the sector, which would benefit consumers potentially lowering costs and improving the affordability of quality health care in the country. Expanded volumes would also enable the corporate players to cross subsidize poor patients more effectively, to do more outreach and extension services, and even establishes themselves in second tier cities and towns. It was also pointed out that through such extension services and set-ups outside major metros, corporate hospitals would be able to make available their equipment and thus expand accessibility of health care.

Some respondents also noted that there would be increased possibilities for partnership arrangements between government medical institutions and private players through management contracts. In their view, the growth of corporate hospitals and the benefits that would accrue from foreign investment for such hospitals in terms of improved practices, better governance, and accountability, would also get transferred to the public sector institutions through such public private partnership arrangements. The view was that the paradigm of doing health care would be positively affected across all kinds of players due to improved standards, greater quality consciousness among health care players, and a greater awareness among consumers of what quality and service mean.

Foreign funding in private hospitals was also seen as promoting opportunities in other areas of the health care sector. One such area was clinical trials outsourcing, which many respondents felt was a growth area that had yet to be tapped. The emergence of major corporate hospitals with foreign funding was perceived to give a boost to this area as pharmaceutical companies would be more comfortable with carrying out clinical tests in such hospitals given their superior patient record and delivery systems. Positive implications are also perceived for research and development and education, as corporate hospitals are expected to invest in these areas. The example of Apollo, which is currently investing in medical, nursing and paramedical education and training as well as in health administration, was cited. Foreign funded hospitals are expected to invest more in continuing medical education through tie-ups with overseas institutions or short-term transfer of personnel. The growth of such hospitals is also expected to spur local manufacturing of medical devices and products, through tie-ups and licensing arrangements, which would ultimately benefit the sector by lowering costs of such inputs.

Negative Impact

The main areas of negative impacted highlighted in the discussions include:

- Higher costs of medical care,
- Unnecessary tests and procedures violating medical ethics,
- Squeezing out of the poor from the market to low quality players,
- Diversion of resources towards curative and high end technology and procedures and away from preventive and chronic ailments and needs of the local population,
- Greater competition for manpower, higher manpower costs, attrition and poaching,
- Pull on resources from smaller players in the private sector and from public sector hospitals,
- Greater divide between the public and private sector in terms of availability and quality of health care and wages,
- Crowding out of local patients for high value foreign patients, and
- Tilting of health care delivery towards higher paying private segments.

Internal brain drain that could arise with the expansion of foreign investment in hospitals and the emergence of larger corporate hospitals. As one practitioner in a public sector hospital noted, it would become harder for the public sector to retain doctors as well as teachers in their affiliated medical colleges, aggravating the already existing trend of doctors moving out of government hospitals and from training towards private practice and the e-flux of paramedics and nurses. In turn, future specialists coming from the public sector would be poorly qualified, which would further affect the quality of training and service available in public sector institutions. The shortage of medical educators in specific domains such as neurology, which are high paying, was pointed out.

Foreign investment would put further pressure on wages and salaries of medical personnel, which are already increasing rapidly at all levels. Thus, expansion of scale with uniform quality would become difficult for large players, for both foreign funded and non-foreign-funded hospitals.

Affordability depends on the socio-economic strata of patients. Low strata people will have to go to government hospitals and have to take the service they get. If it's something serious, they have to sell their land and get money for treatment. The priorities of middle-income people are changing and some are taking medical insurance. Then basic health care can be improved. If some eventuality comes in their lives, they can at least fall back on this insurance. Private hospitals are not affordable for middle class people unless the company pays for it.

Tilt towards Rich

Foreign funded hospitals are perceived to be skewed towards rich people as they would never be in reach of the common man and this is seen to be made worse by the lack of affordable health packages. Foreign investment would possibly aggravate the already existing divide between those who can and those who cannot afford health care. The root problem is the lack of affordable health insurance schemes, which makes the poorer segments more vulnerable to higher costs of health care. Thus the solution does not lie with regulations pertaining to foreign investment *per se* but with the introduction of innovative and affordable health insurance packages, which could include micro insurance and community-based insurance packages which are perhaps managed by community health insurance trusts with government support. Part of the solution may also lie in incentivizing and enabling corporate players to do go beyond metros and to do outreach and extension activities serving a wider section of society. It was also suggested by many that expanded scale and presence of higher paying segments in corporate and foreign funded hospitals could be used to cross-subsidize poorer segments and thus expand the accessibility of health care delivery to all.

Large corporate and foreign funded hospitals are likely to be impersonal and would not provide the personalized care available at smaller establishments. Overall, while there were differing views on the likely implications for the structure of health care delivery and on the possible arrangements that could emerge between the smaller and the larger players, the prevailing view was that poor quality and substandard players are likely to be weeded out with greater foreign investment in hospitals.

The Insight

- Such hospitals are likely to focus on more advanced procedures and specialty areas.

- They are more likely to focus on curative and intervention oriented treatment than on preventive and long-term kind of treatment.
- They are likely to employ a higher ratio of technology to personnel in their health care delivery and thus involve a substitution of human resources with technology and equipment.
- They are likely to invest much more in medical equipment and devices and also in specialized and experienced medical personnel, thus involving a focus on high-end human resources and high-end technology.
- Such hospitals tend to have better systems and processes and usage of IT, which creates a more efficient and professional work environment.
- Foreign funded hospitals pay higher rates to staff at all levels and particularly to senior medical personnel.
- They are more likely to attract overseas doctors and specialists than other hospitals.
- They are more likely to be accredited domestically and/or internationally.
- Their costs are likely to be comparable to or slightly higher than those of non-foreign funded large hospitals.
- Their costs will tend to be higher than for small and medium size nursing homes and hospitals but this is mainly due to greater capital intensity and focus on quality systems and processes and focus on hygiene.
- There could be positive externalities in other areas of the health care sector and some of these could further drive foreign investment in hospitals.
- Foreign funded hospitals could draw away medical personnel at all levels from other hospitals and could adversely impact the quality of medical manpower available to competing institutions.
- There is likely to be closure of substandard institutions, some consolidation of the hospital segment, and new kinds of arrangements could emerge between larger and smaller players as the health care sector evolves.
- There could be greater segmentation between the public and private sector with resource flows towards the latter, greater wage disparity, unless innovative arrangements emerge between the two segments and reforms are undertaken in the public sector hospitals. While there are clearly concerns about the equity, affordability, and market segmentation implications of growing foreign investor presence in India's hospital segment, the root cause lies in structural problems that are already present in the health care sector. Foreign investment and greater corporate presence in hospitals could aggravate such structural problems.

UK's Bupa Health Insurance enters India: question answers

What has encouraged Max Bupa to make a foray in this section?

Health insurance in India—as grown over 35 % per year for the past few years and is set to continue. India has a population of over 1.13 billion and by 2025 it is going to have a middle class of about 600 millions. This is where we see huge demand as 70 per cent of the health care spends is private and 90 per cent of that spend is not insured, it's paid for out of pocket. Most of the existing health policies do not cover full-day care benefits, dental services, vision services, preventative care like free health check-ups, home health services or long-term care, and rarely outpatient services or international cover; which is the need of some consumer segments today.

Most Indians buy health insurance to get tax advantage and as a saving. Do you think this attitude would be a hindrance for your product?

Then we will offer more comprehensive products to ensure that those savings are better protected. However, a health insurance product deals with aspects of people's health and requires detailed explanation compared to other financial products. Hence, we will enable consumers make an informed decision. Secondly, we will assure the quality of the doctors and the hospitals that are on our network. Our network will be selective, but will cover all the main hospitals that a person like you, for instance, would visit. And we will handle all the claims ourselves, so that we can provide a superior service.

How does Bupa's experience in the UK help in the Indian sub-continent?

Max Bupa Health Insurance Company Limited brings Bupa's 60 years of global expertise to India, as well as local market knowledge in insurance and health care by Max India. Bupa is not just an insurance company. It is a health and care company. For instance, we run over 300 homes for the elderly in the UK. We coach people on health in the US. The portal, bupa-healthdialog.co.uk, builds on the knowledge that Bupa has accumulated. Max Bupa Health Insurance Company Limited plans to use some of this expertise in India to develop better services for the Indian consumer.

How difficult was it to design the product when not enough data is available on disease and usage patterns of different socio-economic segments?

It poses a challenge for innovations in product development. To overcome these, we have spent considerable time in research in gaining consumer insights and have developed our products and services based on these.

What would be the uniqueness of your product portfolio?

We would focus on a superior customer experience and the delivery of promise at the moment of truth. Max Bupa Health Insurance Company Limited's vision is to become health care partners and provide its customers expertise for life. For instance, one of the value adds Max Bupa Health Insurance Company Limited intends to offer is under the maternity offer where the new born baby of the insured will automatically be covered for insurance. We will also offer vaccinations as per the World Health Organization recommendations. In India, we will be focusing on wellness and work with our customers in helping them lead healthier lives. We may in future offer primary, secondary and dental cover. Even homeopathic treatment may be covered.

How different would be the Indian product than what is available in the West?

The products available in the Indian market have been designed keeping in mind the need of the Indian consumers. The TNS research has uncovered some interesting facets. Firstly, most people purchase health insurance as a reactive measure to deteriorating health and not proactively during good health not trust that their claims will be processed in time, and without follow-up. Thirdly, value perceptions of health insurance further get eroded due to the fact that they do not see any returns in comparison to life insurance policies—as life insurance sells as an investment product more than as a risk mitigation product. Additionally, it found that there is a need for a high quality health insurance product in the market, which consumers can trust to deliver when the need arises and that health insurance companies can also play a role in helping customers manage their health more proactively.

With the experience in offering specialized health insurance expertise globally, we are confident that we can help raise the standard of health insurance in India when we launch through our products.

What additional benefits would you provide to the customers?

We believe that our success will depend on how happy our customers are. Thus, more transparency in the initial stages means better customer satisfaction at the time of claim reimbursements. It is important that the customer understands what is covered and what is not covered and for what he is paying his premiums. We believe in building relations with our customers that go beyond transactions and this is only possible when we are transparent with them.

Who is your target clientele and why?

The products will be all across the spectrums, the premiums would be ranging from Rs. 3,000 to will also have some rural insurance obligations.

In which cities are you planning to enter first?

We are looking forward to start with the six main cities—Delhi, Mumbai, Chennai, Bangaluru, Hyderabad and Pune. But we also plan to expand our network over 20 cities in the coming three years.

Some health insurance companies have witnessed annual growth of 200-300 per cent. What is your target growth plan?

We are looking to grow profitably in this market.

What is your strategy of selling the product?

We will offer our customer comprehensive family-based products. Our USP is the expertise in delivery of high quality health insurance services to our customers. We train our people for responsible, needs based selling and follow an extensive training process. We will service our customers directly and offer wellness benefits each year that they renew the policy. We are currently also building our network of relationships with quality hospitals for appropriate service.

Why is that you wont tie-up with a TPA? Would not that prolong the time of claims settlement?

We observed that the insurance companies are faceless and the TPA is the one dealing with the customer. We want to own the customer, to build health and wellness around the family. Since most product features can be replicated quite easily the differentiator will have to be service and that can only be given through TPA.

Sources

Business Standard, Weekend Section, July 28/29, 2007, p. I.

CMIE, Prowess database.

CRISIL Research, Annual Review: Hospitals, Industry Information Service, Mumbai, February 2007.

Ernst and Young (2007) and CRISIL Research (Feb 2007).

Ernst and Young and FICCI, Opportunities in Health Care : Destination India, New Delhi, 2007.

Ernst and Young and India Brand Equity Foundation, Report on Health Care, 2004 and 2005.

Express Health Care, Opportunities Galore, 2004.

Government of India, Report of the National Commission on Macroeconomics and Health, Ministry of Health and Family Welfare, New Delhi, 2005.

http://www.expresshealth caremgmt.com/200609/bangalorediscovered01.shtml (accessed on September 1, 2009).

IBEF, www.ibef.org.

International Finance Corporation, conference presentation, New Delhi, 2007.

Technopak, "Health Care Outlook", *Quarterly Report*, Vol. 1, February 2007.

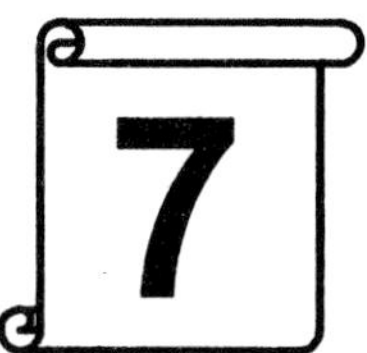

Health Tourism on the Rise in Indian Medical Cities

India's growth story as a medical tourism hub is a relatively newer one. With significant cost advantages, availability of quality medical treatment with the most-advanced medical technology coupled with India's well-known tourist destinations and rich cultural heritage, medical tourism does provide a motive sufficient enough to allure those foreign patients who either want to avoid the long waiting list for medical treatment in the West or, in absence of any health insurance coverage, seek lower cost treatment. India's strength in advanced and life saving health care such as organ transplants, cardio-vascular surgery, etc. as well as in alternative systems of medicine (i.e. ayurveda, naturopathy, etc.) offer significant competitive advantages. Cashing in this opportunity, The National Health Policy 2002 declared that treatment of foreign patients is legally an "export" and deemed "eligible for all fiscal incentives extended to export earnings". Besides, a new category of visa, "Medical Visa" has been introduced by Ministry of Home Affairs, Govt. of India. On the other hand, setting up of Bio-Technology Parks, grant of SEZ status to them, coming up Medicities, entry of private players in health insurance in India along with Indian hospitals looking for international accreditation glitter further hopes of accelerated medical tourism, a growth engine for foreign exchange earnings. However, the poor infrastructure of the country, shabby streets, pity state of our public hospitals shakes our confidence, despairs for this much hype of medical tourism and calls for serious attention wherein much more efforts are needed. Definitely, public-private partnership is one way ahead which can revamp public hospitals and bring them at par with private hospitals. Further, there is still no Medical Tourism Policy either formulated by the Central or any of the State Governments. As the medical tourism industry is growing exponentially, government and the private players need to join hands in order to act as a catalyst to build infrastructure for hospitals, create specialty tourist packages to include medical treatment, promote accreditation and standardization, enable access and tie-ups with insurance companies, provide state of art facilities and improve quality of in-patient care and service to meet the requirements of foreign patients and to attain sustainable competitive advantage.

Health tourism industry is one of the world's largest industries

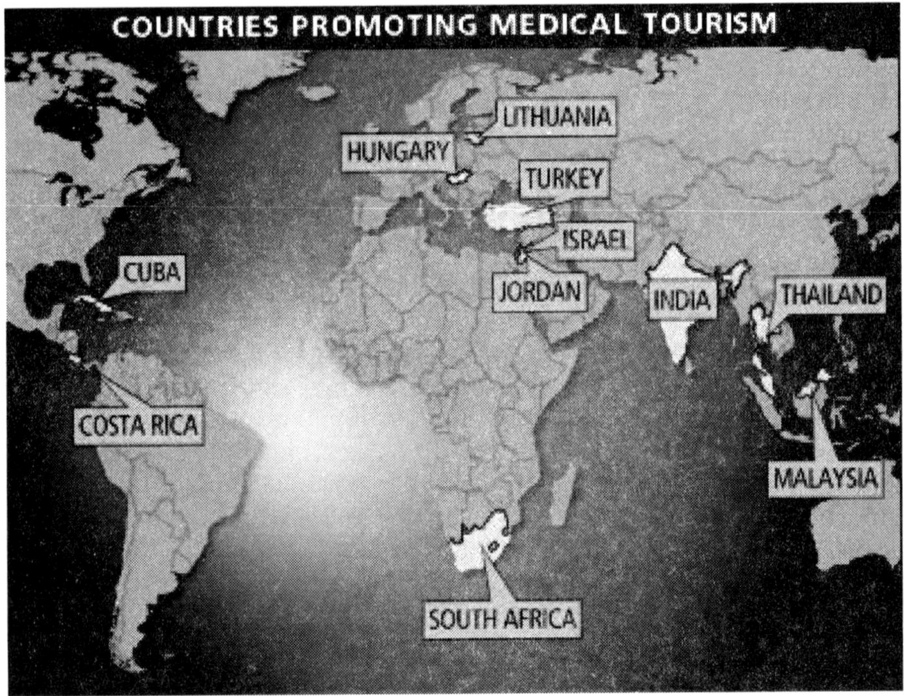

With global revenues of approximately US$ 20 Billion (2005), the medical tourism industry is one of the world's largest industries. India's cost effective treatment makes it an important player in this industry. One of the optimistic outlook in this context is provided by a report entitled, "Health care in India: The Road Ahead", produced by the Confederation of Indian Industry and McKinsey and Co. in 2002. According to it, the medical tourism industry in India is growing at 25-30% annually, contribute upto Rs. 10,000 crore additional revenue to upmarket tertiary hospitals and will account for 3 to 5 per cent of the total health care delivery market and set to become $2 billion by 2012. "A patient opting for medical tourism not only gets the best medical treatment the Indian doctors have to offer, but also as a post-treatment fare, he or she gets to see the best of India's destinations", said Ms Leena Nandan, Joint Secretary, Tourism. Probably realizing this as a big potential, major corporate such as the Tatas, Fortis,

Max, Wockhardt, Piramal, and the Escorts group have made significant investments in setting up modern hospitals in major cities. Many have also designed special packages for patients, including airport pick-ups, visa assistance as well as boarding and lodging. Dr. Prathap C. Reddy, Chairman, Apollo Hospitals Quips, "One way is to get valuable foreign exchange through medical tourism, giving the patient the best of the west and the east; cardiac or neuro surgery with results comparable to the best in the west, while also exposing him to the natural beauty of our country."

US Citizen visits India on health tourism

When James Michael, 35, began trawling the Internet for an affordable option to US health care, the prompt response from an Indian medical city in Bangalore to his enquiries about cervical disc replacement surgery brought him to the hospital recently. Thousands of foreigners are choosing Indian hospitals for complex procedures, not just dental or cosmetic work as was the case when medical tourism started. "Today, India is getting travelers from around 35 countries as against mainly from neighbouring countries and West Asia five years ago," says one CEO. Managing Director, Apollo Hospitals, an early starter in medical tourism, says that, five years ago, 80 per cent of the 'foreign' patients came from South Asia. "Today, it is down to 30 per cent with more patients coming in from a wide range of countries," says Reddy. Reddy says 300,000-odd medical tourists visited India last year, of which more than half are estimated to have headed into wellness centers promoted by locations like Kerala. But there is a clear trend among the rest towards tertiary care. The cost differential is a major attraction. A cardiac bypass procedure, for instance, would cost around $8,500 in India, including stay for one companion in a single room. The US cost: around $100,000. On an average, treatment costs here are 10-20 per cent of US levels.

Health cities draw many tourists

Fortis alone treats close to 2,000 American patients a year now between its Mumbai and Bangalore hospitals, or ten times the Americans it handled in 2005. Both Fortis hospitals are accredited to the JCI or the Joint Commission International, a non-profit US body that sets standards. Health care Global, a Bangalore-based cancer says, "Today, six per cent of our total patients come from abroad and this number is growing at 20 per cent per annum with patients mainly from Africa, Bangladesh, West Asia, Canada and some European countries like Norway and The Netherlands," says Dr B.S. Ajai Kumar, Chairman and CEO, Health Care Global. That a patient with a serious health problem is willing to take a 24-hour flight for treatment indicates a coming of age for the sector, which has been investing in facilities and techniques. Dr G.S. Rao, Managing Director, Yashoda Group of Hospitals, which has units in Hyderabad and Secunderabad and is the first in South Asia to offer rapid arc radiation therapy, cites another factor attracting long distance patients. "We have seen a perceptible increase in patient's inflows with the new international airport coming up in Hyderabad," he says.

The health tourism revenues are rising slowly

Medical value travel is worth $700 million now. "India accounts for no more than 1.2 per cent of the global market by value," says M. Muralidharan Nair, Partner, Business Advisory Services Practice, Ernst and Young (E&Y). Despite the growth potential, he says, the market size in 2012 will be much below $1.5-2.2 billion projected by some studies. The number of international patients coming to India has grown at more than 24 per cent each year since 2002 and over half a million are expected to have visited by the end of 2009. "Medical tourism has transitioned from a cottage industry to an acceptable alternative for elective care that's safe and cost-effective. (See Appendix 'Globalization and Medical Tourism', attached to this chapter).

Fortis group is spreading its wings, but....

Fortis, Apollo and Health Care Global are setting up outposts abroad to catch the tide. Recently, Fortis acquired a strategic stake in Singapore based Parkway Holdings. Malvinder Mohan Singh, Fortis Chairman, told BT: "Singapore is an international medical hub and international patients are an important component for Parkway. Now we could attract patients into our network to service them out of Singapore, Malaysia (where Parkway also has a strong presence) and India."

If an American tourist in India on vacation or work has a heart attack and undergoes an emergency procedure, the tourist's insurer picks up the tab. But the same insurer will not pay for elective surgery here. Then, India has very few JCI-accredited hospitals; just over a dozen. India also needs a deeper pool of highly-skilled manpower attuned to diverse cultures. There is more to it than just providing an American with an Internet connection, to an European a diet brief or an Arab a prayer room.

Attracting the best

- India gets patients from around 35 countries today; five years ago, most were from neighbouring countries and West Asia.
- Foreign patients now taking 24-hour flights to India to seek treatment for life-threatening conditions. Earlier, it was mostly for cosmetic surgery.
- Health care players are investing in the latest technologies, conducting beating heart surgeries and using robotics.
- Some international health care insurance entities have started offering options to cover elective procedures in India.

But the potential for getting more patients from the West is huge: E&Y points out that over half the medical tourists now still are from countries such as Bangladesh, Pakistan and Nigeria, and India has been able to attract only 12 per cent of the medical travelers from the US, UK and West Asia, who account for a quarter of global medical travelers.

How to grow in health tourism

- Speedier grant of medical visa, even visa on arrival.
- Better linkages between health care and tourism.
- Better airports and roads, not just in pockets but at all locations. More hospitals accredited to the JCI.

Setting up of Medical cities in Public-Private Partnership is required to provide quality services to attract potential health care seekers from various countries. Promotion of health care tourism would result in development of associated sectors, such as medical equipment manufacturing, tele-medicine, medical diagnostics, outsourcing of hospital administration and health insurance. There are also opportunities in the infrastructure sectors, due to higher demand for travel (airlines, road/rail transport, hotels, hospitals) and communication (telephone, internet). Newer models of campaigning and promotions provide business opportunities for media and mass-communication segments. With such greater level of opportunities, financial institutions can play an increased role in setting up medical cities in India and abroad. While reflecting upon health care tourism, there are two things to keep in mind. One is that good health is the foundation of any activity, enjoyment and worthwhile living. The second is that a wealth of any country can be judged by several indicators. Of this, health of its citizenry is one of the most critical ones.

Next big success story after software

The Medical Tourism Industry in India is poised to be the next big success story after software. According to a Mckinsey-CII study the market size is estimated to be Rs. 5000-10000 crores by 2012. The key competitive advantages of India in medical tourism stem from the following: low cost advantage, strong reputation in the advanced health care segment (cardiovascular surgery, organ transplants, eye surgery) and the diversity of tourist destinations available in the country. The key concerns facing the industry include: absence of government initiative, lack of a coordinated effort to promote the industry, no accreditation mechanism for hospitals and the lack of uniform pricing policies and standards across hospitals. To realize the industry's full potential, a coordinated effort from the various players—government, private players and the associated sectors is very essential. The government should help in instituting an accreditation mechanism and device policies to facilitate private investment in the sector. An apex body should be formed for the industry in the lines of NASSCOM1 and should focus on building the Indian Brand across the world and promote inter-sectoral co-operation. The private sector for its part, should invest more in infrastructure, horizontally integrate into related services and build joint ventures and alliances with overseas health institutions and insurance players. Finally establishment of MEDICITIES as a public-private partnership model can also give a major fillip to India's quest for success in medical tourism (Gowri Shankar Nagarajan, IIM-B) Medical Tourism refers to movement of consumers to the country providing the service for diagnosis and treatment. During the past few years, the number of people going out of their home country to consume health services has significantly increased. The size of this market is estimated to be $40 billion based on a Saudi Report in 2000. During the past four years, the market grew at a whopping rate of 20-30% and is expected to grow further. Considering this growth the current market size is estimated to be $100 billion. Health Tourism industry offers tremendous potential for the developing countries because of their low-cost advantage. The advantages of medical tourism include improvement in export earnings and health care infrastructure. No doubt, a lot of countries—India, Thailand, Malaysia, Singapore, South Africa, Cuba, Jordan and Lithuania are fighting for a share of the market. In order to realize the full potential of the industry, it is imperative for these countries to develop a strategic plan for coordinating various industry players—the medical practitioners, private hospitals, policy-makers, hotels, transportation services and tour operators.

First World Service at Third World Cost

The main reason for India's emergence as a preferred destination is the inherent advantage of its health care industry. Today Indian health care is perceived to be on par with global standards. Some of the top Indian hospitals and doctors have strong international reputation. But the most important factor that drives medical tourism to India is its low cost advantage. Majority of foreign patients visit India primarily to avail of "First World Service at Third World Cost". India has significant cost advantages in several health procedures making it a preferred destination.

The Case of Cuba

Cuba is one of the earliest successes in medical tourism industry. The country successfully tapped the demand for medical tourism from Latin-American countries. Cuba's success can be attributed to the strategic push provided by government through State-Owned Companies. The government promoted private investment in health care to increase the supply of high quality and specialized health care. Health care was accorded infrastructure status and laws enacted to increase participation of private entrepreneurs. One example is allowing treatment for skin diseases using human placenta that was banned elsewhere.

The government centralized promotion of health services abroad by entrusting the responsibility to SERVIMED—a newly formed public company. SERVIMED coordinated with tour operators and travel agencies to develop health packages. The package included travel in Cuba's national airline, 24 hours assistance, and companion personnel for the patient, repatriation, and post-surgery controls. To support efficient marketing, SERVIMED also opened offices in Argentina, Brazil, Chile, Mexico, and Venezuela. The two-pronged strategy successfully resulted in 30,000 patients visiting Cuba in 1997 for treatment earning US$ 30 million foreign exchange.

The Case of Thailand

A more recent success story is that of Thailand. Thailand is one of the world's leading health care destinations with a forecast of 1 million overseas patients for the current year. The Thai government realized early the need for coordination across various sectors to realize the industry's potential. Hence it developed a common vision, strategic direction, joint-strategy and shared objectives for various sectors in order to facilitate better coordination between the concerned players—the Ministries of Health, Tourism, Foreign Affairs and other bodies like Thai Airways, and Tourism Authority of Thailand.

The Tourism Authority of Thailand (TAT) has played a stellar role in providing integrated marketing Thai tourism abroad. TAT has more than 18 offices worldwide and has won several international credits for developing excellent marketing campaigns targeted at tourists. TAT has so far been extremely successful in marketing Thai health services also. Thailand heavily focuses on hospitality to provide superior consumer experience and building brand equity. For example, the Bumrungrad Hospital in Bangkok provides hospitality services that include: pick up from Airport, language interpreters for 18 languages and an in-house Starbucks and McDonalds to cater to tourists from U.S and U.K.

Thailand built a strong health infrastructure during the economic boom by encouraging private and public participation. In 1996 alone Thailand spent a whopping 7% of GDP on health care. Priority was also given for Foreign Direct investment in health care sector with Thai Government processing 3000 FDI proposals in just four years.

India—Strategic Thrusts for the Future

The role of Indian Government for success in medical tourism is two-fold: Acting as a Regulator to institute a uniform grading and accreditation system for hospitals to build consumers' trust. Acting as a Facilitator for encouraging private investment in medical infrastructure and policy-making for improving medical tourism.

For facilitating investment the policy recommendations include:

1. Recognize health care as an infrastructure sector, and extend the benefits under sec. 80-IA of the IT Act. Benefits include tax holidays for five years and concessional taxation for subsequent five years.
2. The government should actively promote FDI in health care sector.

3. Conducive fiscal policies—providing low interest rate loans, reducing import/excise duty for medical equipment
4. Facilitating clearances and certification like medical registration number, anti-pollution certificate, etc.

The above measures will kick-start hospital financing, which is struggling now due to capital-intensive and low efficiency nature of health care business.

For facilitating tourism the government should:

1. Reduce hassles in visa process and institute visa-on-arrival for patients.
2. Follow an Open-Sky policy to increase inflow of flights into India.
3. Create Medical Attachés to Indian embassies that promote health services to prospective Indian visitors.

Formation of National Association of Health Tourism (NAHT)

The promotion of medical tourism has so far been very fragmented with initiatives by few states and private hospitals. The earlier discussions clearly underline the need for presence of an apex body that can coordinate the promotion of medical tourism abroad. In the Indian context too, this has been successfully demonstrated in the software industry by NASSCOM. It is therefore essential to form an apex body for health tourism—NAHT. The NAHT should be formed as an association of the private hospitals operating in the industry. The main agenda:

1. *Building the India Brand Abroad*: Classify the target consumer segments based on their attractiveness and position the India Brand based on the three main value propositions—high quality service, value for money and destination diversity. An integrated marketing Communications campaign using print media and road shows should be developed.
2. *Promoting Inter-Sectoral Coordination*: The NAHT should take up the responsibility of aligning the activities of various players—Tourism Department, Transport Operators, Hotel Associations, Escorts personnel, etc.
3. *Information Dissemination using Technology*: NAHT should set-up a portal on medical tourism in India targeted at sharing information and enabling online transactions.
4. *Standardization of Services*: NAHT should also focus on establishing price parity for similar kinds of treatments in various hospitals and ensure the hospitals adhere to high hygiene and quality standards.

The action items for private sector are:

1. *Increased participation in building infrastructure*: To achieve its full potential, it is estimated that India needs an investment of Rs. 100000 to 140000 Crores by 2012. Since the government can afford only a third of the amount, the private sector should play an active role to fill the gap.
2. *Integrate Horizontally*: Private hospitals should also plan to integrate horizontally for providing end-to-end health care solutions to consumers. For example, Apollo multi-specialty hospitals is already planning to set-up spas and alternative mediclinics to attract more foreign tourists.
3. *Joint Ventures/Alliances*: To counter increasing competition, Indian hospitals should tie-up with foreign institutions for assured supply of medical tourists. Specifically tie-ups with capacity constrained hospitals and insurance providers will provide significant competitive advantage.

Value Innovation through medical cities

Another successful example of the software industry is the establishment of Export Oriented Software Technology Parks. This model can be successfully replicated in the medical tourism industry by means of MEDICITIES. Each MEDICITY could be a self-sustained health care hub with super specialty hospitals of international standards, ancillary facilities, research institutions, health resort, rehabilitation centers and residential apartments. This model can be floated through a public-private partnership. The government will provide land and ancillary services and the private players will provide infrastructure and services. From the consumer's point of view, the MEDICITIES will offer superior value at affordable prices. From industry's point of view, this will offer significant competitive advantage for India.

The medical tourism industry offers high potential for India primarily because of its inherent advantages in terms of cost and quality. However, the competition is getting heated up and the success in future will largely be determined by development and implementation of a joint strategy by various players in the industry. The government should step in the role of a regulator and a facilitator of private investment in health care. An apex body for the industry needs to be formed to promote the India brand abroad and aid inter-sectoral coordination. Joint ventures with overseas partners and establishment of MEDICITIES will help in India building a significant advantage and leadership position in the industry.

Bengal emerging hub for health tourism

Even till a few decades after Independence, Kolkata was considered to be in the forefront of the health care sector in the country. It was widely felt that the government sector should take on the onus of providing health care facilities, at least at the primary and secondary levels. Private players could, however, come in at the tertiary level, where specialty health care services were required.

The pressure of a burgeoning population coupled with constraints pertaining to resources and available infrastructure ensured that the government sector was found wanting when it came to delivery of health care services. Gradually, the number of people who came to Kolkata from other eastern States and the North-East for medical treatment started dwindling. Indeed, many people from West Bengal, as also from other neighbouring States, headed for South, West and North India for specialized medical treatment.

However, since the mid-1990s, the trend appears to have been reversed. In the last few years, West Bengal has zeroed in on its strategy for the health care sector. A health policy has been formulated towards this end. Among other things, the policy focuses on the importance of PPP in health care and its delivery mechanism. Several latest health care facilities have been set-up by the private sector even as the State Government has been proactive in encouraging public-private partnerships (PPP) in this sector.

The PPP model pursued by the State Government does not involve only the private sector but also non-government organisations and community-based organisations. In the last 10-15 years, several new health care facilities have come up in the city. While there are many health care institutions and allied service providers, there are a few whose names merit special mention. They include:

CALCUTTA MEDICAL RESEARCH INSTITUTE: Set-up in 1969, the Calcutta Medical Research Institute (CMRI) is the first private hospital to be set-up in the city. Since then, the hospital has emerged as a leading multi-speciality tertiary care hospital with ISO 9001:2000 certification. Its pathology laboratory has received NABL accreditation from the Department of Science and Technology, Government of India.

B.M. BIRLA HEART RESEARCH CENTRE: Set-up in 1989, B.M. Birla Hearth Research Centre (BMBHRC) is eastern India's first, dedicated and superspeciality cardiac care facility. The comprehensive cardiac care facility offers complete cardiac care, with the latest digital cath lab, 64 slice cardiac CT scan, EECP therapy, EP study, gamma camera, lifestyle guidance clinic, etc. It provides critical cardiac care for infants and children.

B.P. PODDAR HOSPITAL and MEDICAL RESEARCH CENTRE: Set-up in the posh New Alipore area, B.P. Poddar Hospital and Medical Research Centre is a 220-bedded, multi-speciality hospital that has established itself as a leading edge health care provider in the city. It also offers a learning environment where medical experts come together to promote research and patient care.

ANANDALOK HOSPITAL: Motivated by the spirit of "Manav Seva", Mr D.K. Saraf began his life's journey with utmost dedication nearly two-and-a-half decades ago. Today, Anandalok Hospital, the health care facility he founded, epitomises quality health care at affordable costs.

BASIL INTERNATIONAL LTD: There is no better antidote than nature cure and natural wellness. And this has been well understood by the Mumbai-based Basil International Ltd, which is setting up two resorts that are aimed at promoting wellness, rejuvenation and good health.

NATIONAL INSURANCE COMPANY LTD: Health care insurance policies offer wide coverage and continuous protection against unforeseen health contingencies. For a small price, health care insurance policies help to bring affordability in health care for one and all. National Insurance Company Ltd offers various schemes that include Mediclaim Insurance, Vidyarthi Mediclaim for students, Parivar Mediclaim for families and Varistha Mediclaim for senior citizens.

An increasing number of hospitals are equipped with world-class facilities and it is a known fact that surgeries in India are almost half as expensive as its western counterparts because of next to nothing import duties. "Health care is another issue in the west," added Raghavan, "Patients are on a never-ending waiting list and going to private doctors is not a feasible option for the common man." In case of medical tourism, tour operators often send their prospective clients' medical records to the concerned hospitals. The doctors go through these records and interact via e-mails or have telephonic conversations to build confidence of the patient. Once the patient is convinced, they arrange for travel either themselves or through a travel agent.

"We take care of the patient's entire journey and hospitals too play an integral part in this process. Some even facilitate pick-ups and stay of the relatives within the hospital premises and if advised by the doctors, we incorporate leisure activities in the itinerary," concluded Raghavan.

West Bengal's first medical city is set to come up on a sprawling 100 acres of land near the Durgapur Steel Plant at Kamalpur mouza in this industrial town.

This medical city or township will also house a private medical college on a 25-acre plot, set-up by the Kolkata-based Techno India Group at a cost of Rs. 80-100 crore. Besides, there will be a 350-bed hospital and colleges for nursing, dental, ayurveda and pharmacy. The project, a brainchild of state power minister Mrinal Banerjee, falls under his Assembly constituency. Asansol Durgapur Development Authority (ADDA) CEO, N. Manjunatha Prasad said the DSP had agreed to allot 100 acres for this purpose. After procuring the land, ADDA will hand it over to Techno India.

As ADDA does not possess such huge land, DSP agreed to provide it on Banerjee's request, informed Prasad.

The entire project will be completed within 10 years.

Health cities and Health care expansion brings more jobs

It is the era of health and a booming health care industry is testimony to it. While the Government increases seats in medical and paramedical colleges, private universities are into an expansion mode. Not just conventional medical courses, even students of science courses can now hope for high-end career prospects, all of which portend a much bigger and expansive reach for health care.

The net result: more foreign nationals are now seeking India for its lower cost and reliable medical services. Medical tourism has arrived in India. It has also taught Indian health care industry to become competitive and provide the best not only to the international but to the local patient too.

In the past few years the major super specialty hospitals in Chennai have been playing host to a number of foreign nationals who seek treatment for even difficult procedures. The success in complex surgical procedures has made smaller hospitals also to look upto the examples set by larger corporate hospitals. Rajah Muthiah Medical College Hospital of Annamalai Nagar is expanding its horizons. By next year it will become a super-speciality hospital.

While the medical fraternity concentrates on research, surgeries and procedures, paramedical support systems are also looking up. Hospitals with 50 beds conduct certificate courses for laboratory technicians and larger hospitals with over 200 beds have nursing courses.

Despite major strides in the clinical field, India still imports about 90 per cent of the instruments used by the medical fraternity. This is a neglected area and has currently seen a rising interest and demand to make them indigenously. The country is looking to making a range of instruments from those needed for pathogen detection to automated clinical machines. Developing such instrumentations would need multidisciplinary approach involving biological and medical researchers, clinicians, instrumentation engineers.

Destination India

The Indian success story is the outcome of low cost advantages *vis-à-vis* quality medical treatment. Whereas the cost of treatment in other developed nations especially in the U.S., U.K., etc. is very high, India can provide quality health care at very low cost due to the availability of relatively cheaper but quality manpower, low-priced drugs, and other infrastructure. Whereas a liver transplant costs you 5,00,000 US $ in USA, it can only be done with 40,000 US $ in India. Further, a heart surgery can be done with 5,000-7,000 US $ in India as against 30,000 US $ in USA.

This cost effectiveness does make India a destination where "First World Treatment at Third World Prices" (Gupta, 2004) has rather become a reality to reckon with for foreign as well as Non-resident Indians. Adds Dr. Naresh Trehan, "Now we do over 4,000 heart operations a year, and the mortality, which is an index of how well things are, is 0.8% which is even better than most places in the world. The other thing that we measure is infection rate. Ours is 0.3 % as compared to the world average of 1%."

In terms of advanced medical technology, Indian corporate hospitals now excel in all sorts of critical treatment. Indian surgical techniques are similar to those carried out in the west. Each test is carried out by professional M.D. physicians, and is comprehensive yet pain-free. There is also a gamut of services ranging from General Radiography, Ultra Sonography, Mammography to high end services like Magnetic Resonance Imaging, Digital Subtraction Angiography along with intervention procedures, Nuclear Imaging. The diagnostic facilities offered in India are comprehensive to include Laboratory services, Imaging, Cardiology, Neurology and Pulmonology. The Laboratory services include biochemistry, hematology, microbiology, serology, histopathology, transfusion medicine and RIA. All medical investigations are conducted on the latest, technologically advanced diagnostic equipment. Stringent quality assurance exercises ensure reliable and high quality test results. Studies show that medical technology constitutes around 60 percent of corporate hospital's investment. Hospitals in the country made use of technology to get an edge over their competitors through use of the state-of-the-art technologies (Bhat, 1994). Health care industry is becoming increasingly global in nature.

However, this being India, averages seldom show the complete picture. While the vast majority of population remains poor, there is a strong and vibrant middle class about 300 million strong. This group of consumers is demanding world class quality health care. This demand is essentially driving the movement of private capital towards developing health care institutions. As the middle class becomes assertive, they are demanding and getting better consumer orientation from the emerging health care institutions.

The Government liberalized entry norms in the health care industry for private players in the 1980s. It offers several incentives to private players; such as, land allocation at subsidized rates for new hospital projects.

Over the past two decades, a number of Indian private sector companies have set-up hospital facilities and clinics. Prominent examples include Apollo, Max, Fortis, Escorts and Wockhardt; out of an estimated total of 150 that represent a rapidly growing number of high-end facilities that offer top of-the-line medical treatment.

Private hospitals account for over 32 per cent of hospital beds in India. Besides providing basic health and medical care services, these corporate hospitals often undertake complex surgeries like bone-marrow transplants, open-heart surgeries and kidney transplants.

Another area witnessing increasing corporate presence is diagnostic services. Premier Indian players in this segment include SRL-Ranbaxy, Metropolis Health Services.

The Indian government has recognized the potential of preparing India to be a global health care destination. They are offering special incentives to hospital projects of over 100 beds. Private entrepreneurs, business groups, travel agencies and local governments are catching the trend.

- Travel agencies are increasingly offering "medical tourism" packages.

- Medical cities or "med-cities" are being planned to offer comprehensive health care and other recuperation facilities.
- Additionally, India's costs continue to be attractively low. An open-heart procedure at a top hospital in the country would cost a patient around US$ 5000-7000 as against US$ 50,000 in the US

Cost Comparisons for Medical Treatment in India

Procedure	Cost in the US	Cost in India
Open Heart Surgery	$30,000	$10,000
Liver Transplant	$300,000	$50,000
Orthopedic Surgery	$20,000	$7,000
Bone Marrow Transplant	$300,000	$20,000
Hip Replacement	$20,000	$5,000
Knee Joint Replacement	$15,000	$7,000
Cataract Surgery	$5,000	$1,500
Root Canal Treatment	$1,000	$150
Tooth Whitening	$1,000	$200
Lasik Surgery	$5,000	$1,000

Note: The above numbers are approximations for comparison basis. Exact numbers should be obtained from the service providers.

Some outstanding hospitals in health tourism:

1. All India Institute of Medical Sciences—AIIMS (India)
2. Apollo Hospital (India)
3. Asian Hospital (Philippines)
4. B.M. Birla Heart Research Centre (India)
5. Bombay Hospital (India)
6. Breach Candy Hospital (India)
7. Bumrungrad International Hospital (Thailand)
8. Capital Medical Center (Philippines)
9. CARE Hospitals (India)
10. Christian Medical College (India)
11. East Avenue Medical Center (Philippines)
12. Escorts Heart Institute (India)
13. Hinduja Hospital (India)
14. Indraprastha Medical Corporation (India)

15. Jaslok Hospitals (India)
16. L.V. Prasad Eye Hospitals (India)
17. Lilavati Hospital (India)
18. Lung Center (Philippines)
19. Madras Institute of Orthopaedics and Traumatology—MIOT (India)
20. Makati Medical Center (Philippines)
21. Medical City (The) (Philippines)
22. National Health Care Group (Singapore)
23. National Kidney and Transplant Institute (The) (Philippines)
24. NM Excellence (India)
25. Philippine Children's Medical Center (Philippines)
26. Philippine Heart Center (Philippines)
27. Raffles Hospital (Singapore)
28. St. Luke's Medical Center (Philippines)
29. Tata Memorial Hospital (India)
30. The Bangkok Phuket Hospital (Thailand)
31. Phuket Health and Travel Co., Ltd. (Thailand)
32. The Institute of Cardiovascular Diseases (India)
33. The International Medical Centre (Thailand)
34. Wockhardt Hospitals (India)

Source: Business Standard.

Trends of the Economic Environment of India with Its Impact on the Health Care

Research and Markets announces the addition of new Frost and Sullivan report. Economic Analysis for the Indian Health Care Industry to their offering.

Modernization of the health care systems and greater collaboration with the health care industry to provide innovative drugs, modern medical equipment, better health care services, as well as expand health care insurance are the primary aims of the Indian Government. It has stated in the National Health Policy that it hopes to increase the number of health care centers in remote areas and improve supply of essential health care services by boosting the public health care expenditure to 2.0 percent of the gross domestic product (GDP) by 2010. India is to become one of the largest and fastest growing economies in the world. The GDP and gross capital formation are expected to increase sturdily and the inflation rate is likely to reduce. The Government is also implementing suitable policies to considerably lower the unemployment rate.

Health Care Funding: Needs Greatest Attention

In a letter to finance minister Pranab Mukherjee, Apollo Hospitals group chairman Prathap C. Reddy said India's health care infrastructure is way below what is needed for adequate delivery of services. The overall health care infrastructure in India is very poor when compared with other developing countries, Reddy said in the letter. There exists a huge gap between health care infrastructure facilities available and their demand in the country. India has just 1.5 beds, 0.5 physicians and 0.9 nurses per 1,000 people. These figures are comparable to low-income countries and well below the standards of developing countries. There is an urgent need to add 8,00,000 beds by 2012 with an estimated capital outlay of $20 to $30 million a year for the next decade.

Currently, the sector contributes about 6.1% to the GDP of the country of which the government's contribution is 1.1%. Given its potential for growth and employment generation, the health care sector will become one of the most powerful economic engines for the nation and would contribute to increase in GDP by 2-3%. The sector would provide direct employment opportunities for at least two million people. In order to catalyze quality infrastructure development, the government needs to enable and facilitate the environment by incentivizing the health care sector, he feels.

Besides, the sector seeks a 10-year tax holiday (u/s 80-1B) extension for new hospital projects and 7-year extension for hospitals that are upgrading facilities. Further, industry experts have called for relaxation of GST for the health care sector. Currently, health care services are not taxable under service tax regulations. The present status is likely to be maintained under the new GST regime. Also, supply of goods such as medicines, vaccines, surgical consumables should not be made liable for GST. Basic customs duty for medical equipment under the customs tariff heading should be brought down to 5%. The basic customs duty on inputs required for manufacturing equipment be reduced to 5% across the board, they feel.

Some hard facts:

- It is one of the fastest growing sectors.
- Current industry size is approximately US$ 17 billion.
- Health care spending estimated to double in the next 10 years.
- With the development of the pharmaceutical market, health care sector would grow from US $17 billion to US $50 billion.
- Growth for private participation has been at the rate of 13% annually.
- The industry will grow faster with the expansion of health insurance in the country.

According to forecasts, the GDP growth in the short-term is expected to hover around 6-7%. But, for the short-to-medium term, the projections are at a 10% mark-making India as one amongst the fastest growing economies.

Striking motherhood to infertile medical tourists

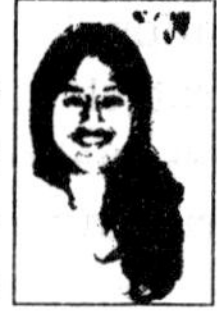

India is fast becoming a land of surrogate motherhood (it's a Rs. 25,000 crore business in India) have raised alarm bells for quite some time. India has become a popular destination for 'rent-a-womb' across the globe because of lower cost (which ranges from one-fifth to one-tenth in comparison with the West), ambiguous law, and availability of poor women willing to rent their wombs. Though commercial surrogacy is allowed in India, experts have pointed out time and again that the guidelines issued by the Indian Council of Medical Research (ICMR) on surrogacy and Assisted Reproductive Technologies (ART) are not adequate to curtail the perils of this burgeoning trade. In the absence of a legal binding between the parents and the surrogate mother to adhere to the 'guidelines' and absence of punishment for violating them, many dubious practices are reported. Many foreign nationals have complained about being cheated by clinics guaranteeing success

Thus, the Government's recent re-iteration on a law by next year on surrogate pregnancy has come as a good tiding. Though the remarks of Women and Child Development Minister Renuka Chowdhury about off-springs of such surrogacy being used for organs trafficking may be a bit far-fetched, the law would definitely bring more clarity and curb the malpractices of reproductive tourism, which seems to have gone out of control. Rent-a-womb practice is fraught with multiple risks. It risks the health of the poor women renting the womb, even affecting Maternal Mortality Rate. Tales abound about rampant exploitation of poor and gullible women who often don't understand what they are getting into or how their lives would be changed. Many foreign nationals have also been cheated by conmen/clinics guaranteeing success. However, what has raised a storm is the ambiguity that prevails over the nationality of the child. Does a child born to an Indian surrogate mother become a citizen of India?

What made everyone wake upto this legal quagmire was obviously the case of German twins Leonard and Nikolas, which raised questions about nationality of such children. The twins born in Anand (Gujarạt), the most favoured destination for rent-a-womb, were forced to be in Jaipur for a long stretch because of Germany's ban on commercial surrogacy. Other similar cases involving citizenship are pending in the Indian court of law.

Other legal question that needs to be addressed is when foreign father of the child becomes single. Such a case emerged when Manji Yamada was born to a surrogate mother a month after her Japanese parents divorced. Her Japanese father could not adopt her, because the Indian law does not allow a single man to adopt a baby girl. It's a pity that innocent bundles of joy suffer because of grown-ups' wish to have their own biological baby at any cost and the legal conundrum.

So, the upcoming law besides ensuring that the poor women lending their womb are not exploited and their health and welfare are not compromised also needs to be crystal clear about citizenship of such children. It would be better that we don't allow commercial surrogacy for nationals whose country bans commercial surrogacy. The law also needs to protect the rights of the infertile couple, so that they are not exploited. Associations like FOGSI must step in to support the Government in bringing in more clarity on this matter.

SOURCES

Rupa Chanda, 'Trade in Health Services', *Bulletin of the World Health Organization*, 2002; 80(2); pp. 158-63.

David Diaz Benavides, 'Trade Policies and export of health services—A Development Perspective', World Health Organization Publication, pp. 53-69.

India Brand Equity Foundation,' India is far Cheaper than Thailand', March.

IDFC Ltd., 'Investing in Private Health Care in India—Funding Robust Business Models', December 2002.

Mueller, H. and Kaufmann, E.L., 'Wellness Tourism: Market Analysis of a Special Health Tourism and Implications for Hotel Industry', *Journal of Vacation Marketing*, Vol. 7(1), pp. 6-17, July 2000.

"The Health Travellers"—Cover Story, Business World India.

'India—Health Care Industry'—India Brand Equity Foundation.

"Prospects for Health Tourism Exports for the English Speaking Carribean"—Consultancy Report, World Bank, SSDS Inc., September 1995.

APPENDIX

GLOBALIZATION AND MEDICAL TOURISM

I. Identification

1. Issue

Globalization has caused many countries to re-evaluate their economical strengths and weaknesses, as well as reassess what products or services in which nations can benefit. One such product and service that has emerged over the past decade is medical tourism. Medical tourism involves the practice of citizens exercising their personal health care choices in less restrictive areas. It is the traveling by candidate service recipients from one institution, jurisdiction or country where treatment is not available to another institution, jurisdiction or country where they can obtain the kind of medical procedures and innovative treatments they desire. Despite the less restrictive policies that encourage this business, these services often can also be offered as a lower-cost and more-timely option.

Because of the nature of this practice and its policies, this phenomenon has only occurred in certain, specific areas around the world. These regions and nations have attractive policies in place and have implemented unique marketing strategies that encourage the medical tourism business. This industry has demonstrated significant impact on these nations' economic health. Unfortunately, other nations, like the United States, have not been as successful in attracting the medical tourism business. Therefore, the issue is to more thoroughly understand, through the analysis of other country's experiences, policies and marketing strategies, why the United States should take advantage of the opportunity to further participate in this emerging industry.

2. Description

Medical tourism is a universal term that encompasses several specialty markets. Included in these specialty markets are health tourism, reproductive tourism, suicide tourism, as well as other niche business opportunities. Tourism, in the sense of this emerging market, is basically traveling from a place where treatment is not available, because of the prevailing rules, to a place where it is available. These rules are not necessarily laws but may also be the personal and moral convictions of the health care provider, institutional policy guidelines, and recommendations by committees. Thus, policy, in some fashion, is the driver of this industry.

Medical tourism is also the most common practice carried out all over world. However, there are other specialty markets within medical tourism that are also emerging as significant businesses. Health tourism is travel in a recuperative climate with natural therapeutic resources. The health tourism business is more specifically known for offering yoga, massage, traditional ayurvedic medicine and spa resorts. Reproductive tourism is the practice of consumers exercising their personal reproductive choices in less restrictive areas by traveling to another jurisdiction or country where the desired medically assisted reproduction procedures and treatments can be obtained. Suicide tourism is a very small branch of medical tourism yet its presence is still notable. This practice, much more so than the others, is tightly structured by policy.

Once consumers commit to travel for their desired medical treatment, often consumers will also take the opportunity to be a tourist in the visiting country and enjoy what it has to offer. Thus, consumers may combine their holiday and medical care into one venture. Medical tourism is comprised of three basic aspects: hospital/health services, hotels and travel/leisure. Thus, with attractive policies and/or the correct marketing strategies, this emerging industry can have significant opportunity for economic growth and infrastructure development for participating nations.

3. Related Cases

As noted, medical tourism is the universal practice with numerous specialty markets within this business. Because this in an emerging industry, extensive research for any particular country or on any individual branch of medical tourism, its policies and marketing strategies are not available. Therefore, all areas comprising medical tourism for many of the participating geographical regions or nations will be addressed. In summary, this case study will address a broad overview of the industry.

II. Policy Impacts

4. Social

The policy behind medical tourism has two distinct functions. In the case of those countries benefiting from medical tourism, standing policy allows for the nation to promote this business to consumers who are willing to travel and have the ability to pay. In essence, policy allows consumers new and different options for their health care needs. Medical tourism policy offers consumers choices. Secondly, this policy can also be enacted to protect the nation and its consumers. In the health care field, ensuring necessary and quality service is of the utmost importance. Therefore, policy, in the medical tourism sense, protects the rights of its participants while also giving consumers more opportunity and choices in their health care.

5. Environmental

While medical tourism focuses on fulfilling health care choices, traveling to a different country or state is also necessary. This is the basic premise behind medical tourism. Thus, by traveling to another geographical area, it is promoting tourism to location. Tourism is being used as a means for providing capital for development and preservation of these geographical areas.

6. Economic

Medical tourism has had significant economic impacts on particular geographical regions and nations. The goal of this industry is to provide economic stimulus to the geographical areas, often developing nations. The objective of this business is to increase jobs, income, and quality of life of the participating nations of medical tourism. This business also promotes infrastructure development to support the industry.

7. Other

Since this is an emerging, competitive industry, countries seek education, advanced skills and training to benefit from this profitable business. Therefore, medical tourism, and the policies around it, has encouraged participants to receive continued education and training. Additionally, this business also requires the use of advanced technology, and this, in turn, encourages participating countries to gain more exposure to these various technologies.

8. Suggested Interventions

While there are several specialty markets of medical tourism that are very controversial, specifically reproductive and suicide tourism, countries are reconsidering and/or analyzing their standing policies. There are consumers who take advantage of these opportunities, as well as opposition from non-market groups who have forced possible policy reform. Thus, these nations must continue to analyze and revise their policies in order to protect the practice of medical tourism and its consumers.

III. Legal Clusters

9. Disclosure and Status/Policy Issue

While there is no main policy issue, policy, or less restrictive policy, is the backbone of this industry. Most often, consumers are willing to travel to receive medical procedures in a geographical location that maintains policies that are less prohibitive than their current location's policies. There are other factors, too, that encourage medical tourism, like time and money. However, if policy is not in place to encourage this business, regions or countries would not be able to participate and benefit from this industry. Additionally, because of their particular standing policies, nations are better able to market themselves to new consumers globally.

10. Forum and Scope/Existing Policy Framework

International: The concept of medical tourism is primarily to encourage travel by consumers globally. Therefore, most countries enact a policy framework that is attractive to world-wide consumers on the basis that if they are willing to travel and pay the necessary fee, consumers are able to receive the health care practice they desire.

National: Medical tourism does not require a consumer to have to cross national borders. Often, medical tourism is evident from state to state or jurisdiction to jurisdiction. In this case, policy encourages consumers to travel from one area to another area where policy is more attractive or less restrictive. This type of medical tourism that markets this practice is more often seen in the specialty market of reproductive tourism.

Regional: Although countries do not tend to formulate policies based on regional expectations, there are certain geographical areas that do benefit more from the medical tourism industry. Southeast Asia has marketed itself as the primary geographical area to cater to medical tourism consumers. Since this has become a competitive business, countries in this geographical area continue to analyze and reform their policies to encourage this practice and rise above their competitors. Additionally, as this industry continues to emerge, this similar phenomenon is becoming more apparent in the European Union as well.

11. Decision Breadth/Stakeholders/Policy Actors

Policy is often shaped by numerous actors. The government plays are large role in outlining medical tourism policy in its nation. However, there are other actors that can affect policy. Health care providers, institutions, special committees, advisory boards, associations, as well as numerous other players, can all impact policy guidelines.

On the tourism aspect of this industry, there are also other actors that can also influence policy. Businesses, recreational organizations, as well other associations and groups can impact policy guidelines that encourage medical tourism.

12. Legal Standing/Legal Regulatory Framework/Suggested Policy Interventions

Although there is no documented legal regulatory framework for the medical tourism industry, there is always a legal liability concern when dealing with the health care industry. The health care industry is a much regulated business entwined with liability issues. Therefore, countries enact policies that address this concern on an individual basis. Because some countries are willing to take on more risk with health care liability, they have been able to emerge as leaders in this industry. Other countries, like the United States, have not been able to benefit as greatly from medical tourism because of increased legal liability and policy.

IV. Trade Clusters

13. Type of Measure

Research states that the economic profit that the medical tourism industry contributes to the nation's gross domestic product (GDP) is the measure of success. This financial revenue can be calculated by health care earnings, as well as the profits from tourism-related activities. Besides the monetary value that is calculated, countries can measure the affects of this industry by the increase in number of tourists, as well as the number of new jobs. Together, countries are able to determine the many influences that the medical tourism industry has on its economy.

14. Relation of Trade Measure to Environmental/Tourism Impacts

Directly Related to Product: The revenue generated from the consumers traveling to the country for their health care needs will go towards building the nation's health care system and tourism infrastructure.

Indirectly Related to Product: Because medical tourism crosses many different types of business sectors, the revenue generated will also indirectly support these other sectors indirectly as well. While this practice will primarily benefit the health care and lodging industries, the service and recreational industries will also profit from this business.

Not Related to Product: The result of the medical tourism industry is far-reaching. Not only will it benefit many different business sectors directly and indirectly, medical tourism can provide an increase in a nation's overall economic health. Revenue generation will increase the GDP. This resultant growth will encourage development of the nation's infrastructure and its people's quality of life.

Related to Process: Revenue generation from this business will hopefully encourage the further development of the infrastructure that is required to carry out the medical tourism product. Development of the health care system, as well as the travel and tourism infrastructure, will benefit the nation and its people on the whole.

15. Trade Product Identification/Trade and Services

The medical tourism product generally provides numerous types of services. First and foremost, medical tourism is providing a consumer with the health care service that they need or desire. In addition, this type of business also offers the consumer the lodging services that they require to participate in this process. Often consumers will also take part in some leisure, recreational or sightseeing activities while visiting the country. Therefore, the tourism industry may also be providing a service to these consumers as well.

16. Economic Data

The medical tourism industry can be a product for any country. However, numerous nations have significantly benefited from this business more than others. The country's that have demonstrated the most significant gains are noted below:

- Medical tourism has contributed approximately $25 million per year to Cuba's economic status.
- India has seen a 27 percent increase in tourists while medical tourism, itself, has demonstrated a 20 percent growth. Additionally, India has attracted 150,000 medical tourists in 2003. By 2012, medical tourism is expected to bring an additional $1.1-2.2 billion in annual revenue.

- o In 2002, Thailand treated more than 600,000 tourists that generated approximately $503 million in revenues.
- o In 2000, Singapore attracted more than 150,000 tourists for medical care which added 0.19 percent to its GDP. By 2012, this island is expected to treat more than 1 million tourists. This figure will complement a 3 percent market share for health care services, generate some $3 billion in revenue, add 1 percent to the GDP and lead to some 13,000 new jobs

17. Impact of Trade Restriction

Because the basis of this industry requires consumers to travel for their health care needs, trade restrictions on travel would impact its capabilities. Among the two most problematic restrictions would be on visa issuing and International Travel Bans to specific regions or countries. Thus, if the consumers are unable to travel to the desired country, the product and service cannot be sold.

18. Industry Sector

As suggested previously, the primary industry sector for medical tourism includes: the health care industry, as well as the international travel and tourism industry. The secondary industry sectors would include: service, information technology and communication industries.

19. Exporters and Importers

In the medical tourism industry, the export is the consumer. Because the consumer comes into the country for their health care needs, they provide foreign currency to the economy. In the end, they leave the country with the desired medical care. It is the hope that there are no real imports and that all of the goods and services are provided domestically.

V. Macro/Environment Cluster/Tourism Policy Clusters

20. Environmental Problem Type/Environmental Aspects

Although the main focus of the medical tourism product is the health care service provided, countries are also encouraging consumers to be tourists. As a tourist, they are enjoying the beauty and recreation of the area. The hope is that some of the revenues from these activities will go into developing the environmental infrastructure, as well as conservation and preservation.

21. Resource Impact and Effect

This type of practice does not really require any substantial amount of environmental resources. Therefore, there are no major impacts or effects of the medical tourism business on a nation's environmental resources.

22. Urgency and Policy Review

On the whole, medical tourism is still in an emergent state. Therefore, this practice has not necessitated any type of real urgency. However, most of the countries participating in this business have launched a global advertising and marketing campaign to varying extents. Each country has unique marketing strategies that target specific markets. Additionally, because each country seeks growth, each has their own unique policies that allow for the attraction of these consumer markets.

23. Substitutes and Alternative Policies

The most common alternative to receiving health care in one's desired country is obtaining one's health care needs in a competitive country. Therefore, countries attempt to make their policies as attractive and simplified as possible to attract the consumer. If not, consumers may find a different country with less restrictive policies to provide them their desired care.

VI. Other Factors

24. Culture

Because this industry is carried out in many different countries around the world with various languages and practices, culture can play a significant role in this business. Nations must be cognizant of culture when marketing to specific target markets. Additionally, consumers must appreciate culture and traditions that may affect their foreign health care experience. Because many of the countries providing this service are developing countries, culture can be very different and varied. All participants in this business must understand and appreciate that culture can play a significant role in the medical tourism process.

25. Trans-boundary Issues

For medical tourism on a whole, overwhelming trans-boundary issues are not present. However, there are two specific markets within medical tourism, reproductive and suicide tourism, which do present trans-boundary challenges. With reproductive tourism, often consumers travel to another jurisdiction to receive a service that cannot be provided at home. Abortions and decisions surrounding in vitro fertilization can be two specific practices that can present challenges to the consumer. This is true for suicide tourism as well. There are issues surrounding the rights of the individual accompanying the consumer. Some countries view this as assistance, which often is prohibited. Therefore, although medical tourism does not present too many trans-boundary issues, specific markets can present challenges and should be more closely analyzed.

26. Rights

For the most part, medical tourism is not affected by one's rights.

However, when dealing with reproductive and suicide tourism, a consumer's rights must be considered. Consumers have rights. However they may be affected by receiving treatment in a foreign country or upon returning to their home country. Consumers must consider their rights, and they make seek treatment in alternative locations if a different area's policies better serve a patient's rights. This could be true for practices or procedures such as abortions, in vitro fertilization, as well as euthanasia. Thus, consumer's rights may play a part in decisions made for the medical tourism product.

27. Policy Implications

Many nations around the world, particularly developing countries, have taken advantage of the benefits of medical tourism. This emerging industry can provide significant economic stimulus for a nation's revenue growth and financial health. It can also stimulate infrastructure development and improve the quality of life of the nation's people. However, nations must position themselves correctly to reap this profit.

Countries must establish attractive policies that encourage medical tourism practice in their country as well as attract consumers to participate in this phenomenon. Nation's often demonstrate less restrictive policies than its neighbours and competitors.

Once a nation has policies in place, they must correctly market themselves. Countries use different and unique marketing strategies, such as lower-cost, more-timely, higher-quality, to promote their services to their target market. Thus, this industry has demonstrated significant impact on the nation's economic health, however, less-restrictive and attractive policies must be in place first. Countries must also market themselves properly to continually enjoy the benefits of this emerging business.

Health Tourism: Medical Cities in Philippines, South Korea

Republic of the Philippines is situated in Southeast Asian region. Its capital is Manila, and it has more than seven thousand islands, making the nation as the world's twelfth most populous countries. The Philippines is home to the most hospitable people on earth, having been very popular because of its hospitality to local and foreign tourists. This attitude is one of the many reasons why a lot of people are thinking about relocating into this Southeast Asian country. The Philippines has about 95,000 or about 1 per 800 people with about 1,700 hospitals where 60% are private totaling 85,000 beds. While the health care of its people has several issues, it is being touted as a destination of medical tourism in Asia.

Health Care in the Philippines

Delivery of health care is a "fragmented system" with a "dysfunctional health workforce," which results in great disparity between health care for the rich and poor. At a forum on the outlook for the Philippines Health in 2010, they spoke on the relation of the number of children in a family with their income level and quality of life, the link between high fertility and poverty, and the fact that rapid population growth impedes human development. Children from large families not only suffer from poor health, but their educational opportunities are also limited. Health care is also affected for the poor. Two-thirds of reimbursements made by Phil-health are to private hospitals that cater to the rich. Health facilities that are accessible to the poor are often not accredited.

Dr. Thelma Tupasi, President of the Tropical Disease Foundation, and a specialist in infectious diseases, pointed out that despite the increase in poverty; there has been a significant decline in TB in the Philippines, where patients are given medication in the presence of health workers, to ensure the medication is taken regularly. Drug prices in the Philippines are among the highest in the world—a situation that increases the risk of poor Filipinos dying from curable diseases because they cannot afford to buy medicines. Health services are fragmented and inefficient. Health management information is rudimentary. The government must enact and implement necessary reforms, with private sector support, for health care reform to succeed.

Health conditions in the Philippines in 1990 approximated to those in other Southeast Asian countries but lagged behind those in the West. Life expectancy, for instance, increased from 51.2 years in 1960 to 69 years for women and 63 years for men in 1990. Infant mortality was 101 per 1,000 in 1950 and had dropped to 51.6 per 1,000 in 1989. In 1923, approximately 76 percent of deaths were caused by communicable diseases. By 1980, deaths from communicable diseases had declined to about 26 percent. Most health care personnel and facilities are concentrated in urban areas. There has been substantial migration of physicians and nurses to the United States. Hospital equipment often does not function because there were insufficient technicians capable of maintaining it.

In 1987 a little more than one-half of the infants and children received a complete series of immunization shots, a major step in preventive medicine. The problem was especially difficult in rural areas. Although very few Filipinos have been infected with acquired immune deficiency syndrome (AIDS), concern about the disease has caused authorities to give it considerable attention. Like many other countries, the Philippines has a problem with illicit drugs. Official Philippine government statistics for 1989 indicate only 1,733 addicts, but the assumption was that the real number was from ten to a hundred times as great. There also was a problem with inadequately tested legal drugs. In 1983, more than 265 pharmaceutical products were sold in the Philippines that were banned in many other countries. The Department of Health succeeded in eliminating 128 of them by 1988. Attempts to eliminate others have been blocked by the courts, which ruled that the department had acted without due process.

Malnutrition has been a perennial concern of the Philippine government and health care professionals. In 1987, the Department of Health reported that 2.8 percent of preschoolers were suffering from third-degree malnutrition and 17.6 percent from second-degree malnutrition. To alleviate this problem, the government targeted food assistance for nearly 500,000 preschoolers and lactating mothers. Nutrition has shown some improvement. In 1955, government statistics estimated the daily per capita available food supply at only 80 percent of sufficiency. In 1986, it had improved to 101.8 percent. In the same period, the consumption of milk nearly tripled and the consumption of fats and oils more than doubled.

Dual health care system

The Philippines has a dual health care system consisting of modern and traditional medicine. The modern system is based on the germ theory of disease and has scientifically trained practitioners. The traditional approach assumes that illness is caused by a breach of taboos set by supernatural forces. It is not unusual for an individual to alternate between the two forms of medicine. If the benefits of modern medicine are immediately obvious—eyeglasses, for instance—then there is little argument. If there is no immediate cure, the impulse to turn to the traditional healer is often strong.

One type of traditional healer that attracted the attention of foreigners as well as Filipinos was the so-called psychic surgeon, who professed to be able to operate without using a scalpel or drawing blood. Some practitioners attracted a considerable clientele and established lucrative practices. Travel agents in the United States credited these "surgeons" with generating travel to the Philippines.

Although medical treatment had improved and services had expanded, pervasive poverty and lack of access to family planning detracted from the general health of the Philippine people. In 1990, approximately 50 percent of the population was listed below the poverty line. A high rate of childbirth tended both to deplete family resources and to be injurious to the health of the mother. The main general health hazards were pulmonary, cardiovascular, and gastrointestinal disorders.

The Philippines has a social security system including Medicare with wide coverage of the regularly employed urban workers. It offers a partial shield against disaster, but is limited both by the generally low level of incomes, which reduce benefits, and by the exclusion of most workers in agriculture. In April 1989, out of more than 22 million employed individuals, a little more than 10.5 million were covered by social security. The government expenditure is constrained by the large fiscal deficit. As a result, poor families' membership of PhilHealth (the national health insurance programme) has been facilitated by a sponsored scheme, and PhilHealth now claims universal coverage, although many poor families remain without PhilHealth cards. PhilHealth implements a National Quality Assurance Program (NQAP) applicable to all accredited providers for the delivery of health services nationwide. This ensures that the health services rendered to the members by accredited health care providers are of the quality necessary to achieve the desired health outcomes and member satisfaction. The main tasks of the NQAP is the implementation of a performance monitoring system which provides safeguards against: Over- and under-utilization of services, Unnecessary diagnostic and therapeutic procedures and intervention, Irrational drug use, Inappropriate referral practices, Gross, unjustified deviations from currently accepted practice guidelines or treatment protocols, Use of fake, adulterated or misbranded pharmaceuticals or unregistered drugs. These practices are grounds for suspension, revocation, denial of accreditation and/or filing of a criminal complaint.

Review of Claims Filed

Phil-Health's work does not end with the reimbursement of claims. It analyzes the profile of the claims submitted for such tell-tale signs of abuse or fraud by the providers through a Utilization Review. Claims profile and data are plotted to identify certain outliers. Through this, PhilHealth is able to identify if the claims for certain diseases are abnormally high for a particular hospital or if the amount reimbursed are higher than the average in the region. In such a case, PhilHealth alerts the provider concerned of the situation. The share of out-of-pocket spending in total expenditure, an important indicator of the inequality of the distribution of health care charges, fell steadily from 1996, reaching 41% in 2000, but rebounded to 48% in 2002, no doubt reflecting budgetary constraints on government expenditure increases. Spending by central and local governments accounted for 41% of total health care expenditure in 2000, up from 35.2% in 1992, but fell back to 30% in 2002, whereas social insurance schemes provided 9% of expenditure in 2002, up from 7.1% in 2000 and 3.8% as recently as 1998. Although government attempts to increase health care spending is limited by fiscal deficit, it is likely that health care will account for a gradually rising share of expenditure over the forecast period. The Economist Intelligence Unit therefore expects the market for health care to offer more potential in the forecast period than in recent years.

The pharmaceutical imports

Local production of pharmaceuticals is limited, so that the Philippines is heavily dependent on imports for supplies of pharmaceutical products and medical equipment, and foreign firms control almost 75% of the market. Drug prices are high compared with other countries, particularly those in the Asia region. The Philippines is a key provider of health care workers and medical staff internationally. A large proportion of overseas Filipino workers are doctors and nurses, and the remittances they send back to the Philippines play an important role in boosting economic growth in the country. During talks with Japan on a bilateral free-trade agreement, the Philippines has pressed Japan to open up its health care sector to Philippine workers. In October 2004, the two countries appeared to reach an agreement that would allow Philippine doctors and nurses to work in Japan, but the upper limit on the numbers of such workers has not yet been agreed. Singapore, Taiwan and South Korea may also open their health care sectors to Philippine workers.

Patients may also increasingly travel to the Philippines in search of cheaper treatment or long-term care. Japan's largest private hospital group, Tokushukai Medical Corporation, announced in September 2004 that it would invest US$ 100 m in the Philippines to set-up a 1,000-bed hospital and retirement home for Japanese in or around the capital, Manila, by 2006. The facility would charge lower fees than equivalent facilities in Japan, and would be staffed by Japanese doctors and nurses. Around 500 retired Japanese live in the Philippines, a figure that the Philippine government expects to increase to around 10,000 over the next three years.

Health care costs

There are three options to cover medical costs in Philippine (a) the State-run Philippine Health Insurance Corporation (Phil-Health), (b) health maintenance organizations or HMOs, both corporate and NGO, and (c) out-of-pocket (Patients have to pay their own way). Phil-Health covers members who are confined in hospitals for at least 24 hours. It covers the cost of treatment and room expenses under specified rates for room and board, drugs and medicines, X-ray/laboratory/other diagnostic tests, and professional fees. Phil-Health also covers limited outpatient services, like day surgeries, dialysis and cancer treatment procedures like chemotherapy. It also covers mothers giving birth upto 4th normal delivery. The excess expenses that are not covered by Phil-Health will be covered by the company's or the individual's HMO, and/or out-of-pocket expenses. The State health insurance corporation, however, does not cover annual physical check-up. It has little preventive health care function, therefore. The focus is on curative health care, when a patient is too sick or too injured to rest at home and needs hospital confinement. Thus, being a Phil-health member alone is not sufficient. One, it does not cover/outpatient consultations; two, it does not cover annual physical check-up; and three, its expense cap may not be enough to cover total expenses for serious diseases. Most medical needs by patients involve ordinary physician visits, like if one has a headache or flu or other body pains. People would prefer to go home later and rest as staying in hospitals is not only expensive, it's also cumbersome and time-consuming for family visits.

HMO card and self-medication

Since many people do not have an HMO card, when they are not feeling well, as much as possible they do not see a doctor and resort to self-medication. A visit to government hospitals and physicians means long queue, while a visit to private physicians and clinics means high costs in physicians' fee and possibly diagnostic tests. So to cut costs or avoid long queuing, people self-medicate and buy medicines that are most popular.

Having a private HMO (many companies do this for their officers and Employees) will save people from unnecessary stress when they sick. Some groups and individuals are not comfortable with allowing more private HMOs because they see such enterprises as principally driven by profit and not by genuine and efficient public service, that is why they lobby for bigger government-run health insurance. This is despite their recognition of the inefficiencies, wastes and corruption involved in many government programs and projects, including the health agencies. A middle ground option is to encourage the emergence of cooperative-type of HMOs.

Phil-Health officials say that their membership coverage is around 80 percent of the population already as of April or May 2009. What they do, they multiply all Phil-Health members, currently at around 17.2 million people, with the average family size of around 4.3 members per household, children or old dependents, and they get 74 million total individuals covered. That is 80.4 percent of the projected 92 million total Philippine population as of middle of 2009. However, there is a miscalculation in this approach. Based on the latest labour force survey by the National Statistics Office (NSO), there were 35 million employed Filipinos as of April 2009. The total Phil-Health membership of 17.2 million, even upto 18 million, is only half of the total employed Filipinos. Thus, 80 percent membership coverage nationwide is impossible.

Hospitals in the Philippines

Most of the government hospitals provide quality health care the same way private hospitals do. Some people have misconceptions that medical advice from doctors in public hospitals is not reliable. What differs the Philippine government hospitals from the Philippine private hospitals is simply the facilities. Most of the public hospitals in the Philippines are not equipped with the latest technologies. As for the private hospitals, there are also a hundred ones located in key cities of the nation. There are also tertiary hospitals that have the latest in medical technologies. However, because they are private hospitals, they are expensive. The Philippines have stand by ambulances for any emergency situation. They also have a hotline number where on can call in times of emergencies. Hospitals are also equipped with the latest in first aid treatments.

Top Philippine hospitals in private sector include, The Medical City, the Medical Center in Alabang, the Asian Hospital, the Makati Medical Center, the Medical City in Ortigas, and St. Luke's Medical Center in Quezon City.

Cost of Medicines and Hospitalizations

Both locals and foreigners can attest to the fact that medicines sold in the Philippines are very much affordable. If you are thinking about visit to Philippines, one of your least worries should be health care. Since the health care system in the Philippines is affordable, and the doctors are well trained, plus nurses can properly aid you, you really never have to worry that much. Communication is never a problem when you are in the Philippines. The people are very hospitable and accommodating, the doctors and medical practitioners are friendly, and the place is really very inviting.

Health Tourism

It is estimated that more than half-a-million Americans traveled overseas for medical and health tourism in 2006. By the end of 2009, this number, according to some experts, may reach several millions. For Americans, the main motivation is financial because of ever escalating health care costs in the United States. Clearly, the global health care industry is expanding with the Philippines poised to capture a chunk of that market. The country's world-class physicians and its modern medical facilities equipped with the latest technology are major factors for the growth of its medical tourism program, according to Cynthia Carrion, undersecretary for sports and wellness tourism. Her department comes under the umbrella of the Department of Tourism which sends an obvious signal to the world that the Philippines means business in this area. Tourism secretary, Ace Durano, says, "The Philippines welcomes guests to take advantage of the value for money offered by our health and wellness tourism program through high quality medical services."

The Public-Private Partnership Task Force on globally competitive Philippines industries (PPPTF) is composed of leaders from many disciplines, including doctors and hospital directors. The latter form an important group focusing on promoting health and wellness and disseminating informational programs. One group is "The Medical City," a private tertiary care hospital that has been working in this field for over 40 years providing complete health and wellness programs for all ages.

According to Cynthia Carrion, a good number of Filipino doctors received their medical training in the United States and interned in U.S. hospitals. Returning to the Philippines, they have shared their knowledge with younger practitioners at some of the country's renowned medical centers such as The Medical City and St. Luke's Hospital.

In addition, Filipinos are inherently caring and compassionate which provides a genuine recipe for success in the health care field, notes the undersecretary.

Why Philippines?

Foreign nationals choose the Philippines as their medical tourism destination for low cost aesthetic and dental procedures. They expect to enjoy the care and compassion that they are familiar with in US, Australian or Middle Eastern hospitals, which are staffed with Western-trained Filipino nurses and physicians. Thousands of Filipino expats visit the Philippines for medical care as well, usually combining the medical procedure with their family visit. A bill was passed in 2006, by the Philippine Congress creating the Medical Tourism Bureau and prompted the nation to start promoting health tourism. Health travelers to the country find this attractive, as they are assisted by highly competent, English-speaking and Western-trained medical staff in over 2,000 hospitals in the country. Philippine health professionals are products of more than 313 health education institutions, and 60% to 80% of whom would eventually work or train abroad and get international medical diplomas. In fact, the Filipinos constitute the second largest group of foreign students that graduated in the medical field from US institutions. Several of these professionals who return home to practice their profession would bring back the latest in technologies, techniques, and expertise and build their own world-class medical practice.

Health Tourism figures

There were approximately 250,000 non-resident patients who traveled to the Philippines for various medical services in 2006. This has grown extensively each year and in the first quarter of 2009, approximately 200,000 medical tourists have been documented as visiting the Philippines for medical care, with figures expected to reach 600,000 by the end of the year. The vast Filipino Diaspora who settled overseas return to the Philippines not only for family visits or vacations but also to undergo minor medical, dental and other health procedures not covered by their medical insurance in their countries of origin. In 2007 alone 180,000 Filipino expatriates visited the country for such purposes and this is expected to increase in the coming years.

Medical education

In the Philippines, dentistry students need to undergo 4 years preparatory and 2 years of practical dentistry. After passing the dentistry board, they would then need another one or two year's specialization study. For physicians, a student would undergo 4 to 5 years pre-med study, then another 4 years of practical medicine and 1 year internship before they can take the medical board exams administered by the Philippines Board of Medicine, which is a special branch of the PRC or the Professional Regulation Commission. After passing, the physician can now be called a General Practitioner, but it would take him several years of medical graduate study if he wants to pursue medical specialization—4 years for most specialized fields and upto 8 years for surgical related specializations like neurosurgery, cosmetic surgeries, etc. The Philippine Medical Association supervises and monitors the practice of medical doctors of all fields, although there are also separate medical associations that are grouped according to the area of specialization.

Accreditation from the Philippines Department of Health

Hospitals in the Philippines undergo periodic accreditation from the Philippines Department of Health. Some of these medical institutions have international accreditation from the Joint Commissions International (JCI) and the International Organization for Standardization (ISO). Privately-owned hospitals located in the National Capital Region or Metro Manila offer the best in medical facilities and luxurious five-star accommodation that are equal to Western hospitals and cater to medical tourists. However, there are clear differences between the private or corporate health facilities as compared to the public health system, which usually do not offer the same quality that patients receive from private institutions. For medical tourists, it is advisable to avail themselves of the medical tourism packages offered by private hospitals and health facilities if they want to get the best health care services available.

Health tourism in Philippines or Organ trafficking?

Some hospitals advertise for global patients: at competitive rates—reserve living Filipino kidney, liver and bone marrow transplants. A web site boasts that the living organs will be transplanted at two unnamed partner hospitals outfitted with "the most advanced Western equipment in the world" and with the "full compliance of the Philippine Ministry of Health". Transplants can be arranged in less than 10 days, according to the site.

Welcome to the brave new world of Philippine transplant tourism, one of the country's few growth industries. It's also a trade coming under tough international scrutiny, due to concerns it sometimes provides cover for illegal human organ trafficking syndicates. The World Health Organization (WHO) recently ranked the Philippines as one of the top five countries in the world for human organ trafficking, along with China, Pakistan, Egypt and Colombia.

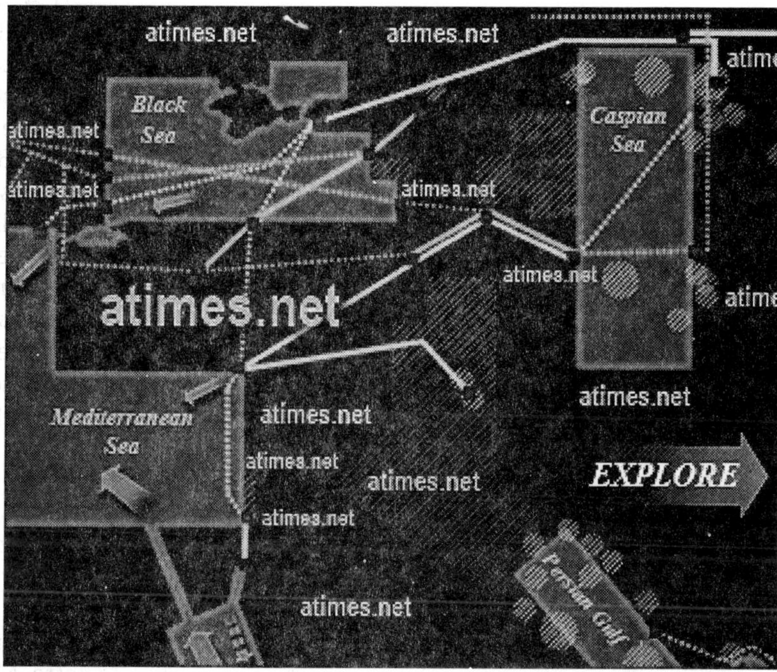

Medical tourism is booming in the Philippines, including among deep-pocketed foreigners who seek organ transplants, most commonly kidneys. About 200,000 health tourists visited the Philippines in 2006, according to official statistics. With this rapid influx, criminal human organ syndicates have seized on the crowds and taken advantage of the government's weak law enforcement to arrange illicit transplants for foreign nationals.

Kidney transplants

The official number of kidney transplants in the Philippines has recently risen dramatically, climbing from 306 transplants in 2002 to 1,046 in 2007, according to records compiled by the Philippine Renal Disease

Registry. Over half of the kidney recipients last year were foreigners, with Middle Eastern nationals comprising 75% of the beneficiaries. Its unclear how many more operations have taken place under the official radar? As the number of foreign national beneficiaries rises, so has the number of non-related living organ donors, a trend which undermines the intent of a 1991 Philippine law that supports cadaver and relative donations. Benita Padilla, president of the local Society of Nephrologists, said what makes the Philippines situation "unique" is that "transplants are done by big hospitals" rather than in back-alley operations, like the other four organ trafficking nations identified by the WHO. Donors are often recruited from poor Filipino communities, particularly in Manila, and paid sums ranging from US$ 2,000 to $ 3,000 per kidney, according to health officials. Brokers have also started scouting for donors in Manila's neighbouring provinces and in central Philippines, according to Padilla.

In April seven men were rescued in a house in southern Luzon after they were found locked up by an organ trafficking syndicate. The men were reportedly held against their will by the criminal gang until it could arrange to sell their organs to foreign patients, according to news reports. It was unclear if they intended to sell the organs to government-accredited facilities or onto underground markets. Some say those are often one and the same in the Philippines. The profit motive for underground syndicates and kidney transplant surgeons is exceptionally high. The website www.liver4you.org advertises liver transplants for $130,000. A foreign patient can expect to spend anywhere between $70,000 to $115,000 for a kidney transplant in one of 20 government-accredited medical facilities. That's a huge increment over the $19,000 to $23,800 hospitals charge lower purchasing power Filipinos for the same kidney transplant procedure. Some 10,000 to 12,500 Filipinos develop end-stage renal disease every year, 50% to 60% of whom are kidney transplant candidates, according to medical sources. However, less than 10% actually receive transplants, usually because of insufficient organ supplies and the failure of local patients to raise sufficient funds for the life-saving procedure.

Unscrupulous scalpels

An administrative order by the Department of Health (DOH) applicable to all local hospitals previously put in place a 10% cap on all transplant procedures for foreign nationals in any given year. That means the official figures of transplants are probably highly understated, some experts say. Enrique Ona, chief of the government-run National Kidney and Transplant Institute, claims that some medical doctors are "responsible" for the underground organ trade in the Philippines. He noted that there are only 24 registered kidney transplant surgeons in the country and that above-ground transplant procedures are conducted in only about 20 licensed medical facilities nationwide.

Those figures raise hard questions about why not a single hospital or medical practitioner has been charged for violating the DOH order, which is binding by law. The DOH has identified eight different medical facilities, including government-run hospitals, for not abiding by the annual cap on kidney transplants for foreign recipients. It has threatened to jail doctors and hospital administrators for upto 20 years in prison if they continue to defy government orders, but so far has not followed up on the threats with legal action.

Under international pressure to combat perceived rampant organ trafficking, the DOH with the backing of President Gloria Macapagal-Arroyo in March issued a new directive banning outright kidney transplants for foreign patients. The policy stated that kidney transplants were not part of the government's medical tourism promotion campaign and aimed to prioritize needy Filipinos as organ recipients. The new ban also aimed to better regulate the local organ donation trade, including government "gratuity packages" for organ donors. A new board chaired by the Health secretary is also set to screen all future transplant recipients. Now, the new directive faces more criticism than praise as signs of compromise creep into the policy's implementation. A group of local doctors has seized on a DOH exemption granted just weeks after the new ban's announcement to eight Israeli nationals who have already, or are scheduled to, receive kidney transplants. One Israeli patient already had a transplant procedure at the government-controlled National Kidney and Transplant Institute. The DOH and the new transplant and donor screening board said that the Israeli nationals were exempted from the ban for "humanitarian reasons" and because they were on the list of beneficiaries long before the policy was announced. The Philippine Society of Nephrologists and others have already accused the DOH of contradicting itself in not immediately implementing the new policy. The lack of DOH transparency, they fear, could work to the advantage of the same organ trafficking syndicates the new policy supposedly aimed to uproot. (Cher S. Jimenez; Business Mirror daily)

The Medical City (TMC)

It is a private, tertiary care hospital, has distilled some forty years of experience in hospital operation and administration in the establishment of its world-class health care complex that serves some 40,000 inpatients and 380,000 outpatients a year. The new site is presently located on a 1.5 hectare property along Ortigas Avenue in the business district of Pasig City, Metro Manila. It is composed of 100,000 sq.m. of floor space and includes two Nursing Towers joined by a Podium, bridge-ways and a Medical Arts Tower. The first 15-storey Nursing Tower with a heliport and a Business Center is currently fitted for 500 beds. The second Nursing Tower provides capacity for an additional 300 beds. The 18 floors of the Medical Arts Tower house 280 doctors' clinics and selected commercial spaces, such as banks, a restaurant, a food court and a convenience store and gift shop. Located within the 6-floor Podium are diagnostic and intervention facilities, as well as support and administrative offices. The 3-basement level parking accommodates over a thousand vehicles for clients and staff. The architectural and interior design of the hospital complex is contemporary yet welcoming with its hotel-like interiors and warm ambiance. Rooms are designed to offer soothing views of the lush gardens below, the Pasig and Makati skylines, and the Antipolo mountains. The complex is equipped with a broad range of state-of-the-art safety and security features, including an advanced Building Management System, for the protection of hospital clients and staff. Bio-safety features are also incorporated into specific patient areas within the complex. This impressive facility is the staging area for the delivery of cutting-edge health services, with centers of excellence in the fields of Wellness services, as well as Cardiovascular, Cancer, Neuroscience and Regenerative Medicine.

TMC's boasts of a distinguished medical staff of some 1,000 physicians, all of whom are experienced, recognized and established experts in their various fields of specialization—Medicine, Surgery, Orthopedics, Obstetrics and Gynecology, Pediatrics, Ophthalmology, Otolaryngology, Anesthesiology and Psychiatry. They are complemented by physicians in other fields of diagnostics and ancillary services—Pathology, Radiology, Nuclear Medicine, Physical Medicine and Rehabilitation, Pain Management, Radiation Oncology and Chemotherapy. All physicians affiliated with TMC, many of whom are internationally trained, pass a strict credentialing and privileging process. The medical staff is supported by a 2,100-strong organization composed of allied medical and administrative staff who has honed their expertise over many years of loyal service to the institution. TMC also serves as a hub of a network of satellite clinical facilities delivering a full range of diagnostic and therapeutic services to ambulatory patients. The satellite network demonstrates TMC's commitment to bring its unique brand of health services right into the communities of its patients.

At the heart of TMC's service philosophy are new paradigms of hospital care as addressing the entire continuum of health needs, and the patient as an equal, informed and empowered partner in the pursuit and preservation of health. TMC has been conferred accreditation by the Joint Commission International Accreditation (JCIA) for obtaining and maintaining the highest international standards of quality for health care organizations. JCIA is widely-recognized as the most prestigious accrediting body for international health care organizations. In its evaluation by JCIA, TMC received perfect scores in standards related to access to care, continuity of care, quality improvement and patient safety, a truly exceptional achievement by any measure. With a renewed commitment towards providing superior health care to individual patients, even as it offers itself as a national resource, to be engaged in the pursuit of social reform and equitable development. The Medical City proves that it is the country's "Capital of Health", the center of all that is new and true about health.

International Hospital

Its centerpiece is a hospital, the ultra-modern International Hospital. Just a 30-minute car ride away from Jakarta, the hospital, which will be built on a 5.50-hectare plot of land, is designed not only to serve local residents but also the entire South East Asian region.

Medical City will establish a medical school within President University, which will turn out young doctors and nurses who will be the stewards of health for populations in this part of the world. It will be supported by the President Research Hospital (PRH), which will serve as a teaching hospital. The University and the PRH will offer a curriculum that will match those of famous medical schools abroad.

Network of satellite clinical facilities

TMC also serves as a hub of a network of satellite clinical facilities delivering a full range of diagnostic and therapeutic services to ambulatory patients. Currently, Satellite Clinics are operational in Antipolo City, Pasig City, Fairview, Cainta, Marikina and Congressional Road in Quezon City and Lipa City. More satellite will be added as the hospital pursues its commitment to expand its network and bring its brand of health services into the very communities of its patient for their easy access. Additionally, Homecare services are offered whenever appropriate, particularly to patients after discharge from confinement. The employees, professional staff and shareholders of TMC draw from their experience of 4 decades to truly live out the organization's mission of "putting patients on center stage and delivering service of greater worth," and in the process exert its leadership in shaping how Filipinos should think, feel and behave about health.

Milestones achieved

The Medical City (TMC) ended 2008 with several milestones that have cemented its position as a leading provider of cutting edge health care solutions and wellness services not only to Filipinos, but to international patients as well. Margaret A. Bengzon, Head of TMC's Strategic Services attributed the bullish performance largely to a combination of service development and aggressive cost management strategies. "We improved our financial strength during this time of economic uncertainty by continuing to invest in product innovation, quality improvement and institutional marketing, while aggressively managing costs to protect and even enhance profits," Bengzon said. "We strengthened and streamlined our supply chain processes, thereby generating significant annualized savings. In addition, we availed of incentives offered by the Board of Investments to expanding health care institutions, and enjoyed considerable tax benefits," Bengzon said.

TMC expanded its Wellness Program—which now includes Fitness, Nutrition, Weight Management, Aesthetic Surgery and Dermatology. Services under this expanded program are being performed at the new Wellness and Aesthetic Center, a plush two-storey structure that has been built above TMC's Podium building. The new facility is a "one-stop shop" for a comprehensive line of diagnostic and therapeutic interventions, and is equipped with its own imaging facilities, a dermatology laser unit, surgery suite and patient rooms.

The TMC Cardiovascular Program was also strengthened with the purchase of a 128-slice CT scan. The first in the country, the premier adaptive scanner delivers highly accurate images while obtaining extremely fast coverage. It is able to perform the most complex and advanced diagnostic examinations for Cardiology and other clinical areas. To attest to the Cardiovascular Program's capabilities, a Transposition of the Great Artery (TGA) Repair was performed successfully on a female infant, the first in the Philippines. The TGA is just one of several advanced surgical procedures that TMC's Cardiovascular Program began offering in 2008. 2008 also marked the year that TMC's Cancer Program fortified its leadership position in the country in offering truly customized Cancer care by adopting a unique multidisciplinary team approach and applying innovative molecular technologies for Cancer prevention, early detection, diagnosis and treatment. Key areas of engagement of the Program are Breast, Colorectal, Head and Neck and Liver Cancers.

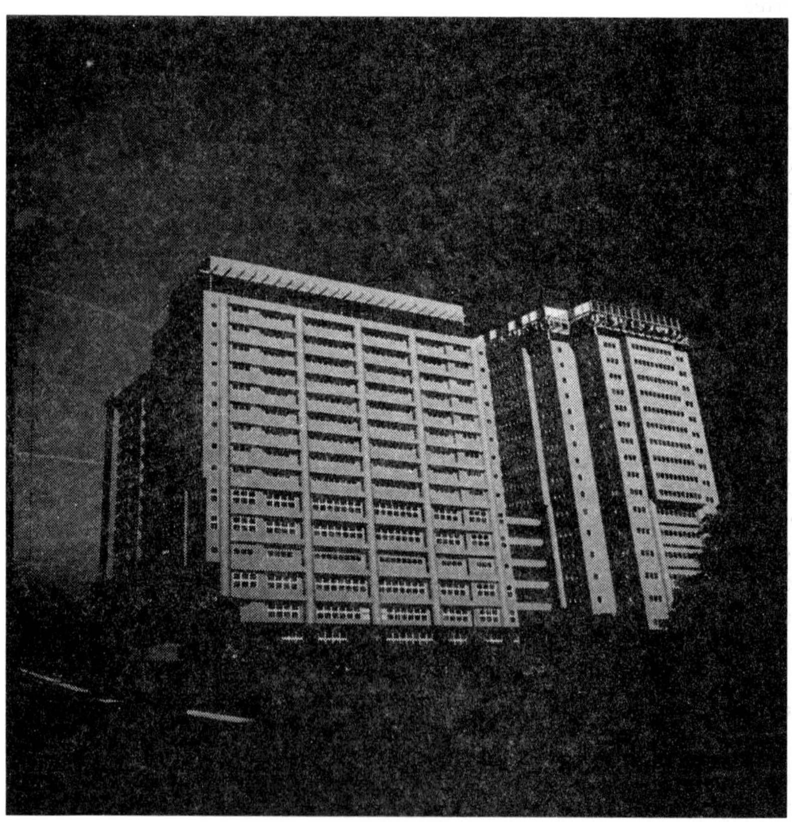

TMC's Breast Clinic provided the first Mammotome Breast Biopsy System in the country, a system that allows computer-guided, minimally invasive biopsies that preserve breast tissue and can be done quickly and safely. Among all private hospitals in the Philippines, the TMC's Colorectal Unit has performed the most number of minimally-invasive, laparoscopic operations for Colorectal Cancer, and has the highest rate of anal sphincter preservations. Similarly, the Unit has treated the most number of Rectal Cancer cases with pre-operative Chemo-Radiotherapy, and boasts of the greatest number of patients in a private hospital setting whose tumors disappeared after employing this treatment protocol.

The Head and Neck Cancer Unit is composed of the strongest multidisciplinary Head and Neck Cancer team in the country, treating the most number of private patients in this field, and performing highly-complex restorative face and voice reconstruction procedures.

The Liver Cancer Unit is likewise situated, boasting of a team of internationally renowned Liver Surgeons, Transplant Surgeons and Hepatologists, as well as fully equipped facilities for Liver Resection and Transplant. The Liver Unit was responsible for the first Selective Internal Radioactive Therapy (SIRT) procedure performed in the Philippines, a procedure that involves the injection of radioactive microspheres into the arteries that lead into the tumor to cut-off its blood supply.

TMC's Regenerative Medicine Program offers revolutionary therapies that harness the body's ability to heal itself, providing unprecedented opportunities to respond to debilitating diseases for which there are few known or no cures. 2008 enhancements included a new clinic and laboratory equipped with the latest technology in cellular study, processing and storage. The Program is indeed a leader in its field, representing the largest scale of operations and delivering the broadest scope of services in the country by far. TMC last year launched its "Talk to Doc" campaign on TV, and print media. In addition, TMC conducted road shows to promote its international patient services in the United States and its territories in the Pacific, the Middle East, Japan, Korea and Taiwan.

TMC also leveraged the World Wide Web to reach out to a broader clientele base with the launch of www.asktmc.com. This interactive website allows web users to conduct a virtual tour of the hospitals facilities, book appointments for services and consultations, research medical and health concerns, and direct medical questions to TMC's cyber doctors. "With our successful strategic thrusts of high-value, high impact service development, accompanied by robust market projection and cost management. The Medical City is truly well-positioned to achieve even steeper trajectories in growth and leadership in the years to come," Bengzon said.

Medical City buys Iloilo-based chain of hospitals and clinics

A Metro Manila-based hospital will invest more than P700 million and the latest technology in health care as it embarks on an expansion to Iloilo City. In a statement, Alfredo R.A. Bengzon, The Medical City president and chief executive officer, said the expansion to Iloilo City and other parts of the country would bring "world-class" medical services to the rest of the country. The Medical City has assumed management and operations of the Great Savior International Hospital in Iloilo City and the Global Medical Network in anticipation of a full purchase before the year ends. It has also acquired sister sites of Great Savior and Global Medical Network in Luzon which includes the Mercedes Medical Center in Pampanga and a network of outpatient clinics in Dagupan, Olongapo and Cavite. These clinics are accredited by Tricare, the worldwide health care program that services retired US military servicemen and their dependents.

The acquisition brings the number of Medical City locations to 18. Its main complex is located on a 1.5-hectare property on Ortigas Avenue in Pasig City.

The Medical City has 40 years of experience in hospital operation and administration, serving some 40,000 inpatients and 380,000 outpatients a year. Mr. Bengzon said they found the Great Saviour network, headed by Evangeline C. Johnson, was ideal for Medical City's expansion plans. Initially, the Medical City has allocated P150 million for the upgrade of the Iloilo hospital building.

Some P600 million will be spent for the acquisition of equipment such as a 4D CAT scan and construction of additional wards. "Some P400 million will be set aside for the Iloilo hospital while the rest will be spent on sister facilities in Luzon," Mr. Bengzon said. Great Savior is a tertiary hospital with a 100-bed capacity. Its sister hospital in Angeles City is a level-two facility with a capacity of 50 beds. Mr. Bengzon said the capacity would be expanded to 200 beds with the construction of another building. Mr. Bengzon also said the acquisition of Great Savior's five clinics in Iloilo City and Luzon would allow the Medical City to serve retired US military servicemen under the Tri-care system. The Medical City will bring to Iloilo a regenerative medicine program which uses stem cell technology in curing cancer and cardiovascular diseases.

Meanwhile, Ms. Johnson denied reports she had sold Great Saviors because it is bleeding financially. She said it was the Medical City that approached her. "No, we're not losing. Just like any entity, we also experienced birth pains but we hurdled past them. Would a top corporation like the Medical City buy a bankrupt hospital?" Ms. Johnson said. Mr. Bengzon said the Medical City also looked into controversies such as the alleged Tricare and Philhealth claims scams involving Ms. Johnson and her medical network but said his group was convinced the hospital and its management had nothing to do with them. The Medical City: Where Patients are Partners Excerpts from a recent interview conducted with Margaret Bengzon, group head strategic services.

Question: The Medical City places much emphasis on a holistic approach to health care as well as a "partnership approach" in treating patients. Can you outline where the origins of these approaches came from and how they have grown over the years? Do you see any changes to this approach or are you satisfied it has worked for The Medical City?

Answer: Forty years of experience have helped us to understand that patient health care can no longer be delivered the traditional way-a one-sided engagement wherein the doctor tells the patient what to do and the patient just obeys. Health care delivery must evolve.

Our patient partnership philosophy stems from TMC's belief that the doctor and patient are at parity.

TMC works hard to train our doctors to understand the patient-partnership philosophy by teaching them how to better engage the patient and understand the patient's lifestyle.

On the other side of the partnership—our Center for Patient for Partnership strives to provide good patient educational materials, support groups and classes for various diseases like diabetes, cancer and strokes that are made available to the general public. By equipping our patients and potential patients with the facts and practical knowledge about their health situation, then they will be in a better position to engage their doctors in a discussion about their health care requirements.

In a recent survey conducted by Scribevision, an independent marketing consultant, 47 percent of their respondents indicated that TMC is the most preferred hospital among the country's top five leading tertiary care institutions and this is attributed largely to our patient partnership approach in delivering health services.

We will continue to espouse this philosophy for the years to come and back this up with the best medical expertise and technological advances that make sense from the patient and business perspectives.

Q: For an American patient to get on a plane and cross the Pacific Ocean for treatment in the Philippines, distance as well as travel time could be a major obstacle. Obviously cost is a great motivation with costs in the Philippines around 60 percent less than the equivalent in the United States. Are there any other reasons that strike you as important, as to why Americans should come to the Philippines and specifically to The Medical City for treatment?

A: Caring for others selflessly is very much in our DNA and this is partly what makes Filipino health care professionals in demand in the Americas, Europe, Southeast Asia and the Middle East.

As such, the natural approach of Filipino health care professionals and providers is very personalized. This is a qualitative trait that cannot be measured in terms of dollars and cents but certainly goes a long way in helping put the patient in the right mindset of healing.

Q: How do you rank the Philippines alongside other major Southeast Asia medical tourism destinations like Thailand or Singapore? And what are the advantages of seeking treatment in the Philippines as opposed to other destinations?

A: The Philippines is on equal footing with the world's best and with the collaboration of the private sector with the different government agencies, the Philippines will see a significant rise in international patient influx in the coming months.

The Philippines is also host to a number of pioneering efforts like in the case of TMC, our main area of innovation is in regenerative medicine - treatments that involve stem cell and molecular biology to address a whole range of needs from staying well to recovering from very serious illnesses including advanced renal failure, cancer, cardiovascular disease, strokes and Alzheimer's disease. This is an area where we are actually ahead of medical institutions abroad.

Last but certainly not least, Filipinos have strong communication skills in English and the country has one of the world's highest literacy rates.

Q: In 2006, The Medical City was awarded the prestigious, JCI (Joint Commission International) accreditation. Has this helped to boost the number of patients that come from abroad? What is the ratio of Filipino versus international patients?

What does The Medical City have to do to maintain the standards that the JCI demands?

A: The volume of our patients is still locally based. While the numbers of international patients are still small, there is a clear trend of steady growth given a more concerted effort by the private and government sectors to boost the country's bid as an international patient destination of choice.

TMC has established dedicated JCI task forces to ensure that we are always in compliance with the JCI directives and initiatives in areas such as access to care, continuity of care, quality improvement and patient safety. We are in the process now of gearing up for re-accreditation by the JCI in 2010.

Q: What is The Medical City doing to attract business from abroad and specifically the United States?

We invest in relationships with credible publications such as The *Washington Times*.

We conduct regular road shows in various cities in the United States, either in tandem with the Philippine Department of Tourism or with international event organizers or even on our own initiative. We recently participated as a major sponsor at the fourth World Health Tourism Congress (WHTC) which was hosted by the Philippines. There were delegates from Arab nations, Europe, Southeast Asia and North America.

We are also building relationships and forming synergies with a number of international partners, i.e. corporate clients, vendors, health care insurance providers and travel agencies specializing in medical tourism.

Q: Lastly, there are so many different titles that an article on The Medical City could have: "The Capital of Health," "A Medical Sanctuary," "Partnering with Patients" are among the few that spring to mind. Which do you like the best? Or perhaps you have another idea for one?

A: The Medical City: Where Patients are Partners.

In estimated more than half-a-million Americans traveled overseas for medical and health tourism in 2006. By the end of 2009, this number, according to some experts, may reach several millions. For Americans, the main motivation is financial because of ever escalating health care costs in the United States.

Clearly, the global health care industry is expanding with the Philippines poised to capture a chunk of that market. The country's world-class physicians and its modern medical facilities equipped with the latest technology are major factors for the growth of its medical tourism program, according to Cynthia Carrion, undersecretary for sports and wellness tourism. Her department comes under the umbrella of the Department of Tourism which sends an obvious signal to the world that the Philippines means business in this area.

Tourism secretary, Ace Durano, says, "The Philippines welcomes guests to take advantage of the value for money offered by our health and wellness tourism program through high quality medical services."

The Public-Private Partnership Task Force on globally competitive Philippines industries (PPPTF) is composed of leaders from many disciplines, including doctors and hospital directors. The latter form an important group focusing on promoting health and wellness and disseminating informational programs.

One group is "The Medical City," a private tertiary care hospital that has been working in this field for over 40 years providing complete health and wellness programs for all ages.

According to Cynthia Carrion, a good number of Filipino doctors received their medical training in the United States and interned in U.S. hospitals. Returning to the Philippines, they have shared their knowledge with younger practitioners at some of the country's renowned medical centers such as The Medical City and St. Luke's Hospital.

In addition, Filipinos are inherently caring and compassionate which provides a genuine recipe for success in the health care field, notes the undersecretary.

The Medical City: Where Patients are Partners.

Excerpts from a recent interview conducted with Margaret Bengzon, group head strategic services.

Question: The Medical City places much emphasis on a holistic approach to health care as well as a "partnership approach" in treating patients. Can you outline where the origins of these approaches came from and how they have grown over the years? Do you see any changes to this approach or are you satisfied it has worked for The Medical City?

Answer: Forty years of experience have helped us to understand that patient health care can no longer be delivered the traditional way—a one-sided engagement wherein the doctor tells the patient what to do and the patient just obeys. Health care delivery must evolve.

Our patient partnership philosophy stems from TMC's belief that the doctor and patient are at parity.

TMC works hard to train our doctors to understand the patient-partnership philosophy by teaching them how to better engage the patient and understand the patient's lifestyle.

St. Luke's Medical Center: A look at the future of health care

The recently inaugurated 629-bed St. Luke's Medical Center (SLMC) at Bonifacio Global City built at the cost of P9 billion surpasses all preconceptions of what a hospital should be. Surely, the primary requisites of highly qualified medical professionals, excellent clinical care, and top-notch medical and diagnostic equipment are in place. But with the addition of world-class design by RR Payumo and Associates, an important collection of Filipino art, and painstaking attention to its clientele's convenience and comfort, the facility sets new standards for the health industry in the region

"This is the future of health care," says Dr. Joven Cuanang, medical director and senior vice president for medical affairs. "Our goal is to be one of the preferred destinations in the world. We benchmarked against the very best medical centers in the United States, Europe, and Asia for excellence in clinical outcome and delivery of care. The whole gamut of services that we offer encompasses health promotion, disease prevention, curative phase, and rehabilitative medicine."

To promote quick and accurate diagnosis, the hospital has invested in the latest high-end technology. State-of-the-art diagnostic equipment include the Philips 3 Tesla Magnetic Resonance Imaging System and a 256-Slice Computed Axial Technology (CT) Scanner. In addition, devices such as an Extra Corporeal Shockwave Myocardial Revascularization System (ESMR), Prone Breast Biopsy System, and Automated Breast Volume Scanner empower physicians to give patients the best medical care.

"St. Luke's Medical Center president Jose Ledesma is very passionate about being up-to-date with the latest technology," confirms Dr. Cuanang. "In the Philippines, we are the leader in this particular field. I daresay that we are, in fact, better in terms of technology than 95 percent of all hospitals in the United States." Adding that the same cutting-edge equipment is available locally only at the St. Luke's Hospital in Quezon City, he quips, "We compete with ourselves."

As an institution accredited by the Joint Commission on International Accreditation, the world's most prestigious accrediting body for international health care organizations, St. Luke's has its fair share of medical tourists. Dr. Cuanang estimates that five to eight percent of patients at the St. Luke's Hospital in Quezon City come from abroad. Still, he emphasizes, "The more important aspect is serving our own countrymen. There is no need for Filipinos to go abroad for medical concerns because here is a hospital that can offer the same services, the same expertise, and the same level of customer care. Without the need for foreign travel, cost of care is significantly reduced."

Perhaps, however, what sets St. Luke's Medical Center above other health care organizations is its resolve to achieve excellence in customer care. This is developed using the Four Seasons template for luxurious service, so that the entire hospital staff is even more attentive towards maintaining efficiency and a pleasant hospital environment. "We train all our people, from the security guards to the cleaners—to be customer care officers. Our aim for both St. Luke's hospitals is to give our patients a delightful experience even if, or especially because, they are sick." With 60 customer care officers on call to attend to the patients' various needs, the institution seeks to establish life-long relationships based on dependability and trust.

"We are very passionate about maintaining quality." This is the rationale for the hospital's Center for Quality and Patient Safety. To keep up with the latest world standards, eight senior staff members were sent for courses at the Institute of Health Care Improvement in Cambridge, Massachusetts. "We adhere to international patient safety codes."

For even more comfortable hospital stays, patients at St. Luke's in Bonifacio Global City are provided computers with free Internet connection in their suites, 24/7 concierge service, an area designated for shopping and dining, a grand lobby, landscaped decks, and even a piano bar. While individual suites are tastefully furnished, patients who are especially particular about luxurious accommodations can be ferried to the hospital by helicopter and stay in the 157-square-meter presidential suite that goes for P50,000 a night.

However, most impressive was the Bonifacio Global City hospital's vast collection of Filipino art. During our quick tour of the facility, we took careful notice of sculptures by Ramon Orlina and Daniel dela Cruz, paintings by Bencab, Angel Cacnio, Elmer Borlongan, Jose John Santos, and photographs by Wig Tysmans. There are numerous artworks that still need to be displayed and Cuanang has taken it upon himself to find places in the hospital for these.

"My greatest gratification is that the patients get well and that they are happy with the service," says the neurologist who regularly spends 12-hour work days for clinical practice and administrative duties. "Why do I put up paintings in the walls of St. Luke's? My philosophy is that you must take extra effort to make the environment in the hospital setting delightful. This hospital, after all, is a showcase of the best in healing and the arts. As a center for excellence in the medical arts and the finest in Filipino art, we are creating a destination that will be the embodiment of the best in the Philippines."

Other Hospitals in Medical Tourism

- **Philippine Heart Center—Quezon City**
  Established in 1975, the Philippine Heart Center is regarded as one of the most active cardiac care treatment and surgery center in the Asia-Pacific region. Located in a 2.7 hectare facility with two hospitals and a medical arts building, the institution offers various cardiac, cardio-pulmonary and cardiovascular procedures for both local and international patients.

- **Asian Hospital and Medical Center—Muntinlupa City**
  Established only in 2002, the Asian Hospital is the first major private health facility in the south of Metro Manila. Success came quickly, as in 2005 it received an award as the Most Outstanding Modern Hospital. It offers world-class treatments and facilities catering to both local and international patients seeking various health services including Cardiology, Cosmetic Surgery, Dermatology, Executive Health Screening, Oncology, General Surgery and Urology among others.

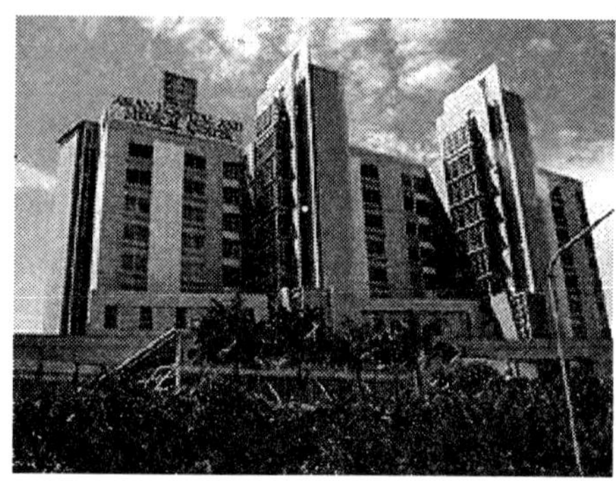

- **American Hospital Chain**
  Cardiovascular Hospitals of America, a U.S. hospital chain, reportedly will build a state-of-the-art, medical tourism center in Cebu City in the Philippines. The Antara News-Asia Pulse quoted Dr. Philip S. Chua, CHA's vice-president for Far East operations, that the proposed American Medical Center Cebu will be accredited by the Joint Commission International, U.S. Blue Cross/Blue Shield and U.S. Medicare agencies. He said the facility will serve as dedicated center for medical tourism in the country. Chua said medical tourism is growing into a major industry in Malaysia, India, and Thailand. He said the Philippines can expect to do better, given its resources, talent and knowledge of the English language.
- **Manila Doctors Hospital—Ermita, Manila**
  Established in 1956, this ISO-certified health facility is a private tertiary hospital that offers various health and medical services catering to local and international patients. Among the services offered are Industrial Medicine, Nuclear Medicine, Radiology, Rehabilitation Medicine, Special Diagnostics, Laboratory Medicine and other Clinical services.

The following procedures are more common among non-Filipino medical tourists:

- Aesthetic procedures

- Cosmetic surgery
- Dentistry
- Dermatology
- Eye Surgery and Ophthalmology
- Fertility Treatment
- General Surgery
- Hair Transplantation
- Rehabilitation
- Weight Loss Surgery
- Stem Cell Therapy

The following are cost comparisons between medical procedures in the Philippines and equivalent procedures in the United States:

	US Hospitals	*Philippines*	*Average Savings*
Medical Procedures			
Coronary Artery Bypass Surgery	$70,000 - $133,000	$11,500 - $17,500	83% - 86%
Heart-valve Replacement	$75,000 - $140,000	$14,000 - $21,000	81% - 85%
Laparoscopic Gastric Bypass	$35,000 - $52,000	$2,000 - $3,500	92% - 94%
Hip Replacement	$33,000 - $57,000	$5,000 - $7,600	84% - 86%
Knee Replacement	$30,000 - $53,000	$5,200 - $7,700	82% - 85%
Prostate surgery (TURP procedure)	$10,000 - $16,000	$1,500 - $2,700	83% - 85%
Liver Transplant	$290,000 - $310,000	$120,000 - $150,000	51% - 58%
Kidney Transplant	$200,000 - $250,000	$23,000 - $25,000	88% - 90%
Plastic and Reconstructive Surgery			
Tummy Tuck (Abdominoplasty)	$6,000 - $10,000	$3,000 - $4,000	50% - 60%
Face Lift (rhytidectomy)	$10,500 -16,000	$3,500 - $4,500	66% - 71%
Breast Augmentation (Mammoplasty)	$7,500 - $8,500	$3,000 - $3,500	58% - 60%
Breast Reduction	$8,000 - $10,000	$3,000 - $3,200	62% - 68%
Complete Liposuction (lipoplasty)	$13,000 - $14,000	$3,000 - $4,000	71% - 76%
Nose Surgery (Rhinoplasty)	$5,500 - $6,500	$2,000 - $2,500	61% - 63%
Eye / Ophthalmology			
Cataract surgery	$1,500 - $2,500	$800 - $900	46% - 64%
General and Cosmetic Dentistry			
Dental Implant	$3,500 - $5,500	$500 - $600	85% - 89%

Malpractice Laws in the Philippines

In the Philippines, there are adequate provisions in the Philippine Revised Penal Code for medical malpractice that would protect patients against medical negligence and incompetence from erring or criminal physicians. On top of this, the Republic Act #9173 or the Philippine Nursing Act of 2002 has also been passed by Congress to guarantee the delivery of basic health services through adequate and competent nursing personnel in the country. Significant awards have been awarded to victims of confirmed medical malpractice cases as well as fines meted out by the Department of Health on erring physicians. However, according to the Philippine Medical Association in a Medical Malpractice Workshop conducted in 2005, such medical malpractice incidence account only for a mere 0.00003% of the total number of affected patients. The Philippine Congress and the Senate continue to file bills related to medical malpractice and health care liability, although the medical sector continue to oppose passing of these resolutions, stating that these are detrimental to the health care industry in the country.

Pros

- Prices of medical procedures are very cost-effective.
- Medical staffs are trained to international standards, and many doctors are trained in Western countries.
- Hospitals catering to health tourism have state-of-the-art facilities.
- English is widely spoken among the medical staff, and by the general public.
- 5-star hotel room accommodation are available at very affordable prices
- There are several choice vacation destinations in the Philippines that are perfect for fast and relaxing recovery after a medical procedure

Cons

- Flight times from the US, Canada and Europe are long and may not be conducive for patients with certain medical conditions.
- There are clear differences in the levels of quality and offered health care services between private health institutions and public health providers. Good medical tourism packages are offered mostly in private institutions and are not available in public hospitals or clinics.

Traveling to the Philippines

All major airline carriers travel to the Philippines directly from major cities in the USA, Canada, the Middle-East, Europe and the rest of Asia.

Average estimated travel time in hours

From/To	*Philippines*
New York	18
Los Angeles	15
Miami	19
Montreal	17
Quebec	16
Toronto	17
Sydney	8
Riyadh	10
Dubai	9
Oman	9
Kuwait	10
Singapore	3

The following are the visa requirements for entry or stay in the Philippines:

- Foreign nationals from the USA, Canada, UK, Australia, Kuwait, UAE, Saudi Arabia, Asian countries, and other countries specified in a list released by the Philippine Department of Foreign Affairs can enter the country without a visa for a period not exceeding 21 days provided they have a 6-month valid passport and a return ticket. Visitors who wish to stay longer are required to have a visa.
- Foreign nationals from Afghanistan, Bangladesh, India, Iran, Iraq, North Korea and other countries not in the list are required to have a visa even if the stay is less than 7 days.
- Holders of Brazilian and Israeli passports can enter without a visa and stay for a period not exceeding 59 days.
- Holders of Hong Kong Special Administrative Region, British National Overseas, Macao-issue Portuguese passports, and Macao Special Administrative Region passports can enter and stay without a visa for a period not exceeding seven days.

South Korean medical tourism

Seoul, Korea is one of the emerging leading destinations for medical tourism and global health care in the world. The 1st Asia Medical Tourism and Global Health Care Congress took place in April 13-15, 2010 in Seoul, Korea as a joint initiative between the Medical Tourism Association (MTA), Korean Health Industry Development Institute (KHIDI).

The 1st Global Health Care and Medical Tourism Korea Congress featured 800 attendees from over 25 countries and focused on the high quality of health care available in Asia. It also brought together the stakeholders involved in Asian medical tourism for intense networking event and educational opportunities. Seoul City intends to boost tourism as one of its top priority tasks for 2010, and the metropolitan government is ambitiously seeking to attract 10 million foreign tourists this year. The city will try to attract more Chinese tourists as their number is expected to rise due to a loosening of visa regulations. It is seeking to boost the medical tourism industry, and hopes to increase the number of medical tourists to 52,000 from 37,000 recorded in 2009, out of a total of 50,000 for all South Korea.

The city plans to offer a range of support programs for foreign medical tourists and improve related rules and regulations to reinvigorate medical tourism. It will also seek to intensify publicity efforts to attract more foreign patients. The city plans to develop a set of special tourism products targeting Chinese tourists, which will enable them to visit major tourist attractions where they can experience Korean food, culture and advanced technology. For 2010, it seeks to attract 1.8 million Chinese tourists. Last year, 1.34 million Chinese people visited Seoul. In 2010, Korea is expecting to attract around 60,000 medical tourists and the target is to attract 140,000 in 2015. Korea's cosmetic surgery clinics are packed with foreign patients. In the past, the patients were largely from China, Hong Kong and Singapore, but recently they have diversified and now they come from Indonesia, Saudi Arabia, the UK and the USA.

Foreign visitors spent more than US $60 million in Korea for medical treatment during the first nine months of 2009. The Bank of Korea says health care travel revenue between January and September jumped 29 percent from the same period last year while health-related outbound travel expenditures recorded a 35 percent drop at $69 million. Medical tourism has increased rapidly as the quality of medical treatment in the country improved and the Korean won weakened against other currencies in early 2009. Foreign patients in Korea reportedly spend twice as much money as regular Japanese tourists. Cosmetic surgery among Asians reflects the "Korean Wave." Cost is not an issue, as they are willing to pay upto three times more for surgery in Korea. Asian women from China, Taiwan, Vietnam, Singapore and Hong Kong are flocking to Korea for facial bone contouring and cosmetic surgery on their eyes and noses. Asians from other territories want to look more like popular Korean actors and musicians, and they are willing to travel and pay upto three times more than they would in China.

Daegu Medicity Korea

Daegu Medicity is the new name for Daegu hospital association. It will utilize Korea's top information technology and cutting edge medical equipment. South Korea's LG Electronics and Daegu Metropolitan City will join hands to develop the medical industry of Daegu. Daegu's medical facilities are well known esp. in the field of cancer, hospice, medical robotic equipment and advanced medical care. This city has strong medical infrastructure, 5 medical colleges, 11 general hospitals, 15 dental clinics, 9 oriental medicine clinics, 22,000 medical personnel including 5000 doctors.

LG Electronics announced on March 31 that its CTO Woo-hyun Baek and Mayor Bum-Il Kim of Daegu signed a partnership agreement at the City hall on the 30th to build up Daegu's medical industry. Under this partnership, the two parties will cooperate in the following areas; promotion of the smart-care service pilot project (remote treatment and care services for patients with chronic illness using IT); founding of the High-Tech Medical Complex and fostering the local medical equipment industry; and establishment of medical industry policies. According to Mayor Kim, the successful inducement of the Daegu-Gyeongbuk High-Tech Medical Complex has contributed to making Daegu a true "Medicity" and LG Electronics' health care solution and business experience will be helpful in this context. CTO Baek showed confidence in bringing success to the smartcare service pilot project through active cooperation with Daegu Metropolitan City.

Thailand is in the forefront of Medical Tourism. It has improved health care for its citizens also. (See Appendix 3 at the end of the book: Health System in Thailand).

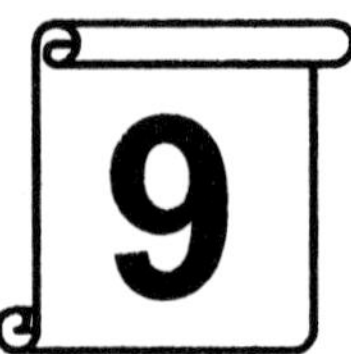

Proposed Model of Medical City in India: A Dream or Reality

It has been stated by experts that Medical city model of health care can work in this country. Medical cities would not only provide world class medical treatment to the citizens of India but would also attract a large number of health tourists from the globe, far and near. The medical city will not limit its activity to administering only medical and surgical treatment. It will provide, administer and supervise primary health care as well. It will train and educate the necessary medical, paramedical and nursing personnel to fulfil the needs of other hospitals in the region. In addition it will be a centre of research for generic medicines and pharmaceuticals, biotechnology and stem cell research and an epicenter of medical and health conventions. It will also interact with the community to make them aware and to provide services for prevention of disease and development of health and fitness of the community. Since India is short of 30 lakh hospital beds as per CII study, setting up of large medical cities with 5000-10000 beds would be a good beginning to meet the demands. For this involvement of corporate houses and foreign collaboration will be required. This entails making the health care sector an attractive avenue of investment. Since procurement of land has become the most ticklish issue all over the country, this has to be facilitated. The role of Government is paramount in these two matters. The government has also to act as a regulator and supervisor and oversee the process of accreditation and implementation of quality control and fair delivery of the committed facilities.

In addition, the medical city should have holistic approach with provision for CAM as well as spiritual healing. (See Appendix attached to the chapter: Global Hospital and Research Centre, Mount Abu).

Why medical cities are the in thing!

Most Public hospitals being overburdened and corporate hospitals being well managed but extortionist in their approach, both have their own problems. Resultantly, the country is suffering from stark contrast; inadequate health care for the public at large on the one hand and excellence in surgery and infrastructure in the corporate hospitals for the 'chosen few' on the other hand. For a huge country like India with health care the current buzz, it is hardly surprising that medical cities seem to be surfacing on the horizon. A chain of Medicare cities all over the country can improve the health care for countrymen, provided a balance is reached viz. well managed cluster of hospitals but with a motto of service for the people of India/world.

The recommendation: Chandigarh Administration to set-up Medical city

The author working as honorary advisor to the Chandigarh administration, through the tourism department had conceived and recommended the setting up a Medical city. This model implied setting up of similar medical cities in various parts of the country to improve the health care of the nation and to promote health tourism for revenue generation. The name recommended was Chandigarh Medicare City (CMCC). The name CMCC was coined on the pattern of Dubai Health Care City (DHCC). The author studied the model of DHCC and advised to adopt a modified, enhanced and improved model of DHCC, in setting up the CMCC. Dubai Health Care City (DHCC), has taken a monumental step towards becoming a regional center of excellence for health care delivery. The Center has Harvard Medical International (HMI) and Mayo clinic as its partners, besides others. The example of Bumrungrad hospital, Thailand, the best hospital from Medical tourism point of view, as a management-model for the proposed Medicare city may also be considered. This will also require modification as per local needs, resources and to showcase the best before the world.

CMCC can be a unique facility and serve as a model of Medicare for rest of the country. Thus, the announcement of Chandigarh Medicare city has not come too soon, whereas the city-beautiful is catering to the medical needs of 600 lakh citizens of the region.

Chandigarh has credibility in health care sector

As a locus of political and economic stability and being a vibrant city, Chandigarh is in a position to serve the region's needs for high-quality health care, and to be a model for institution-building in the region. The CMCC administration has to commit itself to the principle of accessibility for all, to professional and academic development, and to international recognition for quality of care as well as patient privacy, rights, and satisfaction. This entails world class infrastructure, world class faculty and accreditation with JCI.

At Chandigarh the intention is to have a multi-superspecialty hospital with expertise in 20 medical disciplines and 8-10 sub-specialties in each, besides making it a centre of training for the trainers and centre of international medical conventions. Since this will be a unique centre providing world class surgical/medical services, this will attract international patients as well, in good numbers. Keen to take advantage of low-cost health care in India, the US is pushing its insurance firms to draw up attractive medical tourism packages with Indian hospitals to facilitate travel and treatment for its citizens there. The cost of services will have to be reasonable and affordable at this centre, to become people-friendly institution.

Concept of a medical/health city

The concept of a medical or health city entails a cluster of hospitals, a holistic health care centre; a large hospital sprawled across hundreds of acres of land? Certainly. But it doesn't end here. In simpler terms, the difference between a hospital and a medicare city is as vast as the difference between a corner shop and a mega store. In what could be the beginning of a medical renaissance, Medicare cities could change the way medical education and research and development is conducted in India, taking it from public to private to corporate.

The cluster of towers; one each for one superspecialty

The cluster should have at least the following wings, each given on royalty to a top hospital group/corporate house. If paucity of land is the issue, it can grow vertically; each block being a skyscraper so that world class and adequate facilities can be created.

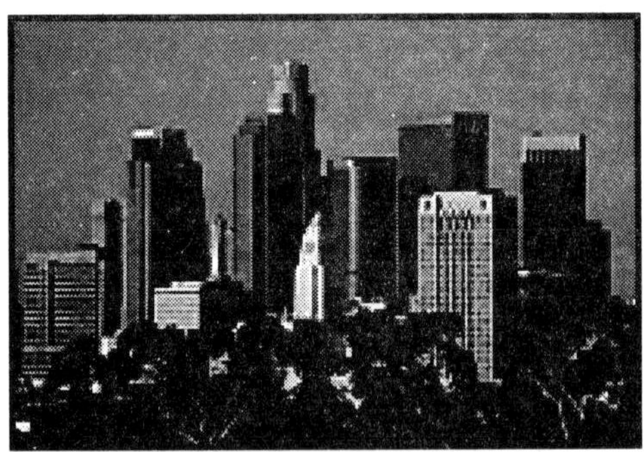

- Oncology—Tata, Mumbai
- Cardiology—Narayana, Bangalore
- Cosmetic and reconstructive surgery—Ambani-Kokilaben medical centre, Mumbai
- Orthopedics and Neurosurgery, sports and rehabilitative medicine—Wockhardt
- Ophthalmology—Mayo clinic
- Pediatric and gynecology—Harvard medical International

- o Geriatrics and obesity, multiple organ transplant, stem cell centre—Apollo
- o Dental and oral surgery block—Manipal group
- o Centre of training of the trainers: medical/nursing/paramedical education, tele-medicine, NRIS
- o Primary Medicare centre—free service on the pattern of Sri Ramachandran hospital, Chennai
- o Imaging and laboratory wing—Fortis
- o Convention centre, cafeteria, underground parking, - Chandigarh administration/P. builder
- o Pharmacy and clinical research—Niper

This will have an estimated outlay of $5 billions and can yield a revenue of $ 1 billion per year to begin with.

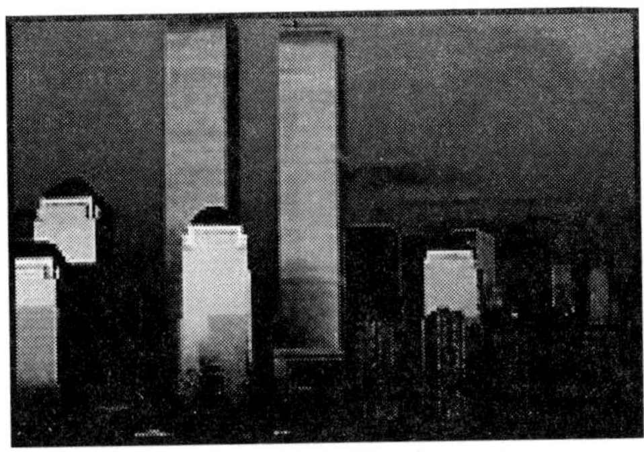

Indian Medical city; a concept

- o People traveling across borders for health care needs
- o Only ambulatory care can be really linked to tourism
- o Tourism is recreation linked. Is health recreation linked?
- o Serious ailments e.g Heart Surgery, Joint replacements, etc. which can be treated in Indian Hospitals without any waiting can not be linked with Tourism
- o Worlds largest after retailing
- o Global health care revenue US$ 2.8 trillion
- o India's health care industry worth US$ 17 billion; to grow by 13% per annum for next 6 years
- o In 2004, India treated 1.8 Lac patients. This is to grow substantially at the rate 25-30% in 2005
- o Medical tourism could account for 3-5% of the total health care delivery market
- o India is rated amongst the world's "must see top ten destination" by Conde Naste (international magazine)
- o A study by CII Mckinsey estimates that country could earn 5000-10,000 crore by 2012

- o Health procedures across world show 200-800% cost difference SAARC, AFRICAS, MIDDLE EAST
- o No advance care available e.g Afghanistan, Nepal and Bangladesh, etc.
- o Limited specialized care

WEST

- o Long waiting—UK
- o Insurance unaffordable leading to semi-insured and uninsured population—US
- o Private hospitals very expensive

Quality

Large pool of doctors, nurses and paramedics

Strength — Over 650,000 doctors;
— Highly skilled experts; and
— Possess English-speaking skills.

Comfort Level

- o NRI doctors recognized as amongst best in adopted countries (First World)
- o Usage of English
- o Indian Nurses increasingly getting international exposure

Value Proposition

Quality medical services at 1/10th costs:

- o Complicated surgical procedures possible at 1/10th the cost
- o Increase in use of Computerized Hospital Information Systems
- o Software technologists facilitating tech revolution in health care
- o State-of-the-art medical establishments of great repute

India's cost effectiveness

- o A cataract surgery costs a fraction of the cost in India as compared to abroad, i.e. (most common)

Cataract surgery

USA—2,000$, India—450$
UK—14,00$

- o Lasik surgery
  USA/UK—3,000-5000
  India—850 $
- o No waiting period

Procedure	US	UK	Burmungrad Bangkok	Max Health care	Raffles Singapore
Angioplasty	30000	21000	5000	4000	5000
Angiography	2500	2000	1100	400	800
Hip replacement	19000	13000		6000	6600
Knee replacement	27000	16000		6000	6000
CABG	30000			6400	9600
Lasik		2250	750	400	

The prices are in US $.

Lower Medication cost

- o Strong Pharma Sector and gaining world recognition
- o Fast emerging as major Drug R&D Center
- o Strong Generic drugs business
- o Low cost of drug development in India
- o No waiting

Tourist Interest

- o 5000 year old civilization
- o Renowned for Historical, Cultural and Religious diversity
- o Diverse geographical landmarks; vast coastline
- o Traditional arts and crafts
- o Vibrant democracy: Freedom for citizens; empowered women population

Future focus

- o Uniform Medical Education Standards
- o Industry Accreditation Standards
- o Mandatory Accreditation of all Colleges and Hospitals
- o Target-oriented Infrastructure Investment
- o More Medical, Nursing colleges and Hospitals
- o Regulatory Bodies with Teeth
- o Government soft loan to Private Players

- o Tax Holiday and Further Duty Roll Back
- o Apex Industry body under Union List
- o Greater Industry and Govt. Interaction
- o Medical Insurance Reforms
- o Seamless Single-Window Facility to Tourists
- o Government sell India as Medical Tourism Destination
- o GDP Growth
- o Employment in Health Care Sector
- o Employment in Tourism Industry
- o Overall Growth in Commerce
- o Reversal and Arrest of Brain Drain
- o Stimulus to Pharmaceuticals Industry
- o Growth in Insurance Industry
- o Better medical facilities for larger population
- o Catalyzes India to the Club of Global Leaders

Holistic and Spiritual Healing

India has been a world leader in propagating wellness through Yoga, Ayurveda and spiritual healing for a long time. The hospitals in various cities that are known as centers of pilgrimage speak of synergy between religious and wellness tourism. The author visited Mt. Abu in Rajasthan to study this aspect of health tourism and was impressed to see several hospitals and projects being run under 'Global hospitals' under the umbrella of Brahmkumari. They claim that many ailments that are amenable to surgical treatment or are not curable ordinarily can be treated with holistic healing and lifestyle modifications. Some details are given in the appendix attached to this chapter.

Countries with Excellent Medical Cities

Singapore Medicine

- — A multi-agency government initiative involving Singapore Tourism Board, the Economic Development Board and International Enterprise, Singapore
- — Aimed at developing Singapore into one of Asia's leading destinations for health care
- — Positioning Singapore more than a center for the treatment of illness:
  - o Destination where visitors can select from wide range of services to enhance their health and well-being
  - o Includes health screening, medical wellness, aesthetic and anti-ageing programmes

Thailand

— Attracts maximum Americans and western expatriates across South East Asia

— Bangkok, a center for medical tourism
  - o Its International Medical Center offers services in 26 languages and recognizes cultural and religious dietary restrictions

— The medical tour companies that serve Thailand often put emphasis on the vacation aspects
  - o Offering post-recovery resort stays

— Is successful in tapping the health tourism market
  - o Good infrastructure
  - o Aggressive international marketing in conjunction with tourism authority

- Over 60,000 cardiac surgeries done per year with outcomes at par with international standards
- Multi-organ transplants like Renal, Liver, Heart, Bone Marrow Transplants, are successfully performed at one-tenth the cost.
- Patients from over 55 countries treated at Indian Hospitals.

INVESTMENT REQUIRED TO BRIDGE THE GAP IN NEXT 10 YEARS

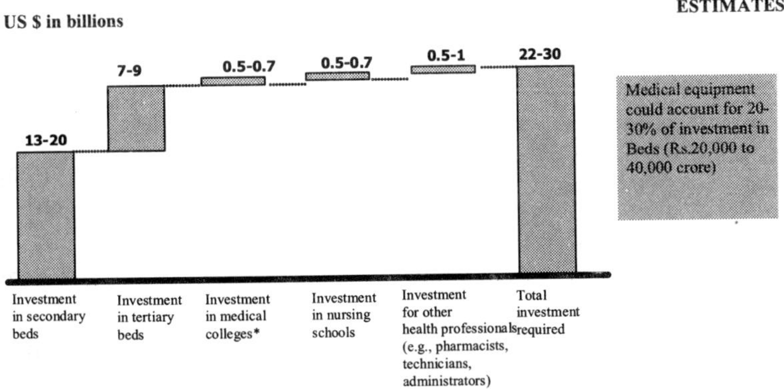

* Excludes investment in bed capacity to avoid double count with investment in secondary/tertiary beds

(Source: CII-McKinsey & Company Report 2002)

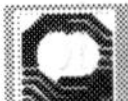

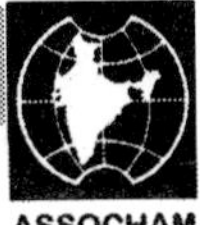

ASSOCHAM

Chandigarh Medical City Project; Bureaucratic perspective

Official sources said here that the Medicity Project has been conceptualized with elements of public private partnership in view and the selected partner will be tasked with setting up an ultra-modern health care facility with a superspecialty hospital and a multi specialty genera! Hospital at the core. The vision, innovation and dynamism of the partner-consortium or a single company are central to the project. The Administration would thus provide an opportunity for the establishment of a Medicity into which the latest international best practices would flow.

The expressions of Interests for the project were called in the month of February 2008 and 19 applicants expressed interest in the project. The Administration had asked them to submit details regarding their concept and their track record in terms of operational and financial viability, etc. The Medicity Project is in fact envisaged as one where the participation of eminent experts and distinguished citizens will help choose the best contender.

Official sources clarified that by far the revenue model for the Medicity has not yet been finalized. It is only after the revenue model has been decided upon that technical presentations can be scheduled, followed by calling of the financial bids. For this an independent consultant, HDFC has been engaged. The consultant has been asked to design a revenue model based on the project features. However, the project is still at the formative stage, with no decision having yet been finalized on these issues.

Under the Medicity project, a superspeciality hospital and a multi-speciality genera! hospital are to be set-up either as two different units or as an integrated hospital with many common facilities. Over all, 25 per cent of the beds are to be reserved for 'poor-free' patients, 30% beds for general patients and 45% for private patients. The Medicity is free to have even more liberal criteria than the ones above. A system of in-built safeguards is being designed for this Project.

The Chandigarh administration would enter into a MoU laying down all the technical parameters and defining in detail the social obligations cast on the Medicity partner in near future. A system of annual social audit will be a part of the project.

The fulfilment of social obligations under the Medicity will be closely observed and governed by a Board of Governors with eminent citizens, medical experts, NGOs, social workers, etc. as members, to sustain the implementation of the social commitment as per the terms and conditions laid out in the MOU for the Medicity, official sources told.

An Administrative Officer from the Chandigarh Administration will also be tasked with day to day monitoring of the social obligations. This MOU is under finalisation, and the inputs of a legal experts and the consultant will also be taken.

One of the most significant safeguards proposed under this project is that the land is to be given on Licence for a period of 33 years in the first instance, extendable further only on the satisfaction of the Chandigarh Administration.

Thus, the Medicity would not involve a sale or transfer of ownership of land. The ownership of the land would continue to vest in the Chandigarh Administration. Stiff penalties including resumption of land are a normal part of such a Licence agreement.

The ownership of the land would continue to vest in the Chandigarh Administration. Stiff penalties including resumption of land are a normal part of such a Licence agreement.

Official sources claimed that the Chandigarh Administration's endeavour is to cater to the future health-care needs of the citizens, with social commitment at the cornerstone of the Medicity. Building more Government Hospitals poses challenges of funding, staffing and management.

The time lag of 10-15 years before such a facility can be planned, designed, built and operational zed can prove costly in terms of public health goals.

The project has, since been scrapped.

Concept of Fortis—Health care group about the Medical City at Chandigarh

The "Fortis Health Care Medicity" will be an entity that has the size, critical mass and capability to develop into a world-wide centre of health care delivery and learning similar to the leading medical institutions of the USA like John Hopkins and Mayo Clinic. An institution, which has exceptional doctors, the best facilities, the latest equipment ensuring cutting-edge research and exceptional treatment. A destination, where patients come not only from India but also from the Middle East, South and South East Asia and later from the developed world due to its superior quality of services and cost effectiveness. An institution, which attracts the best medical students and researchers and in turn helps create world-class doctors. A platform that offers exceptional capabilities in conducting clinical trials and analysis for central laboratory services and research in Bio-Services.

Fortis Health care medicity will thus be an organization that envisages to transform and add value to the practice of medicine; set highest standards for teaching and research in the arena of Medical and Bio Sciences in the country. With individual centres of excellences in different facilities, Fortis Health care medicity will comprise of:

- Medical care facilities for all diseases—tertiary care super-specialty hospitals conforming to international scale and standards.
- Education and training facilities for all types of medical and health personnel.
- A full-fledged medical college for undergraduate and postgraduate courses that would over time be affiliated to the leading medical schools/institutions of either USA or Europe.

- A dental college for undergraduate and postgraduate courses.
- A nursing college.
- College of Technical Training in different disciplines of Medical Services.
- Facilities for primary and applied research in medicine.
- Bio Sciences and Clinical Trials.
- A Rehabilitation Centre-*cum*-Medical Inn for outstation patients and relatives.
- A commercial centre for catering to the needs of patients, relatives and staff in the campus.

At the outset, it is pointed out that the Medicity Project is the subject matter of CWP No. 2553 of 2008 titled Harmeet Singh Grewal *vs.* Union of India and others, pending before the High Court of Punjab and Haryana, with the next date of hearing fixed for 12th December. The matter therefore, is subjudice. The entire process of decision making is, consequently, under the scrutiny of the court and a detailed report on any decisions taken so far will be presented before the court on the next date of hearing. Therefore, questions touching upon the necessity of such a project, the Medicity concept, the revenue model under this project and other operational details are already the subject matter of this Writ Petition and form a part of the comprehensive reply filed by this Administration before the court. They are therefore not being touched upon at this juncture. The Medicity Project is proposed to be set-up on a site measuring 44.8 acres near village Kishangarh. The objective of the Medicity is to offer citizens a wide array of world class health services right in the heart of the city.

Thus, the Project is still at the formative stage, with no decision having yet been finalized on these issues. There have been apprehensions expressed in certain quarters that the PPP model may not work well in practice. The Administration is conscious of the fact that the selected partner has to discharge his social commitments under the project with full dedication. Based on the technical and social commitment parameters of the Medicity, the following aspects are worth noting:

The superspeciality hospital and a multi-speciality genera! hospital will be set-up either as two different units or as an integrated hospital with many common facilities. Over all, 25% of the beds will be reserved for 'poor-free' patients, 30% beds will be reserved for general patients and 45% reserved for private patients. The Chandigarh Administration's criteria will be used label a patient as entitled to free treatment ("poor-free"). The Medicity is free to have even more liberal criteria than the ones above. Poor patients would be provided free OPD consultation and admission including routine investigations. The charges for investigation and treatment in the general ward would be comparable with PGIMER, Chandigarh rates. For the 45% beds earmarked for private patients, the Medicity partner is free to lay down his own schedule of rates. Whatever route is chosen the following overall arrangement all will be effected.

- o 25% beds will be reserved for poor (FREE) patients.
- o 30% beds will be reserved for general category patients.
- o 45% beds will be reserved for private patients.

These form part of the Technical Parameters recommended by a Committee of medical experts for this project.

A system of in-built safeguards is being designed for this Project.

- o A comprehensive Memorandum of Understanding laying down all the technical parameters and defining in detail the social obligations cast on the Medicity partner will be signed by the Administration with the finally selected Medicity partner.
- o A system of annual social audit will be instituted.
- o The fulfilment of social obligations under the Medicity will be closely observed and governed by a Board of Governors with eminent citizens, medical experts, NGOs, social workers, etc. as members, in order to sustain the implementation of the social commitment as per the terms and conditions laid out in the MOU for the Medicity.
- o An Administrative Officer from the Chandigarh Administration will also be tasked with day-to-day monitoring of the social obligations.
- o Despite such carefully planned safeguards, however, if the selected partner does not comply with any clause with of the MOU, there are enough legal and procedural provisions that can be invoked to make sure that there are no violations.
- o This MOU is under finalization, and the inputs of a legal experts and the consultant will also be taken.

One of the most significant safeguards proposed under this project is that the land is to be given on Licence for a period of 33 years in the first instance, extendable further only on the satisfaction of the Chandigarh Administration. Thus, the Medicity would not involve a sale or transfer of ownership of land. The ownership of the land would continue to vest in the Chandigarh Administration. Stiff penalties including resumption of land are a normal part of such a Licence agreement.

At this point in time, issues regarding what should the annual Licence fee be, what should the upfront project fee be, what should the revenue sharing engagement be, etc. are all being looked into by an independent consultant, and hence have not attained finality. Therefore, any reporting on this issue can at best be described a conjecture or speculation and is thus totally premature.

Based on the reserve price (yet to be fixed) there will be a system of inviting sealed financial bids in the presence of the Medicity Committee. The factor of market forces will also naturally come into play. Issues such as what is the need of a Medicity for Chandigarh, why should the Medicity

Project be allotted to one single partner and not to several individual partner, are all the addressee in the detailed reply filed by the Administration in the above cited court case.

The Administration's Endeavour is to cater to the future health-care needs of the citizens, with social commitment at the cornerstone of the Medicity. Building more Government Hospitals poses challenges of funding, staffing and management. The time lag of 10-15 years before such a facility can be planned, designed, built and operational zed can prove costly in terms of public health goals.

Though the division bench of chief justice Tirath Singh Thakur and justice Hemant Gupta gave the liberty to the petitioner, Harminder Singh Grewal, to challenge the fresh EOI as and when issued, it steered clear of the moot issue regarding the "validity and the very concept" of the project. This means that UT could go ahead with the project at the new site in Rajiv Gandhi Chandigarh Technology Park even though it has to begin the tender process again.

Dismissing reports that land had been under-valued to ensure undue advantage to vested interests, UT senior standing counsel Anupam Gupta told the bench that the new site would result in more land for the project.

"The valuation of land is still to be done and thus reports appearing in a section of media are baseless," he added. Stating the administration didn't want to change eligibility criteria for the project, he claimed major health players, including Fortis, Max and Apollo, had shown interest in it, ruling out any malafide on the part of UT.

"A very strange culture of governance by photostat has evolved in UT administration where even before ink has dried on an officer's note and before the note reaches the administrator, it reaches media and gets published," Gupta responded to the petitioner's reference to news reports highlighting advisor Pradip Mehra's objections to Medicity.

The order came in the wake of petitioner's assertion that since UT had shifted the site, it ought to reinvite EoI for the same. Following this, justice Hemant Gupta asked the senior counsel to explain the reasons for this and if administration was ready to issue fresh expressions. Anupam Gupta informed the bench that UT had no hassles in doing so. He added the project-site was changed as "the administration plans to set-up a huge warehousing project in Raipur Kalan".

Media hype!

Health care services in Chandigarh get a shot in the arm, with the Megacity project moving from the conceptual blue print stage towards implementation, with the formal invitation of expression of interest being issued on 7 September 2008. Spread over 45 acres, the Medicity would see a long-term lease agreement awarded to one selected party or a consortium of investors, which will be governed by a MoU, incorporating essential features in line with the vision statement and ethos of the city. Modeled around a Public-Private Partnership model, it would have a modern health care facility with a super-speciality hospital. Users would be local residents and/or visiting NRIs which is why medical tourism, wellness therapies and holistic health will be its key features. However, surplus generated from it will go into running the various charity components of the Medicity.

Scope of Megacity Project

- *Superspeciality hospital-cum-recuperatory centre*: Will specialize in cardiology and oncology; recuperatory centre attached to hospital will be ideal for NRIs and foreigners; facilities like helicopter evacuation, tele-diagnosis and tele-medicine will be on offer.
- *Nursing College*: Will empower girls to train in a profession that is in demand locally and overseas; the initiative is in response to gender bias that Northern region has for long harboured with families preferring a son to a daughter, accounting for high rates of female foeticide, girl child neglect, dowry and lack of education; the project will provide free nurses training every year to a batch of 600 girls; through strategic tie-ups in Europe and America, they will be suitably placed.
- *Research Centre*: Cutting-edge research in Thalassemia and Sickle Cell Anaemia will be conducted (Punjab-Chandigarh region has high incidence); centre will engage in seminal research and pioneer new treatment techniques; reliable pre-marital counselling, prevention, treatment and sustenance will be provided.
- *Holistic Medicine Research Centre*: Medical knowledge in Ayurveda, Homeopathy, Siddha, Yoga, Unani and Naturopathy will be carried out through innovative research, case documentation and standardization of medical practices.
- *Multi Speciality Charity Hospital.*
- *Medical College*: Will equip students to emerge as fully trained doctors, who provide counselling, combat evils like female foeticide, run IEC campaigns for mass health education and design modules in preventive health.
- *Dental Hospital-cum-College.*
- *Terminal care centre/hospice*: Centre will provide palliative care to terminally ill while offering alternative therapies.

Transparent, inviting public comment/suggestions

While making details available of various stages in the project finalization, Raji P. Srivastava, project director, said that various committees have been formed to finalize location, lease details and process of allotment, all of which are shared with the public.

Selection Committee headed by the Adviser will have home secretary and finance secretary viewing live presentations by applicants along with member/s of the public, fulfilling the overarching objective of inclusive development.

APPENDIX

Global Hospital and Research Centre is unique, not only in it's energy and ambience, but it's eco consciousness. Most hospitals invoke a sense of fear, anxiety and tension, but here when you walk in the healing begins. The order and efficiency of the organization, the tranquility of the staff instills a sense of calm, of hope and well-being. The holistic approach which incorporates alternative healing techniques addresses the health of the whole being. If and when I need care I can't imagine a better place to get it, unfortunately it is a very long way north as well south India. "Is this a hospital?" is the first thought that enters the mind of many of our visitors.

What the President of India said: Global Hospital Mount Abu

The mind and body, both have to be treated in an ailment as the two are integrated. You cannot treat one and ignore the other. In particular, student who dream of becoming doctors should give attention to this fact. They will learn that the human body is not a mechanical system; it is a very intelligent organism with a most intricate and sensitive feedback system. The human system is indeed an integrated life package made of psychological and physiological systems. Realizing this, I integrated the two laboratories Defence Institute of Psychological Research and Defence Institute Physiological and Allied Sciences under one Director in 1999 when I was in DRDO. I am happy that the SIRIS has recognized the importance of mind body working together and have organized one hour out of eight hours for meditation in the industrial complex. Today, when I am in this environment, I would like to talk on the topic *"Healthy life results from lifestyle practices"*.

During the last ten years, I have participated and addressed several conferences on Coronary Artery Diseases (CAD) and possible solutions. Every time, it is indeed a great experience to interact in this important area. During this period, I have come across number of specialists in CAD, compared to any other health area. This may be due to my having more friends in the cardiac care field, some of whom are experts in open heart surgery, bypass surgery, some in interventional cardiology some of them in combination. I have seen and witnessed the whole mechanism of the heart surgical operations, treatment of patients and above all, I have interacted with many patients. Also more than five years, I had been in touch with experimental results of three dimensional lifestyle intervention research on Dilwallahs at Mount Abu.

Now I would like to present the findings of a research study jointly conducted by DRDO (Defence Research and Development Organisation) and Global Hospital, Mount Abu on lifestyle intervention on cardiac patients. I was participating in this programme.

Mind-Body-Synergy Studies

Studies on optimization of mind-body-synergy had commenced in the

Defense Research and Development Organization in 1993 by integrating two laboratories namely the Defense Institute of Physiology and Allied Sciences and the Defense Institute of Psychological Research. This enabled creation of mind-body-synergy in understanding problems faced by humanity. Studies were started in three areas, namely, breast cancer, HIV/ AIDS and coronary artery disease. The aim of the studies was to validate the hypothesis that mind-body-synergy could provide a solution to global health problems.

Health has to be treated not as the absence of disease but the feeling of complete physical, mental and social well-being. Generally, the conventional health care system pays attention to only physiology. We need to pay attention to holistically to mind, body, social and spiritual.

DRDO—Global Hospital Initiative

Keeping this in mind the DRDO took the initiative of formulating a project in collaboration with the Global Hospital and Research Centre, Mount Abu an institution of the Brahma Kumaris. They added a spiritual environment to take care of total heart health. In addition, this project involved a partnership from many hospitals and research institutions spread in different parts of the country, wherein cardiologists, endocrinologists, physiologists, fitness experts and spiritualists worked hand-in-hand for more than ten years to understand if this integrated mechanism can provide an antidote to the expanding global heart problem.

Effect of Positive and Negative Thoughts

Friends, we know well that thoughts whether positive or negative are well-defined electro-chemical events with physiological consequences. Thoughts, in the brain are converted into matter, which I understand reach all fifty-sixty trillion cells of the body in the form of neuro-peptides. If thoughts are distressing, full of worry, anger, ego or anxiety, the brain starts pouring stress hormones, which in turn increases the load on the heart and can set in coronary artery disease. If, we can reverse this process by creating an environment of positive thoughts, peace and happiness, this can minimize the load on the heart, which should lead to reversal of the disease. The main hypothesis was by adapting a healthy lifestyle of low fat high fibre vegetarian diet, moderate exercise and stress management through meditation, we can decrease load on the heart which in turn should reverse or halt the disease process. It has been recognized that keeping mind and body busy through beautiful minds is another way of Yoga.

Study Design

This hypothesis was tested in more than five hundred and eighteen patients, who had angiographically proven coronary artery disease. Two trials were carried out, Mount Abu Open Heart Trial in which patients served as their own controls and Abu Healthy Heart Trial in which hundred and twelve patients received a healthy lifestyle, whereas hundred and five patients served as control and did not receive the healthy lifestyle intervention. In fact, the control group was also prescribed the same diet and exercise but was not given instructions on meditation. Most of these patients had advanced coronary artery disease involving all three heart arteries and had coronary artery intervention. These patients were tracked over a period of ten years by the Global Hospital and DIPAS. I had an opportunity to be with the research group for 5 times during the review process of patients (Dilwallahs).

Lifestyle Intervention

The lifestyle given to these patients was very simple and elegant. In fact, they received a traditional Indian diet having lots of fiber, fruits and sprouts which I understand was a staple diet of every Indian family about five decades ago. The exercise given was simple; a brisk walk both in the morning and evening hours (5 km in one hour). The major component of the intervention was stress management through meditation. The three dimensional preventive methods heart is: (1) high fibrous vegetarian diet, (2) aerobic exercises—30 to 60 minutes, (3) meditation, apart from meeting the medicinal requirement and progressive reduction based on periodic tests. The main efforts were to empower patients with information and education on heart disease and how they themselves can control or reverse it.

Angiographic Evaluation

I understand that angiographies were coded and analyzed by a panel of independent angiographers. The outcome appears to be quite rewarding. Like any medical treatment, a visibly marked improvement in cardiac health of these patients could be seen within seven days of the commencement of the intervention. Their requirement of drugs prescribed by their cardiologists decreased markedly. The symptoms of chest pain and uneasiness reduced. Their capacity to exercise improved dramatically. I understand that after six months of intervention, some of the patients were even able to take to swimming. The so-called bad cholesterol, stress hormones profile reduced. The psychological or mental health showed considerable improvement. The heartbeat became very rhythmic and natural. The brain waves especially the Alpha wave, which I understand is an indicator of mental tranquility increased dramatically. In fact, the increased Alpha waves could be recorded both during eye closed and eye open conditions, suggesting that while they were doing their routine work mental tranquility was well maintained.

When their angiographies were repeated the control group showed an increase in artery blockage whereas the group, which received lifestyle intervention, showed a substantial decrease in artery blockage. Thus, this experiment clearly gives us ample evidence to confirm the hypothesis about the efficacy of lifestyle intervention in promoting sustainable healthy hearts.

I am happy to know that over 2500 doctors and over 5000 teachers from different parts of the country and abroad have been trained on three dimensional approach to heart care. Also, the treatment has been accepted by hospitals like CARE Hospital, Hyderabad, Medwin Hospital, and Government Hospital, Raipur for application among their patients. Very soon I am sure, this will be accepted by all the members of heart care community and the members of this international Congress should facilitate early induction of three dimensional approach throughout the world.

Light of the Soul

Conscience is the light of the Soul that burns within the chambers of our psychological heart. It is as real as life is. It raises the voice in protest whenever anything is thought of or done contrary to the righteousness. Conscience is a form of truth that has been transferred through our genetic stock in the form of the knowledge of our own acts and feelings as right or wrong. Conscience is also a great ledger where our offences are booked and registered. It is an unbiased witness. It threatens, promises, rewards and punishes, keeping all under its control. If conscience stings once, it is an admonition, if twice, it a condemnation. Cowardice asks, "Is it safe?" Greed asks, "Is there any gain in it?" Vanity asks, "Can I become great?" Lust asks. "Is there pleasure in it?" But conscience asks, "Is it right?" The answer could be lack of meditation. I am sure, the yoga meditation practice by the employees at SIRIS Yoga Meditation Centre will guide them to use their conscience and be always righteous. My greetings and best wishes to all of you.—Dr. APJ Abdul Kalam

Mount Abu area is backward and deprived

Western Rajasthan is one of the least privileged areas of India. Much of it is desert, water is in short supply and the illiteracy rate is very high. The majority of the population is deprived of basic health measures. This situation began to change in 1990 in the District of Sirohi (where Mt. Abu is situated) with the establishment of the J. Watumull Memorial Global Hospital and Research Centre initiated by the Brahma Kumaris.

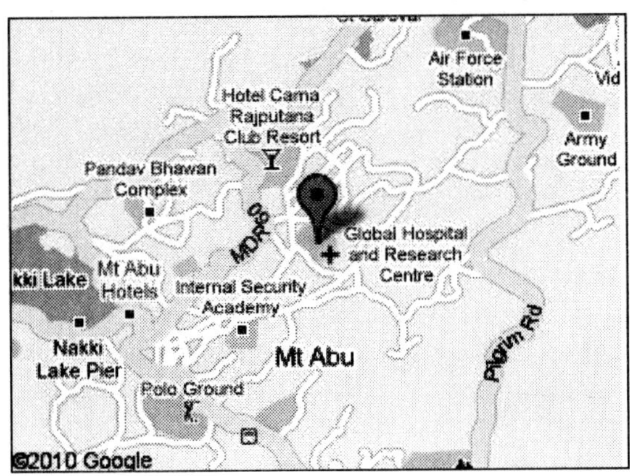

"A novel approach in holistic healing" is what many visitors comment about J. Watumull Global Hospital and Research Centre. Our founder trustees include an industrialist, a surgeon and a spiritual leader. In 1989, eminent head and neck cancer surgeon from Dr. Ashok Mehta visited the Brahma Kumaris in Mount Abu and believed they were an ideal, like-minded group of people he could partner, to implement his vision of a model Hospital focusing on Holistic Health Care.

The project was adopted by our founder mentors, Mr Khuba Watumull and Mr. Gulab Watumull of Mumbai and Hawaii (U.S.A.) respectively, and named J. Watumull Global Hospital and Research Centre, in memory of their late father, B.K. Nirwair, officer-in-charge of the Brahma Kumaris International Headquarters at Mount Abu was appointed Managing Trustee of the hospitals' governing board, the Global Hospital and Research Centre Trust.

Our founder Trustees envisaged that a multi-disciplinary secondary care hospital at Mount Abu would help bridge the existing deficiency in available health services in district Sirohi, Rajasthan. At the time, four hospitals with combined bed strength of 457 served the district's roughly 7,00,000 strong population. Besides offering medical services through out-patient clinics and ward admissions, the hospital was expected to focus on Outreach health care, Medical research, Vocational education in paramedical streams and the promotion of health awareness.

J. Watumull Global Hospital and Research Centre is a hospital, albeit with a difference. The brain child of an industrialist, a surgeon and a spiritual leader, Global Hospital, as it is popularly called, is a centre for holistic health care. It combines the best that modern medicine has to offer with complementary medicine systems like Ayurveda, homeopathy, magnet therapy, yoga and so on.

How did Global Hospital come into existence?

In 1989, eminent head and neck cancer surgeon from Mumbai, Dr Ashok Mehta visited the Brahma Kumaris in Mount Abu. His positive

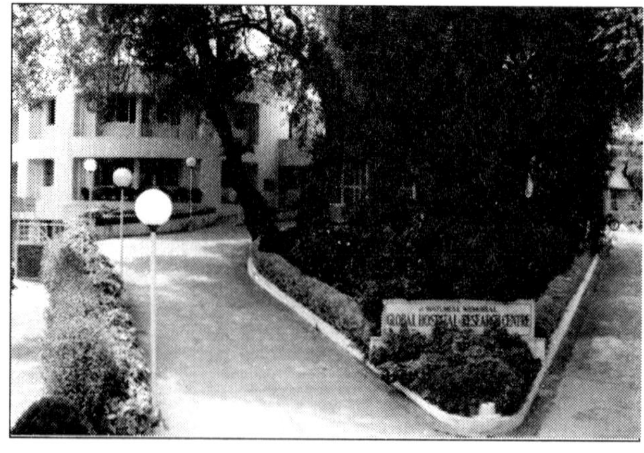

experience led him to believe that the Brahma Kumaris represented a like-minded group of people he could partner to implement his vision of a model hospital focusing on holistic health care. The project was adopted by our founder mentors, Khuba Watumull and Gulab Watumull of Mumbai and Hawaii (U.S.A.) respectively, and named J. Watumull Global Hospital and Research Centre, in memory of their late father, B.K. Nirwair, officer-in-charge of the Brahma Kumaris international headquarters at Mount Abu was appointed managing trustee of the hospitals' governing board, the Global Hospital and Research Centre Trust.

Serving the community

Our founder trustees envisaged that establishing a multi-disciplinary secondary care hospital at Mount Abu would help bridge a yawning gap in health services in district Sirohi, Rajasthan. At the time, four hospitals with a combined bed strength of 457 served the district's roughly 700,000 strong population. It therefore comes as no surprise that besides offering medical services through out-patient clinics and hospitalisation, the hospital has since then, expanded its operations to focus on community outreach programmes, medical research, vocational education in paramedical streams and the promotion of health awareness.

Hospital Services

J. Watumull Global Hospital and Research Centre offers free out-patient clinic consultations to all, irrespective of caste, economic status, gender or religion.

We charge patients who have the capacity to pay for out-patient procedures such as dental treatment, and diagnostic tests like audiometry, ECG, blood tests and so on.

Clinics dedicated to allopathy include:

- Cardiology
- Dentistry (supported by a dental lab)
- Dietetics and fitness
- ENT (supported by audiometry testing, offers a wide range of ENT surgeries)
- General Surgery (includes general surgery, laparoscopic surgery, surgery of the pancreas, urology surgery, etc).
- Gynaecology and Obstetrics (offers miscellaneous surgical procedures)
- Medicine
- Neuropsychiatry
- Ophthalmology (includes miscellaneous surgeries)
- Orthopaedics (includes joint replacement surgery)
- Paediatrics (supported by immunisation room)
- Physiotherapy
- Plastic Surgery

We also offer complementary medicine therapies. These include acupressure, acupuncture, ayurveda, homeopathy, magnet therapy and yoga therapy. Wherever possible, we encourage patients undergoing allopathic treatments to simultaneously take benefit from alternative medicine therapies.

Synergy of Mind and Body and Synergy of Religious Tourism and Health Tourism can Work

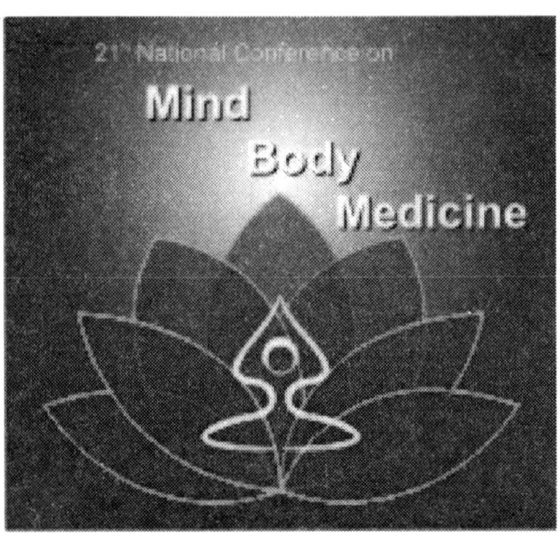

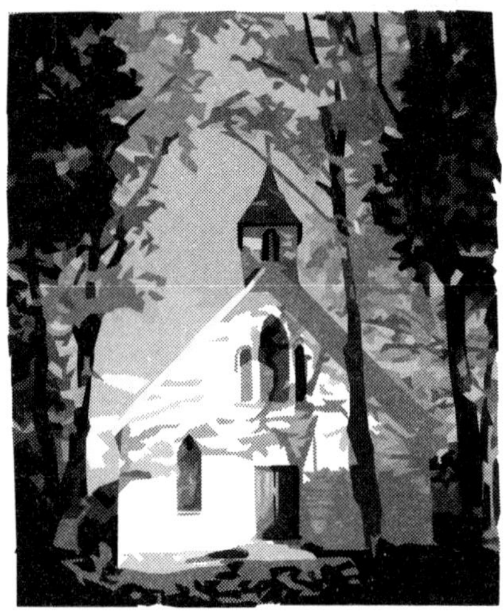

Imaging: Our radiology department is well-equipped with a C-Arm for intra-operative imaging, colour Doppler, mammography, orthopantomogram, sonography and X-ray machine. Special procedures like barium study, intravenous urography and myelography are also available.

Pathology: We offer a wide range of laboratory investigations in our biochemistry, clinical pathology, cytology, haematology, histopathology, microbiology and serology sections. Each sub-department has equipments facilitating testing procedures, such as a semi-automated biochemistry analyzer, fully-automated electrolyte analyzer, blood gas analyzer, coulters, Elisa reader, automatic Elisa well-washer and automatic tissue processor and microtome.

Other equipment that aids diagnosis in specific departments includes an audiometry machine (ENT), 2D Echo cardiography, computerised ECG and TMT machines (cardiology), bio-feedback therapy and EEG machines (neuropsychiatry) and an auto-refractometer, autoperimeter, ultrasound A and B equipment and direct and indirect ophthalmoscopes (ophthalmology).

The licensed blood bank attached to our pathology laboratory is a source of life-saving blood for victims of road traffic accidents occurring in the hilly terrain around Mount Abu, as well as a life support measure for surgery and anaemia patients seeking indoor treatment.

The blood bank is fully equipped with collection monitors, tube sealer and temperature regulated refrigerators.

In order to comply with the stringent regulations controlling the supply of safe blood, blood donors are fully examined and blood is screened to exclude the presence of HIV, HBsAg, HCV, syphilis and the malarial parasite prior to transfusions.

The Global Hospital Blood Bank lays much emphasis on encouraging voluntary blood donation. To this end, it conducts blood donation camps and organises programmes to motivate voluntary donors at regular intervals.

In-Patient Department

Our hospitals' bed strength is 102, spaciously laid out in four wards, including general rooms, twin-occupancy rooms, single occupancy AC and non-AC rooms and deluxe suites.

Patients are constantly supervised by their admitting consultants, well supported by a team of resident doctors and nurses.

Our indoor department also houses a dialysis unit, where regular treatments are offered by cheerful staff to chronically ill patients.

An eight-bed intensive care unit (I.C.U.), which forms an essential part of our indoor services, is well equipped with three ventilators and a multi-parameter central monitoring system.

What makes J. Watumull Global Hospital and Research Centre a novel hospital is that its intensive care facilities for monitoring serious patients are offered irrespective of a patient's paying capacity. Hence, well-to-do and poor patients both avail of high quality of care in our I.C.U.

Operation Theatre

Our main operative departments are ENT, general surgery, ophthalmology, orthopaedics, and plastic surgery. Operations are conducted in three operating suites supported by a minor operating room and post-operative recovery room.

We would be delighted to have a chance to serve you or a loved one, should you be unfortunate enough to need surgery of the kind we offer. Allow us to point out the benefits of undergoing surgery at Global Hospital, as well as share the major surgeries we conduct in each of our operative disciplines.

Why would you choose to have surgery at J. Watumull Global Hospital and Research Centre?

- our operation theatre complex is world class. It boasts of central air-conditioning, laminar airflow ventilation systems, excellent lighting, post-operative monitoring equipment for patients' vitals and adheres to stringent cleanliness guidelines,
- surgery at Global Hospital is cheaper than most private hospitals in your city,

- we do not conduct surgery on a commercial basis, by which we mean that we conduct a healthy mix of paid surgeries for patients who can afford modern health care and free surgeries for the economically underprivileged,
- since our mindset is not purely commercial, we do not compromise on the quality of medications or implant used,
- in the case of rehabilitative surgeries like joint replacement, the hospital package charge includes the cost of daily post-surgery physiotherapy sessions, which actually determines the outcome of surgery. It makes it so much easier to have a facility like physiotherapy come to the patients bedside, instead of having to commute to the facility as you would have to in a city, and
- especially from February to June, and September to November, Mount Abu provides a perfect climate for the rehabilitation of patients thanks to its clean, air and noise pollution-free environment.

We present details of common surgeries conducted with the approximate charges for each mentioned alongside. These charges relate to deluxe room occupancy for the mentioned hospital stay.

ENT

Tympanoplasty, that is, surgery for the reconstruction of the middle ear to correct deafness and stop discharge. Approximate treatment charges inclusive of a hospital stay of one week is rupees 16,000.

Stapedectomy, surgery to correct conductive deafness due to otosclorosis. Approximate treatment charges inclusive of a three day hospital stay is rupees 24,500.

Rhinoplasty or cosmetic nose surgery. Approximate treatment charges inclusive of a four day hospital stay is rupees 27,000. However, a patient would need to have the nose plaster removed after a fortnight, for which he/ she may need to revisit the hospital, if this cannot be done where you live.

Surgery for thyroid and parotid swellings calls for treatment charges of approximately rupees 30,000 inclusive of a hospital stay of one week.

The charges of surgery to excise head and neck tumours depends on each case, as the tumour may be benign or malignant. Email us for more details.

GENERAL SURGERY

Surgery for the removal of an abcess (cyst/lump/swelling) will require a two day hospital stay for which the approximate treatment charges are rupees 5,000.

Phimosis will require a four day hospital stay for which the approximate treatment charges are rupees 9,000.

Surgery for inguinal hernia will require a seven to ten day hospital stay for which the approximate treatment charges are rupees 12,500.

Surgery on an ingrown toenail will require one day hospital stay for which the approximate treatment charges are rupees 4,000.

Surgery of a fissure will require two to four day hospital stay for which the approximate treatment charges are rupees 9,000.

Surgery of a fistula will require two to seven day hospital stay for which the approximate treatment charges are rupees 11,000.

We also offer specialised laparoscopic and urology surgery on prior appointment basis in association with visiting specialists.

GYNAECOLOGY

Abdominal hysterectomy charges rupees 18,500 inclusive of eight day stay (Indication: fibroid ovarian cysts with fibroid, adenomyosis, unhealthy cervix, carcinoma uterus and cervix).

Vaginal hysterectomy charges rupees 18,500 inclusive of eight day stay (Indication: prolapse uterus).

Cystocoel and recto coel repair charges rupees 18,500 inclusive of eight day stay (Indication: prolapse of bladder and rectum).

Myomectomy charges rupees 20,000 inclusive of eight day stay (Indication: fibroid in uterus especially in young patients in whom facility has to be preserved).

Ovarian cystectomy charges rupees 18,500 inclusive of eight day stay (Indication: ovarian cysts, cancer ovaries).

Caesarian section charges rupees 18,000 inclusive of eight day stay.

OPHTHALMOLOGY

Phaco cataract surgery with foldable IOL (intra-ocular lens) using imported lenses of international quality standards, such as Acrysof by Alcon, Tecnis by AMO, and Dura lens by AMO (non-foldable). The approximate treatment charges which includes a hospital stay (single room) of four days is rupees 15,000.

Small incision cataract surgery (SICS) with IOL implant. Again, patients can choose from the same range of high quality imported lenses. The approximate treatment charges which includes a hospital stay of four days is rupees 13,000.

Phaco and trabeculectomy (which is glaucoma surgery) with IOL implant. The approximate treatment charges which includes a hospital stay of four days is rupees 16,000.

Glaucoma surgery—also called trabeculectomy—charges are approximately rupees 8,500 which includes a hospital stay of ten days, as regular post-operative checks are mandatory. If required, patients can also undergo Laser Iridotomy during their stay (extra charges).

Paediatric squint surgery charges are approximately rupees 8,000 which includes a hospital stay of five days.

Paediatric ptosis surgery charges are approximately rupees 6,000 which includes a hospital stay of five days.

ORTHOPAEDICS

Our orthopaedics department offers surgery for trauma, degenerative joint disorders and congenital limb deformities. Email us for approximate costs.

We also offer knee and hip joint replacement surgery and neurosurgery on appointment basis in association with visiting specialists.

Community services

The village outreach programme has been an essential part of the hospital services since 1991. The outreach team conducts regular visits to ten adopted villages providing basic health care and medication.

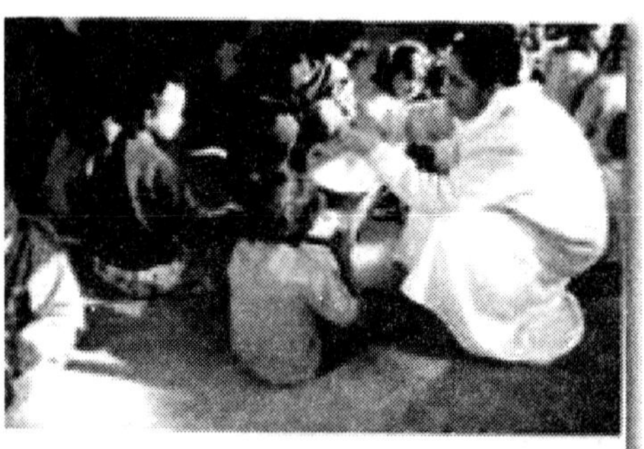

Patients requiring indoor treatment are encouraged to travel back to the base hospital with the team. The health service focuses on mother and child care, malnutrition, skin diseases and tuberculosis.

The ten villages forming the village outreach programme circle are Aarna, Chandela, Jaidra-Kyaria, Jawaingaon, Nichalagarh, Oriya, Salgaon, Takiya, Uplagarh and Utteraj.

Supplementary nutritional (mid-day snack) projects are also run in twelve village primary schools. The village outreach programme has taken up the training of village women in sewing skills in an effort to make them economically self-reliant.

The village outreach team is indebted to the Global Harmony Foundation, Hong Kong Indian Womens' Association, Sindhi Nari Sabha of London and others who have contributed to various village outreach programme endeavours.

Our community ophthalmology project was kick-started in 1997 thanks to support from the Ministry of Health, Government of India under its National Programme for Control of Blindness. Over the years, the project has changed the lives of thousands of villagers afflicted with cataract or glaucoma causing blindness by offering sight-restorative surgical procedures.

The project is presently being implemented by the ophthalmic staff stationed at J. Watumull Global Hospital and Research Centre, Mount Abu and at the P.C. Parmar Global Hospital Eye Care Hospital at Abu Road. Community coordinators from these units travel extensively seeking to garner support from village leaders and local social organisations, such as the Rotary International and the Lions Club, to reach out to more patients.

The recurring expenses incurred towards arranging field screening camps to identify mature cataract cases and the subsequent hospitalisation charges of villagers needing surgery is partially met through Government support. Private donors, charities and individuals, help close the gap between the expenses incurred and nominal charges recovered from patients who can afford the cost of health care.

G.V. Modi Rural Health Care Centre and Eye Hospital

The G.V. Modi Rural Health Care Centre and Eye Hospital at Abu Road was built in 1994 with support from the Modi family of Surat, our patron—Robin Ramsay of Australia, and Government funding received under the National Programme for Control of Blindness.

The hospital was established as a general health centre, also housing a laboratory, X-ray unit, pharmacy, dental clinic, and most important, an eye clinic that would function as a referral *cum* post-operative check-up clinic for the many eye patients seeking surgery for cataract, glaucoma and other blindness causing illnesses.

Since then, the ophthalmic unit has been shifted to the Global Hospital Institute of Ophthalmology. The G.V. Modi Rural Health Care Centre presently houses a family medicine-*cum*-geriatric medicine clinic, a blood collection centre and a pharmacy. A visiting neuropsychiatrist and dermatologist also offer their services at the centre on a weekly basis. Since the centre is located adjacent to the Shantivan Complex of the Brahma Kumaris, which is visited by thousands every year, it offers a number of health check-up packages and counselling services for the benefit of these tourists.

Paediatric Ophthalmology

Project Nayanraj, launched in 2006, is a 3-year partnership between J. Watumull Global Hospital and Research Centre and Orbis International Inc. aimed at improving the paediatric ophthalmology infrastructure and outreach activities in districts Jalore, Pali, Sirohi and Udaipur in Rajasthan and district Banaskantha in Gujarat.

At the outset of the project, Orbis International Inc. sponsored the acquisition of essential paediatric ophthalmology equipment thus commissioning a fully-equipped paediatric eye care department at the P.C. Parmar Foundation Global Hospital Eye Care Centre, an extension wing of our sister concern the Global Hospital Institute of Ophthalmology at Abu Road. It is also assisting in training staff in paediatric ophthalmology.

Our ophthalmic staff implementing this project has a target of screening 80,000 school and pre-verbal children for ocular diseases, especially focusing on childhood ailments like amblyopia which need early detection. Children having refractive errors are being given free spectacles. Both sight restorative surgery such as congenital cataract and trauma, as well as non-sight restorative surgeries like squint and ptosis are conducted.

Besides, 1000 school teachers and 54 ophthalmologists/paediatricians/general practitioners are being trained in screening techniques so as to diagnose and manage paediatric ocular health problems at a primary level. Most importantly, 10,000 mothers and guardians are being educated about methods to prevent the occurrence of ocular diseases in children.

It is commonly seen that poor village people who lead a hand to mouth existence do not visit a health care centre until their disease takes a turn for the worse. Can you blame them? At the lower end of the economic ladder, taking a day off to visit a doctor—especially one who is located a day's trek away—can mean keeping your family hungry. This is why if you desire to make a difference to the health status of rural poor, you need to reach out to them in their surroundings.

We have discovered that contact is best established through a revolving clinic staffed by a caring doctor and well equipped with essential medicines. This reality led us to partner the K.P. Sanghvi Charitable Trust of Pawapuri Tirthdham (Sirohi) to launch a community services project targeting remote villages not served by a government-funded Primary Health Centre. We are grateful to the Children's Hope India (USA) for meeting the cost of medicines distributed by one of these mobile clinics.

Since its commissioning in April 2004, the project has grown to include four mobile clinics which together visit over 40 villages on a rotational basis. During the fiscal 2008-09, the clinics conducted 31663 field consultations and referred 563 patients to our hospitals at Mount Abu or Abu Road.

School Children

In 2004, the support of an anonymous corporate donor and Children's Hope India (USA) enabled us to launch a comprehensive school upliftment programme in primary and secondary government schools located in far-flung villages and in the municipality of Mount Abu. The programme has three major components—health, nutritional supplements and educational aids.

Under the auspices of this programme, we conduct extensive health check-ups on the school children. Children needing spectacles or hearing aids are suitably equipped. Children are also explained the basics of personal and dental hygiene. Regular follow-up visits ensure that children needing medicine or hospitalisation are taken care of.

A nutritional component of this programme involves the distribution of supplements—biscuits, seasonal fruit, a mix of groundnuts and black gram and a glass of milk—twice weekly. A novel part of this programme is a nutricandy that is distributed daily to all school children.

Students are also distributed educational aids, books and uniforms, while the schools are provided sports materials and classroom teaching aids.

Smile Train

May 2006 represented a major milestone in the history of J. Watumull Global Hospital and Research Centre. The hospital was accepted as a partner of the Smile Train, a New York-based charity with global operations. The Smile Train works to offer needy children and adults free cleft lip/palate surgery through its wide network of partner hospitals.

Two Smile Train accredited surgeons follow stringent protocol covering the operative procedure and after-care to ensure the best surgical results. Our cleft surgery department is very active—it performed a total of 533 operations during the fiscal 2008-09.

Brigadier Vora Clinic and Jyoti Bindu Diagnostic Centre

The Brigadier Vora Clinic and Jyoti Bindu Diagnostic Centre was established at Vadodara (Baroda) in 1993.

It houses a family medicine clinic, a laboratory and basic imaging diagnostic services. Thanks to the cooperation of city specialists who offer part-time honorary services, it offers free consultations in various medical disciplines. The clinic also organises health awareness programmes in schools, at community centres and for groups in the police department.

Future plans on the anvil include further development of the laboratory facility and arranging medical consultation programmes in rural areas bordering the city centre, so as to benefit the weaker sections of society.

P.C. Parmar Foundation Global Hospital Eye Care Centre

The excellent response of the community to the Global Hospital Institute of Ophthalmology resulted in the construction of a new eye wing adjacent the existing centre.

The creation of this new facility, named the P.C. Parmar Foundation Global Hospital Eye Care Centre, was supported by the Parmar Foundation, Orbis International Inc. and New World iCare Pvt. Ltd. Launched in 2007, it houses specialist ophthalmic clinics, private hospital rooms and an area to teach ophthalmology.

The commissioning of this unit has drawn a large number of paediatric and adult patients requiring advanced eye surgery.

Radha Mohan Mehrotra Global Hospital Trauma Centre

The Radha Mohan Mehrotra Global Hospital Trauma Centre, a trauma unit at Abu Road constructed with support of the Radha Mohan Mehrotra Medical Relief Trust, was launched in 2007.

The centre offers emergency specialist medical care to trauma patients—road accident and medical emergencies—around Abu Road. It is equipped for emergency and routine surgery in the disciplines of general surgery and orthopaedics. If need be, the centre refers serious cases to J. Watumull Global Hospital and Research Centre at Mount Abu or to nearby cities.

Laboratory and imaging diagnostic devices both as support services for surgery and for the routine diagnosis of residents in the vicinity of the centre are also available. A neurosurgeon is attached to the centre on a 'visiting basis' and a critical care ambulance equipped with wireless control equipment to ensure prompt attention to cases rushed to the centre is also a vital part of our trauma set-up.

Research Center

Neuropsychiatry

Our neuropsychiatry department carried out a retrospective study for overseas meditation practitioners who visited the international headquarters of the Brahma Kumaris spiritual institution in 1994-95, to assess the efficacy of Rajayoga meditation to overcome psychoactive substance abuse/dependence.

A group of three hundred and eighty foreigners including two hundred and sixteen Europeans, having a maximum of eight kinds of substance abuse/dependence for a duration ranging from two months to forty years were interviewed. Data was collected using a structured questionnaire.

The majority of the meditation practitioners (93%) abstained completely from all the substances within one month period of practice of Rajyoga Meditation, without taking concurrent psychiatric treatment. This emphasizes the use of Rajyoga Meditation as an effective method to overcome substance abuse/dependence.

Other research studies conducted by the department of neuropsychiatry are Effects of Rajyoga meditation in treating neurotic illnesses and Changes in Physiological Parameters—EEG, muscle tension, etc.—after Rajyoga practice.

Coronary Artery Disease

In 1997, we launched a research project focused on determining the effect of lifestyle changes - specifically a vegetarian wholesome diet, moderate aerobic exercise and stress control by Rajyoga meditation.

The project was co-partnered by the Defense Institute of Physiology and Allied Sciences and the Morarji Desai National Institute of Yoga, and sponsored by the Central Council for Research in Yoga and Naturopathy. Other collaborating medical institutes were the J.J. Group of Hospitals and Grant Medical College (Mumbai), U.N. Mehta Institute of Cardiology (Ahmedabad), G.B. Pant Hospital (Delhi), V.S. Hospital (Ahmedabad) and Care Hospital (Hyderabad).

We invited patients suffering from coronary artery blockages to Abu for one-week sessions at intervals of six months. Patients were introduced to lifestyle changes, and their blood test and physiological parameters and the extent of reversal of atherosclerosis (blocked arteries) was monitored during their stay. They were encouraged to keep up the meditation practice back home.

Over 500 patients volunteered to participate in this research. The data collected over five years was analyzed to evaluate the efficacy of the treatment as a permanent cure for cardiac patients. The positive research results have resulted in our keeping up with our coronary artery disease programme.

Sickle Cell Anaemia

In 2006, the Indian Council of Medical Research approved our three-year project proposal to determine the prevalence and distribution of sickle cell anaemia among scheduled tribes (Garasias) of Sirohi district, Rajasthan.

This project is being implemented by our consultant paediatrician as principal investigator and consultant gynaecologist and chief of the village outreach programme as co-investigator.

The project also aims to study the clinical and haematological profile of sickle cell disease, and where possible, to study the effect of preventive measures like penicillin prophylaxis, hematinics (folate), vaccination and health education.

College of Ophthalmology

The expansion in ophthalmic services at Abu Road includes the establishment of a College of Ophthalmology, as part of a new eye wing, thanks to support from New World iCare.

The school will continue to offer the Diploma Ophthalmic Techniques course, though the number of seats per batch will be increased to fifteen. The College has also applied for accreditation with IGNOU to conduct a BSc in Optometry course.

It is also proposed to commence a three year DNB postgraduation specialization in ophthalmology course for doctors, conducted in affiliation with the National Board and thus considered equivalent to an MS in ophthalmology.

Besides, several short-term courses of a few weeks duration are planned for ophthalmic doctors—in Community Ophthalmology aimed at equipping doctors and project managers in the techniques and methods of going about community work; Phacoemulsification, the latest technique in cataract surgery and Glaucoma Diagnosis and Management.

Ophthalmic Techniques

Since 1999, we offer a three-year Diploma in Ophthalmic Techniques in association with the Federation of Ophthalmic Research and Education Centres. This course is conducted from both the J. Watumull Global Hospital and Research Centre at Mount Abu and the Global Hospital Institute of Ophthalmology at Abu Road.

Nursing Assistants

Our nursing assistant's course is delivered from a training centre created in 1997 with assistance from the Dr Bhanuben Mahendra Nanavati Foundation of Mumbai and the Dutch Government.

BSES M.G. Hospital

In the year 2002, the Global Hospital and Research Centre Trust entered into a public-private (sector) partnership (PPP) with the BSES and the Brihanmumbai Municipal Corporation (BMC).

The BMC allocated land for a hospital at Andheri in Mumbai, the BSES covered the cost of constructing and equipping the hospital building while the management of BSES M.G. Hospital as it is called, was taken on by the Global Hospital and Research Centre Trust.

This 100 bed multi-disciplinary hospital has posted encouraging results ever since it was commissioned. The hospital offers out-patient clinics in the disciplines of cancer, cardiology, child guidance, chest medicine, dentistry, diabetes, ENT, endocrinology family medicine, GI endoscopy, gynaecology, homeopathy, medicine, nephrology, neurology, ophthalmology, orthopaedics, paediatrics, pain management, physiotherapy, psychiatry, sports medicine, surgery and urology.

It also offers diagnostic, indoor and operative facilities. It has a well equipped laboratory, imaging department, blood bank and pharmacy. The hospital conducts health check-ups and specialty clinics which bring together a number of consultants to proffer advice to large number of patients. Much emphasis is placed on organizing medical camps for underprivileged sections of society and continuing medical education programmes.

APPENDIX I

HEALTH IS WEALTH

RAVI GUPTA, EDITOR RAVIGUPTA@CSDMS.ORG

The Ministry of Health has admitted that there is hardly any upward transmission of information from around 24,000 Primary Health Centers (PHCs) taking place. The Ministry is dependent entirely on newspaper reports for information and assessment during the outbreak of diseases in many parts of the country. It has been found that it takes nearly a year for information to travel from PHC to the Ministry. The government has concluded that such disease surveillance is meaningless and its data was only for the consumption of government files.

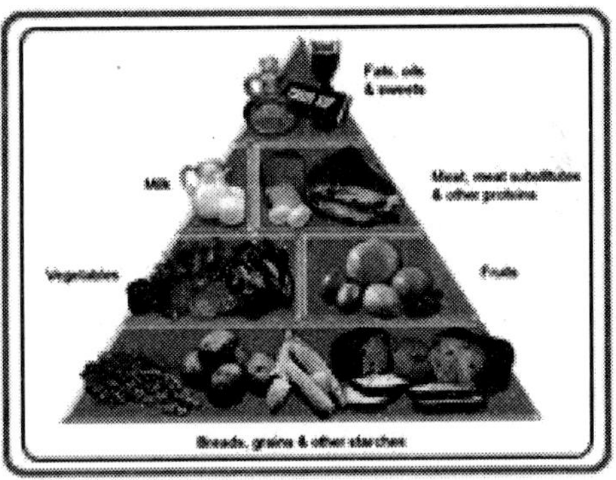

Two important fields need attention, that are so close to each other and yet so far apart in a developing country like India. The US and the UK provide lessons as to how these two fields can develop synergy between themselves and to the benefit of the society at large. Health GIS applications are an important area of activity at the National Centre for Health Statistics of the US government. The National Spatial Data Infrastructure (NSDI), the United States Geological Survey (USGS), Census and many other databases, which are important for improved public health surveillance are widely used by the health departments. Recently, the UK national mapping agency signed an agreement with National Health Service (NHS) of UK for developing customized geographic information products for the health community. OSCAR, which tracks precise details of every motorable road in Britain, and ADDRESS-POINT, which can pinpoint any postal address instantly, are already popular among the emergency services run by the health authorities.

The GIS and the health community in India are living in two separate watertight compartments. Both need each other. The map sector of the country will find a large market for its products and services in the Health sector. The health sector will make a quantum leap in its service delivery using maps for better planning and decision-making. But both are not able to talk to each other due to rigid institutional framework. The limited and sometimes non-existent commercial orientation of the government organizations (like Survey of India, Indian Council of Medical Research, etc.) in the country also led them to ignore the opportunities offered by new technologies like GIS. As a result, they continue to operate with antiquated technology and have little incentive, let alone funding to upgrade.

Merely an absence of disease does not necessarily mean that you are healthy. It's true that sometimes diseases strike us when we least expect them, even when we do everything right as far as staying healthy is concerned. Indeed, a wise man once truly said "Health is Wealth", for there is nothing worse than feeling ill at ease. Illness and diseases not only make you dependent on others, they also rob you of your zest for life. Why not take measures to ensure a long, happy, self-sufficient and healthy life? Here are a few tips to help you do just that!

Follow the Pyramid

We mean the food pyramid. A food pyramid basically tells you what to eat most and what to scrimp on. At the base of the pyramid are things that you should consume the most like cereals and pulses. As the pyramid tapers-off to its peak, it tells you about the things you should eat sparingly like oils and fats. In the middle of the pyramid are food items to be consumed moderately like fruits and veggies followed by milk and meat products. Keep this in mind when you eat or plan your meals.

Regular Checks

Never underestimate the power of monitoring your health. A major part of staying well is consistency in health and that can only be figured out if the indicators of your health are regularly monitored. These indicators are Sugar Levels, Blood Pressure, Haemoglobin Count, Urine Analysis, Cholesterol and Lipid Profile, Liver Function Test, ECG, and Chest X-Ray.

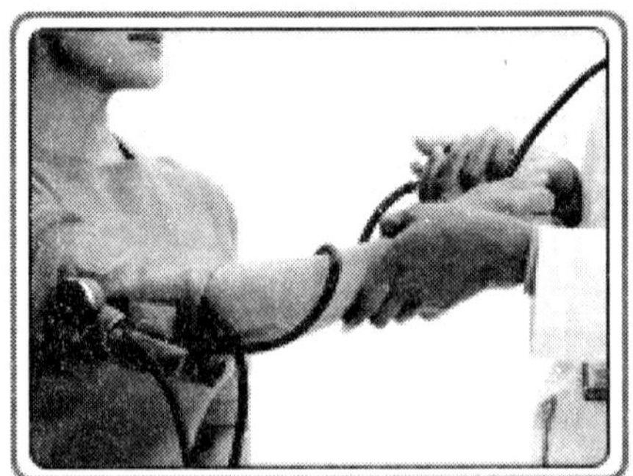

Many hospitals such as Apollo Hospitals have comprehensive health check-ups that cover all these tests and more. These tests become all the more important as you age.

Sweat It

There is no alternative to exercising and you don't just need to do it when you gain a few extra pounds. Exercise keeps you active and energetic

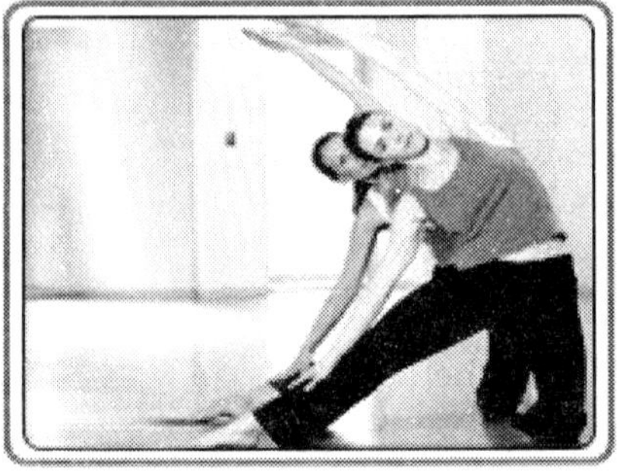

and it is great for the joints. However, be careful of over-straining yourself. Consult a physician or fitness trainer to figure out a fitness plan that is best suited for you. And do remember to wear the right outfit and footwear while exercising, else you may injure yourself. Keep moving and don't allow yourself to be glued to a chair all day.

Water Rules!

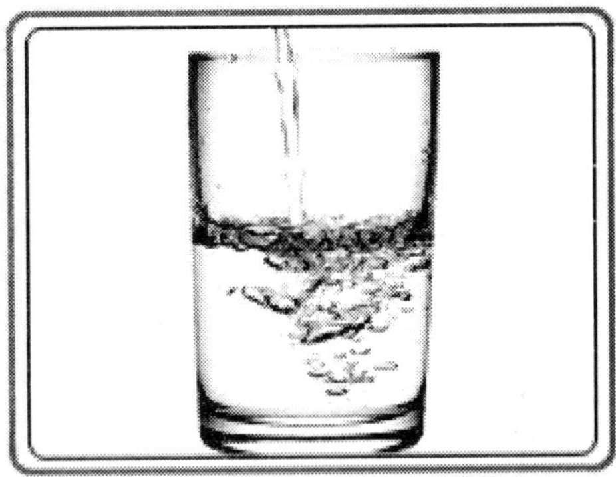

Keep your body well-hydrated by drinking a lot of water throughout the day. Water is actually a miracle drink that aids many of your bodily functions like getting rid of toxins, eliminating wastes, regulating body temperature, lubrication of body joints, assisting in digestion processes, and much more. This is one drink you should indulge in all day and every day!

Relax

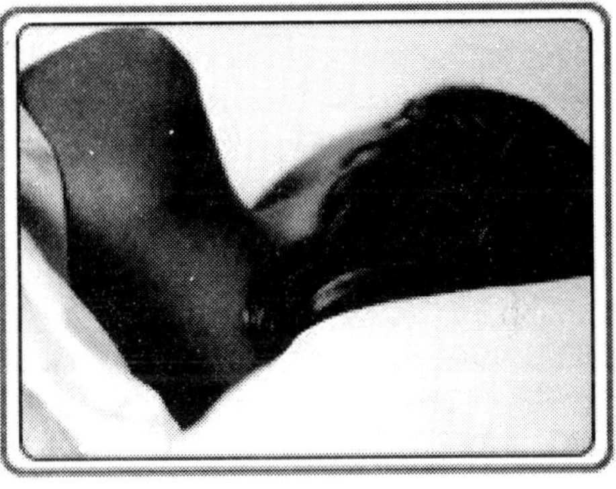

Stress leads to many physical and mental disorders. Keep it at bay with deep breathing, leisurely strolls, meditation, chanting, and listening to music. Other ways to relax include socializing, traveling, talking to friends, or basically doing anything that pleases you and makes you feel good. Happiness has got different meaning to different people. Some people think that they may live happily if they have more money. But, health is wealth. Without money you cannot recover health. Try to earn some money for your health. So, do not spoil your health for earning more wealth. It is enough if you earn money for your livelihood and save some money for your future.

Excessive wealth is also harmful. So, by spending your wealth little, you have to take medical insurance policy, to safeguard your health. Life is not merely to be alive but to be healthy and wealthy. You will also accept that the greatest wealth is health. Health and wealth are like two sides of a coin. Wealth buys success, career and leisure. The young man of today is ready to work for 24 hours a day, all the 7 days without break, to earn wealth. But where will it end. Can he sit and enjoy after earning wealth or will he become mad when the stress and strain make him to boil. He may collapse while earning money. Everyday we hear about new disease. Stress is a new disease which the young generation is going to face, since earning money within a short period is the criteria for them. Many people earn wealth at the cost of their health. But, where is the time for them to enjoy the hard earned money. They have to sacrifice their entire life to recover the ill-health.

Manage stress

You should formulate your life in such a way to live with happiness without much stress and strain. Your career, physical fitness, relationship with others, financial position, spiritual aspect, the environment everything should be adjusted towards your health and earning little wealth. Changes are often to be made in your lifestyle to accommodate to the trend of modern world. You have to adopt a positive approach and allot time for everything. You should also be ready to adapt yourself for any change. If you feel that your approach is wrong or involves much strain, you have to rethink whether to continue or alter your approach. You can do your day-to-day activities also in an enjoyable manner. You can spend sometime with little kids, as a relaxation. You can park your car at a distance and go for a walk. You can observe people who come across in your life and try to help them in someway to keep them and yourself happy.

Public health

It is "the science and art of preventing disease, prolonging life and promoting health through the organized efforts and informed choices of society, organizations, public and private, communities and individuals." (1920, C.E.A. Winslow) It is concerned with threats to the overall health of a community based on population health analysis. The population in question can be as small as a handful of people or as large as all the inhabitants of several continents (for instance, in the case of a pandemic). Public health is typically divided into epidemiology, biostatistics and health services. Environmental, social, behavioural, and occupational health are also important subfields.

There are two distinct characteristics of public health:

1. It deals with preventive rather than curative aspects of health.
2. It deals with population-level, rather than individual-level health issues.

The focus of public health intervention is to prevent rather than treat a disease through surveillance of cases and the promotion of healthy behaviours. In addition to these activities, in many cases treating a disease may be vital to preventing it in others, such as during an outbreak of an infectious disease. Hand washing, vaccination programs and distribution of condoms are examples of public health measures.

The goal of public health is to improve lives through the prevention and treatment of disease. The United Nations' World Health Organization defines health as "a state of complete physical, mental and social well-being and not merely the absence of disease or infirmity."

Objectives

The focus of a public health intervention is to prevent rather than treat a disease through surveillance of cases and the promotion of healthy behaviours. In addition to these activities, in many cases treating a disease can be vital to preventing its spread to others, such as during an outbreak of infectious disease or contamination of food or water supplies. Vaccination programs and distribution of condoms are examples of public health measures. Most countries have their own government public health agencies, sometimes known as ministries of health, to respond to domestic health issues. In the United States, the front line of public health initiatives are state and local health departments. The United States Public Health Service (PHS), led by the Surgeon General of the United States, and the Centers for Disease Control and Prevention, headquartered in Atlanta, are involved with several international health activities, in addition to their national duties.

There is a vast discrepancy in access to health care and public health initiatives between developed nations and developing nations. In the developing world, public health infrastructures are still forming. There may not be enough trained health workers or monetary resources to provide even a basic level of medical care and disease prevention. As a result, a large majority of disease and mortality in the developing world results from and contributes to extreme poverty. For example, many African governments spend less than US $10 per person per year on health care, while, in the United States, the federal government spent approximately US $4,500 per capita in 2000.

Many diseases are preventable through simple, non-medical methods. For example, research has shown that the simple act of hand washing can prevent many contagious diseases.

Public health plays an important role in disease prevention efforts in both the developing world and in developed countries, through local health systems and through international non-governmental organizations. The two major postgraduate professional degrees related to this field are the Master of Public Health (MPH) or the (much rarer) Doctor of Public Health (DrPH). Many public health researchers hold PhDs in their fields of specialty, while some public health programs confer the equivalent Doctor of Science degree instead.

History of public health

In some ways, public health is a modern concept, although it has roots in antiquity. From the beginnings of human civilization, it was recognized that polluted water and lack of proper waste disposal spread communicable diseases (theory of miasma). Early religions attempted to regulate behaviour that specifically related to health, from types of food eaten, to regulating certain indulgent behaviours, such as drinking alcohol or sexual relations. The establishment of governments placed responsibility on leaders to develop public health policies and programs in order to gain some understanding of the causes of disease and thus ensure social stability prosperity, and maintain order.

Early public health interventions

Public health nursing made available through child welfare services in U.S. (c. 1930s). By Roman times, it was well understood that proper diversion of human waste was a necessary tenet of public health in urban areas. The Chinese developed the practice of variolation following a smallpox epidemic around 1000 BC. An individual without the disease could gain some measure of immunity against it by inhaling the dried crusts that formed around lesions of infected individuals. Also, children were protected by inoculating a scratch on their forearms with the pus from a lesion. This practice was not documented in the West until the early-1700s, and was used on a very limited basis. The practice of vaccination did not become prevalent until the 1820s, following the work of Edward Jenner to treat smallpox.

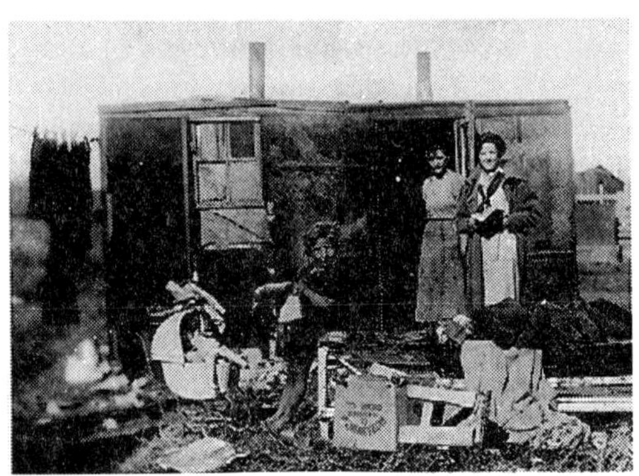

During the 14th century Black Death in Europe, it was believed that removing bodies of the dead would further prevent the spread of the bacterial infection. This did little to stem the plague, however, which was most likely spread by rodent-borne fleas. Burning parts of cities resulted in much greater benefit, since it destroyed the rodent infestations. The development of quarantine in the medieval period helped mitigate the effects of other infectious diseases. However, according to Michel Foucault, the plague model of government efforts was later controverted by the cholera model. A cholera pandemic devastated Europe between 1829 and 1851, and was first fought by the use of what Foucault called "social medicine", which focused on flux, circulation of air, location of cemeteries, etc. All those concerns, born of the miasma theory of disease, were mixed with urbanistic concerns for the management of populations, which Foucault designated as the concept of "bio-power". The German conceptualized this in the Polizeiwissenschaft ("Science of police").

The science of epidemiology was founded by John Snow's identification of polluted public water well as the source of an 1854 cholera outbreak in London. Dr. Snow believed in the germ theory of disease as opposed to the prevailing miasma theory. Although miasma theory correctly teaches that disease is a result of poor sanitation, it was based upon the prevailing theory of spontaneous generation. Germ theory developed slowly: despite Anton van Leeuwenhoek's observations of Microorganisms, (which are now known to cause many of the most common infectious diseases) in the year 1680, the modern era of public health did not begin until the 1880s, with Louis Pasteur's germ theory and production of artificial vaccines.

Other public health interventions include latrinization, the building of sewers, collection of garbage followed by incineration or disposal in a landfill, providing clean water and draining standing water to prevent the breeding of mosquitos. This contribution was made by Edwin Chadwick in 1843 who published a report on the sanitation of the working class population in Great Britain at the time. So began the inception of the modern public health. The industrial revolution had initially caused the spread of disease through large conurbations around workhouses and factories. These settlements were cramped and primitive and there was no organised sanitation. Disease was inevitable and its incubation in these areas was encouraged by the poor lifestyle of the inhabitants....

Modern public health

As the prevalence of infectious diseases in the developed world decreased through the 20th century, public health began to put more focus on chronic diseases such as cancer and heart disease. An emphasis on physical exercise was reintroduced. In America, public health worker Dr. Sara Josephine Baker lowered the infant mortality rate using preventative methods. She established many programs to help the poor in New York City keep their infants healthy. Dr. Baker led teams of nurses into the crowded neighbourhoods of Hell's Kitchen and taught mothers how to dress, feed, and bathe their babies. After World War I many states and countries followed her example in order to lower infant mortality rates. During the 20th century, the dramatic increase in average life span is widely credited to public health achievements, such as vaccination programs and control of infectious diseases, effective safety policies such as motor-vehicle and occupational safety, improved family planning, fluoridation of drinking water, anti-smoking measures, and programs designed to decrease chronic disease.

Meanwhile, the developing world remained plagued by largely preventable infectious diseases, exacerbated by malnutrition and poverty. Front-page headlines continue to present society with public health issues on a daily basis: emerging infectious diseases such as SARS, making its way from China (see Public health in China) to Canada and the United States; prescription drug benefits under public programs such as Medicare; the increase of HIV-AIDS among young heterosexual women and its spread in South Africa; the increase of childhood obesity and the concomitant increase in type II diabetes among children; the impact of adolescent pregnancy; and the ongoing social, economic and health disasters related to the 2004 Tsunami and Hurricane Katrina in 2005.

Since the 1980s, the growing field of population health has broadened the focus of public health from individual behaviours and risk factors to population-level issues such as inequality, poverty, and education. Modern public health is often concerned with addressing determinants of health across a population, rather than advocating for individual behaviour change. There is a recognition that our health is affected by many factors including where we live, genetics, our income, our educational status and our social relationships—these are known as "social determinants of health." A social gradient in health runs through society, with those that are poorest generally suffering the worst health. However even those in the middle classes will generally have worse health outcomes than those of a higher social stratum. The new public health seeks to address these health inequalities by advocating for population-based policies that improve health in an equitable manner.

Schools of public health

In the US, the Welch-Rose Report of 1915 has been viewed as the basis for the critical movement in the history of the institutional schism between public health and medicine because it led to the establishment of schools of public health supported by the Rockefeller Foundation. The report was authored by William Welch, founding dean of the Johns Hopkins Bloomberg School of Public Health, and Wycliffe Rose of the Rockfeller Foundation. The report focused more on research than practical education. Some have blamed the Rockfeller Foundation's 1916 decision to support the establishment of schools of public health for creating the schism between public health and medicine and legitimizing the rift between medicine's laboratory investigation of the mechanisms of disease and public health's non-clinical concern with environmental and social influences on health and wellness. Even though schools of public health had already been established in Europe and North Africa, the US had still maintained the traditional system of housing faculties of public health within their medical institutions. However, a year following the Welch-Rose report, the Johns Hopkins School of Hygiene and Public Health was founded in 1916. By 1922, schools of public health were established in Columbia, Harvard and Yale universities. By 1999 there were twenty nine schools of public health in the US, enrolling around fifteen thousand students. Over the years, the types of students and training provided have also changed. In the beginning, students who enrolled in public health schools had already obtained a medical degree. However, in 1978, 69% of students enrolled in public health schools had only a bachelors degree. Public health school training had evolved from a second degree for medical professionals to a primary public health degree with a focus on the six core disciplines of biostatistics, epidemiology, health services administration, health education, behavioural science and environmental science.

Education and training

Schools of public health offer a variety of degrees which generally fall into two categories: professional or academic. Professional degrees are oriented towards practice in public health settings. The Master of Public Health (M.P.H.), Doctor of Public Health (Dr. P.H.) and the Master of Health Care Administration (M.H.A.) are examples of degrees which are geared towards people who want careers as practitioners of public health in health departments, managed care and community-based organizations, hospitals and consulting firms among others. Master of Public Health (MPH) degrees broadly fall into two categories, those that put more emphasis on an understanding of epidemiology and statistics as the scientific basis of public health practice and those that include a more eclectic range of methodologies. A Master of Science of Public Health (MSPH) is granted to students who do extra studies in research, and often have had little health background before entering the degree.

Academic degrees are more oriented towards those with interests in the scientific basis of public health and preventive medicine who wish to pursue careers in research, university teaching in graduate programs, policy analysis and development, and other high-level public health positions. Examples of academic degrees are the Master of Science (M.S.), Doctor of Philosophy (Ph.D.), and Doctor of Science (Sc.D.). The doctoral programs are distinct from the M.P.H. and other professional programs by the addition of advanced coursework and the nature and scope of a dissertation research project. The Association of Schools of Public Health represents Council on Education for Public Health (CEPH) accredited schools of public health in the United States, Puerto Rico, and Mexico.[Delta Omega is the honorary society for graduate studies in public health. The society was founded in 1924 at the Johns Hopkins School of Hygiene and Public Health. Currently, there are approximately 50 chapters throughout the United States and Puerto Rico.

Public health programs

The 1963 poster given below, featured CDC's national symbol of public health, the "Well-bee", encouraging the public to receive an oral polio vaccine. Today, most governments recognize the importance of public health programs in reducing the incidence of disease, disability, and the effects of aging, although public health generally receives significantly less government funding compared with medicine. In recent years, public health programs providing vaccinations have made incredible strides in promoting health, including the eradication of smallpox, a disease that plagued humanity for thousands of years.

An important public health issue facing the world currently is HIV/ AIDS. Antibiotic resistance is another major concern, leading to the re-emergence of diseases such as Tuberculosis. Another major public health concern is diabetes. In 2006, according to the World Health Organization, at least 171 million people worldwide suffered from diabetes. Its incidence

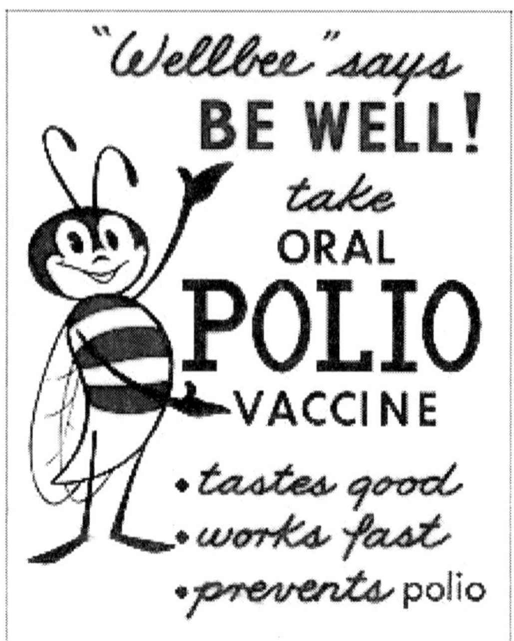

is increasing rapidly, and it is estimated that by the year 2030, this number will double. A controversial aspect of public health is the control of smoking. Non-communicable diseases caused by smoking have been threatening public health because it requires a long-term strategy for improving unlike the communicable diseases which take a shorter period to be improved. The reason for this is because communicable diseases have been at the top as a global health priority while non communicable diseases have been at the bottom as a global health priority. The global health system needs to find a way to even out communicable and non-communicable diseases. Also, these health problems are heavily framed by private sectors that most of the time benefits from being involved in our global health issues. At the same time, many of these decisions, regarding health problems, are made by industries who emphasize on technological solutions. Governments of all nations need to focus more on proactive solutions rather than relying on private actors to do the job, which they do only to their advantage. Simultaneously, global health policy-making is increasingly aligned with industrial and trade policies, and is being done hand in hand with business, thus weakening the firewalls necessary for effective regulation and normative actions both at national and global levels. Many nations have implemented major initiatives to cut smoking, such as increased taxation and bans on smoking in some or all public places. Proponents argue by presenting evidence that smoking is one of the major killers in all developed countries, and that therefore governments have a duty to reduce the death rate, both through limiting passive (second-hand) smoking and by providing fewer opportunities for smokers to smoke.

Opponents say that this undermines individual freedom and personal responsibility (often using the phrase nanny state in the UK), and worry that the state may be emboldened to remove more and more choice in the name of better population health overall. However, proponents counter that inflicting disease on other people via passive smoking is not a human right, and in fact smokers are still free to smoke in their own homes.

Prevention is Not Only Good Health Policy, It's Good Economic Policy in USA (KENNETH THORPE)

The current debate around how to best control burgeoning health costs, has pushed the issue of prevention to the forefront. By shifting our health care to be more pro-active and prevention-oriented, we can make a major impact on common and costly chronic diseases such as diabetes. In turn, this will help to secure the financial stability of our health care system and continued economic growth and prosperity.

Over the past century, the burden of disease among Americans has shifted from acute and infectious illness to chronic disease. With more than 75 cents of every dollar in this nation spent on patients with chronic disease, prevention offers the opportunity not to spend more money—but spend smarter. By embracing prevention, we can help more Americans lead healthier, active lives free from disease, so that they can avoid costly complications and hospitalizations, and remain productive in their communities and workplaces.

Prevention today involves a lot more than flu shots, cancer screening, and annual checkups. It is a pro-active strategy of disease avoidance and mitigation that should be embraced throughout and beyond the health system. In the context of chronic illnesses such as asthma, cancer, depression, heart disease and diabetes, prevention runs the gamut from lifestyle changes to screening for risk factors and symptoms, to early intervention to slow or reverse disease, to active management of already present cases. The case of diabetes—one of the fastest growing and most-threatening chronic conditions in the U.S.—provides perhaps the most compelling example of our opportunity. For most individuals who progress to type 2 diabetes, the disease can be prevented or delayed significantly by following a well-established routine of diet and exercise. The potential impact of such an approach is enormous, both in terms of lives saved, and dollars saved. Consider the economic impact alone. On average, diabetes patients have medical expenditures 2.3 times higher than those of other patients of the same age. With the incidence of diabetes expected to double worldwide by 2030, it is not only a medical necessity but an imperative to identify those at highest risk and implement disease prevention strategies.

Recent advances in diagnosis

Fortunately, we now have the tools to do just that. Recent advances in understanding the biological complexity of human disease have transformed our ability to predict and prevent the onset of chronic diseases such as diabetes. Where previously we had one somewhat inadequate tool for measuring diabetes progression—the fasting glucose test — today we have sensitive diagnostic tests capable of measuring a wide range of biological processes implicated in the advance toward diabetes. As a result, physicians can identify those patients at highest "near-term" risk for diabetes — and target intervention efforts to them.

Stratifying those truly at highest near-term risk among the 57 million Americans now considered to be "pre-diabetic" would streamline diabetes prevention, and allow physicians to focus their efforts on those most in need — thus transforming preventive medicine from a means to protect the general population to a truly personalized effort to fight disease in at-risk populations. This fundamental shift would pay substantial long-term dividends in reduced medical expenditures, improved patient quality of life and improved workplace productivity. Economic research unveiled at the most recent American Diabetes Association meeting shows that such a prevention strategy would be cost-effective in the near-term, and actually save the health care system money over the long-term. Likewise, the Diabetes Prevention Program administered in community based settings—a well-recognized "gold standard"—illustrates that cost-savings can be achieved in two to three years. Effectively adopting such a strategy requires a new approach throughout the health care system, from physicians whose familiarity or comfort with new technologies çan be slow to develop; to professional organizations who can be slow to adopt changes that deviate from the status quo; to private insurance companies and government health plans, whose reimbursement support for physicians and patients who adopt such tests and prevention strategies into clinical practice is critical.

Progress on prevention

Health reform opens the door to making true progress on prevention. On the other side of the door lies better health for our entire population—and a healthier, more vibrant economy. To get there, we must embrace policies that make it easier for patients to actively prevent and manage disease—as well as those that encourage health care providers to collaborate on care of chronically ill patients and take steps towards paying for outcomes and not just volume of services. These types of "game changers" are required to set us on the right path for our health and our economy by providing better results for all our health care spending.

Comments by critics on US health care reforms

A smart person will see the catastrophic destruction of health care in America and realize he/she is on his/her own. The smart person will therefore be highly motivated to stay healthy and out of the clutches of health care. The not-so-smart person will not have the same reaction, leaving them vulnerable to the short-comings of the system, now increased geometrically by the combination of less talent in the ranks and more people demanding salvation as promised. Remember, prevention is free.

Early detection is very expensive. Lots of mistakes, too. The advantages of preventive medicine are overrated. The public believes that these tests, such as mammography, are lifesaving, when their true benefit is much more modest. I do not accept that preventive medicine reduces health care costs. There are some experts who have argued that preventive medicine might increase costs by extending people's lives. Will mammography save women in their 40s who are at average risk of breast cancer? Perhaps, but much fewer than the public believes. (Michael Kirsch, M.D.)

Some time back, Health Affairs published an article about a study done in the Netherlands which claims that preventive care probably increases costs because it extends lives. Smokers, for example, die seven years sooner than healthy people and, according to the study, incur lower lifetime medical costs than healthy people. People who live to old age often get expensive diseases like Alzheimer's, Parkinson's, etc. I don't expect it to save health care dollars for the system, however. Indeed, it is more likely to cost money.

In my own case, I'm on medical therapy for heart disease and have been for the past ten years since my CABG. The cost of the drugs, based on Drugstore.com prices, is a bit over $3,300 per year. If I were born 30 years earlier, I probably would have died of a heart attack in my early 50's. While that's obviously not so good for me, my health care costs would have ceased upon my death. Heart disease, cancers, and some other conditions which were once death sentences are now chronic diseases that can be managed, often at considerable cost. Medical management, along with stents and other devices all cost money, sometimes a lot of money. Moreover, many of us develop heart disease due to genetic factors despite sound lifestyle choices. With respect to cancer, aside from not smoking, there is no evidence that any of the other good lifestyle choices including maintaining a normal weight, getting enough exercise, eating plenty of fruits and vegetables, consuming enough fiber, have any discernible effect on whether a given individual will develop the disease or not.

I think it is disingenuous, at best, to try to sell preventive care as a health care system cost saver which many of our politicians are trying to do. If you talk about medico-technical prevention (mammograms, screening colonospcopies, PSA, whole body scans, etc.), it is definitely overrated in the US (although some do make sense). If you mean addressing western civilization problems such as sedentary lifestyle and high caloric processed diet, it likely will pay-off, since treating 2 decades of DM II is likely more expensive than medi-care expenses for a healthy non-agenerian, and I believe there is a statistical model study supporting that. I truly believe that Pres. Obama would have a chance to be a trendsetter by living and preaching a healthy lifestyle, but so far it looks like he misses the chance (like many others). Dr. Thorpe correctly observes that we are undergoing a national "debate about how to best control burgeoning health costs." He places great reliance on "recent advances in understanding the biological complexity of human disease [which] have transformed our ability to predict and prevent the onset of chronic diseases such as diabetes." He seems to be saying that we should focus on getting the medical providers and payers to adapt more quickly to new screening tests so that intervention can occur sooner.

Forget the new tests, think of the savings if patients were to receive correct screening and follow-up care based on existing technology. It has been estimated that patients receive recommended care barely 50 percent of the time.

Overall, participants received 54.9 percent of recommended care (95 percent confidence interval, 54.3 to 55.5). This level of performance was similar in the areas of preventive care, acute care, and care for chronic conditions. The level of performance according to the particular medical function ranged from 52.2 percent (95 percent confidence interval, 51.3 to 53.2) for screening to 58.5 percent (95 percent confidence interval, 56.6 to 60.4) for follow-up care.

Our results indicate that, on average, Americans receive about half of recommended medical care processes. Although this point estimate of the size of the quality problem may continue to be debated, the gap between what we know works and what is actually done is substantial enough to warrant attention. These deficits, which pose serious threats to the health and well-being of the U.S. public, persist despite initiatives by both the federal government and private health care delivery systems to improve care.

No simple solution

What can we do to break through this impasse? Given the complexity and diversity of the health care system, there will be no simple solution. A key component of any solution, however, is the routine availability of information on performance at all levels. Making such information available will require a major overhaul of our current health information systems, with a focus on automating the entry and retrieval of key data for clinical decision-making and for the measurement and reporting of quality. Establishing a national base line for performance makes it possible to assess the effect of policy changes and to evaluate large-scale national, regional, state, or local efforts to improve quality. (McGlynn, et al., The Quality of Health Care Delivered to Adults in the United States, NEJM, June 26, 2003.)

In order to effect change we need performance measurement and transparency, something the medical-industrial complex has resisted. We need a serious change of attitude, not a technological breakthrough.

Prevention is best seen in the context of risk assessment, which converts the population-based approach to a patient-centered view. Instead of stratifying prevention by cohorts, we need to have tools that allow each individual's particular risk profile to be assessed, and identify the most important health concerns that can be prevented or mitigated. Prevention applied to a person = risk assessment + appropriate intervention +

measurable goals for process and outcome. True Prevention is stopping disease before it arises. One randomized controlled study, presented November 16, 2009 at the American Heart Association's annual meeting, found that heart disease patients who practice TM have 47% lower rates of heart attacks, stroke and deaths compared to similar patients who don't practice meditation. The 9 year study was funded with a $3.8-million grant from the federal government (NIH) and was conducted at the Medical College of Wisconsin in collaboration with the Institute for Natural Medicine and Prevention, at Maharishi University of Management in Fairfield, Iowa. Dr. Robert H. Schneider, MD, Institute Director and lead author, has received over $25 Million in funding from NIH for his Transcendental Meditation research. A major study is under way with the Ho-Chunk tribe in Nebraska to verify their observation that TM is the only observed effective intervention for Native Americans with diabetes. Eighty percent of Native Americans have diabetes. Individuals typically report normalized sugar levels within a few weeks or months with reduced or eliminated insulin need accompanied by multiple beneficial side effects.

Wellness programs

Employers could potentially save approximately $5,000 over 5 years for each employee by introducing proven health promotion programs into employee wellness programs." Mitigating the impact of the financial crises is only one beneficial side effect of creating healthy, happy, creative and productive employees. The conservative projected saving of $5,000 is based. More than 700 scientific studies conducted at 250 independent universities and medical schools in 33 countries during the past 40 years has verified the holistic benefits of the Maharishi Vedic Approach to Health. This prevention-oriented system employs forty approaches including the Transcendental Meditation (TM) program (http://www.tm.org/research-on-meditation), diet, daily and seasonal routines, herbs, and toxin removal life in harmony with Natural Law.

Multiple studies analyzing insurance records of health care utilization have documented cost savings by preventing disease from arising in the first place with non-medical interventions. (http://www.doctorsontm.com/reduced-health-care-costs). One study: The Transcendental Meditation group and Non-TM group payments to private physicians had similar growth before the intervention. After learning the Transcendental Meditation technique, the TM group made an abrupt change and decreased while the Non-TM group continued to grow. The TM group averaged an additional 14% less payments each year for 5 years with 55% less payments compared to the Non-TM group in the 6th year. (Herron, R.E. Cavanaugh, K. Can the Transcendental Meditation Program Reduce the Medical Expenditures of Older People? A Longitudinal Cost Reduction Study in Canada. *Journal of Social Behaviour and Personality*, 2005; 17: 415-442.)

Penny wise....

I used to work with a fellow who'd had a major heart attack. He'd bring a huge steak and cheese or a meatball sub. He enjoyed one of those every day telling us that it didn't matter what he ate because of the drugs he was taking for his heart to keep his lipids in check. I guess it didn't matter to his heart about that gut it was trying to pump blood through. That's not my idea of prevention. A fundamental shift would pay substantial long-term dividends in reduced medical expenditures, improved patient quality of life and improved workplace productivity. "In order to effect change we need performance measurement and transparency".

True prevention lies in one's own control in diet, exercise and avoidance of environmental influences. Changing our habits to a healthy lifestyle would have a dramatic reduction on the financial burden of care, but I'm not sure policy changes will bring about these types of changes. Prevention of chronicle diseases starts with health promotion for all people: lifestyle-intervention. More exercise, less smoking, drugs and alcohol, healthier food, safer sex, safer traffic that provides a healthier population! The problem is: our environment (physical and psychosocial) seduces us to live unhealthy. It's not easy for all people to live your life healthy. Especially if your economic status is low. In Europe they try to go further than community-based prevention. Together with the local government and the food industry they try to make changes in the environment: to reduce the seduction of too less exercise, and too much fat food. It's a slow process, it will take decades, but it is for the long-term! "More exercise, less smoking, drugs and alcohol, healthier food, safer sex, safer traffic: that provides a healthier population!"

Better lifestyle choices

Millions of smokers would probably love to quit and have tried unsuccessfully numerous times but, for whatever reason, can't. Exercise takes time, effort and discipline. For the non-athletic among us, it's not fun which makes it a slog. A lot of healthier foods don't taste very good. On the positive side, seatbelt use is upto 84% and traffic fatalities in the U.S. are at the lowest level on record based on deaths per 100 million miles driven. Doctors can advise, exhort and cajole their patients until the cows come home, but better lifestyle choices, for the most part, need to come from within ourselves. Screening tests to find problems at an early stage when they are easier and less costly to treat are a different matter. We need doctors for that, and the lower income segments of the population need some help in paying for them. On the negative side, its hard to know how many issues are identified that never would have caused any harm yet result in additional, often expensive, testing and treatment.

If we want to nudge personal behaviour in the right direction, we would impose high taxes on cigarettes, alcohol and unhealthy foods while offering financial incentives in the form of insurance discounts or rebates for people who don't smoke or quit smoking, maintain a healthy weight and keep their blood pressure and cholesterol within recommended limits. (Barry Carol, Nov. 25, 2009).

The battle for the prevention of diabetes will not be won by the medical profession, it will be won when we change our food policy that allows advertising junk food to children and which subsidizes HFCS and beef production through subsidizing corn. High calorie/high sugar/high carbohydrates/high fat has become engrained in our food culture because it's easy and cheap for corporate America to sell food that way, while they pass the costs onto the health care system. The current debate around how to best control burgeoning health costs, has pushed the issue of prevention to the forefront. That's right where it should be. The only kind of "preventive medicine" that generally universally says money is immunizations. For almost all kinds of preventative medicine, it depends on several factors that go into a cost-benefit/cost-effectiveness analysis.

Lower-class obese people have plenty of kids in their teens, 20s, and 30s before they have a chance to die in their 50s and 60s. If bad-health people live to be 58 on average, and good-health people live to be 116, that doesn't change the fact that bad-health couples can have 3 kids each and good-health couples might only have 1 or 2. MD as HELL may indeed be correct in the comment about trying to save people from themselves. Our Team (Ex Physiologist, Physical Therapists and MD's) have put together a FREE site that provides a daily prescription of what we deem the lowest level of movement needed to obtain basic benefits of "prevention." It gets some use, but nowhere near what it should/could. We thought we were going to radically change the lives of so many but have found the behavioural side very challenging!

Hype of fancy packaging and labels

Ironically, one of the problems with wellness and health in the USA is the vast array choices. A lot of the products and services that are offered are nothing more than fancy packaging and labels. From yoga and pilates to acupuncture and chirpropractors, it is nice to see that a variety of health and wellness options are available. However, like anything else, education and careful discretion is advised. Don't believe the hype—do your research and you can find good, inexpensive wellness options almost anywhere. I've started using somibo.com—a good site where you can find lots of health and wellness businesses and read and post-reviews on them.

Prevention does not just mean better screening for chronic conditions and cancers. I believe it does begin with lifestyle changes—eating healthy, exercising, reducing stress, wearing seat belts, etc. However, this is, indeed easier said than done. Yes, it must be difficult for doctors to try to convince patients to make healthier choices, but what happens when patients do not even have choices because of circumstances and environment? We must consider the additional factors that could contribute to the difficulty of making healthy choices, especially when socio-economic status is concerned. What if people want to eat healthy, but the closest and most convenient place to buy food is the local fast food restaurant? A single mother juggling 2-3 jobs probably does not have much time to cook the healthiest dinner for her kids (not to mention, may not be able to afford the freshest ingredients—the reality is, healthy food is expensive). What if they want to be physically active, but the neighbourhood they live in is unsafe for jogging and a gym membership is just unaffordable? If we want to advocate prevention in health care, it seems necessary to address not only healthier attitudes, but environmental and social issues as well to see the patient not only as a single, isolated entity, but to take them in their context and community. In doing so, we must discover what prevention means in their context and how it can be applied where they live.

Need for more Primary care physicians

Also, on the physician's end, if there is to be any call for prevention as a means of lowering health care costs, it seems that there must also be a call for more primary care physicians (PCPs). An increasing number of specialists are having a difficult time finding work because there are too many specialists and not enough patients who require their services. Meanwhile, PCPs are swamped with patients, allotting maybe 15 minutes per visit and probably find it difficult to address preventive strategies in such a short amount of time. If patients don't get preventive counselling from their PCPs, by the time they get to a specialist, it's just too late. More PCPs may mean more time per patient, and therefore more opportunity to address preventive strategies, which would hopefully lead to a healthier nation. With many medical students swayed by the promise of prestige and financial return of going into a specialty, perhaps some serious measures must be taken to encourage those pursuing medicine to consider primary care.

Health politics and health policy

It is hardly novel to say that there is a sense of malaise in the NHS. Problems come out in any conversation across the health system—problems with staff retention, targets, micromanagement, impatience, and expectations as well as with waiting lists, "superbugs" and dirt on the wards, and overburdened GPs, specialists, dentists, and nurses. This malaise comes despite the large sums of money entering the health services of the UK, despite the vocal commitment of Labour governments across Britain, and despite the goodwill towards the health services from its practitioners, its patients, and its wider publics. It might be one of the most-loved institutions in Britain, but something seems to be going wrong.

The best indicator of an organization with a management structure in trouble is constant reorganization. The literature on organizational theory, public or private, leaves little doubt that reorganization is dysfunctional. It is distracting, expensive, and blocks improvement or initiative while staff try to find and occupy new roles and start up or shut down different organizations. The UK health services have been in a maelstrom of structural reorganization for two decades. Meanwhile, in their everyday activities, they have been subjected to a variety of top-down forms of managerialism that try to impose objectives and management styles on them in a peculiar (and not particularly realistic) imitation of private-sector organizations (Pollitt, 1993). At present, that means targets, star ratings, "earned autonomy," "traffic lights," and league tables, but the barrage of central interventions outlives particular initiatives and governments. And many within the NHS insist that it erodes morale and effectiveness, distorting managerial priorities and sapping professionals' sense of autonomy and responsibility.

The problem of friction between politics and the health services, and bad health policy, is structural. The political system, behaving predictably, produces regular outcomes that gradually erode the organizational stability, coherent goals, and sense of self the NHS requires. It has powerful enabling conditions that allow politicians to try to micromanage the health services.

NHS UK ; hall mark of low-cost interventions

The particular structure of Westminster democracy and the NHS itself lower the costs of political intervention. While major interventions in health policy require serious political mobilization in any country (Tuohy, 1999), the UK system is particularly open to seemingly politically low-cost interventions in everything from individual disease treatment to organizational structure. The first section of this chapter presents the "multiple streams" model of policy-making applied to UK health policy. It stresses the processes that lead to policy outcomes large and small, and points up both their inherent unpredictability and their substantial disconnection from the health services themselves. The second section examines the institutional makeup of the UK political systems and health services in order to identify what factors put the political system and the health services in such unusually close contact and that so reduce the costs of political intervention. These lead to the conclusion, which considers various changes that might reduce the amount of friction between democratically elected politicians, health services managers, and the professionals who treat the patients.

Government in the UK—"is that we are putting billions of pounds into health and we don't see what we're getting" noted a high-level UK politician in a February 2003 interview. The sentiments are common among politicians. In addition to the disenchantment with public-sector organizations that pervades contemporary thought, politicians in the UK are feeling that the considerable sums of new money put in by Labour should have produced more of an effect than they have. Measures of throughput in the health services have not risen in line with expenditure, there are worries the money will be wasted, and politically sensitive indicators such as waiting lists stubbornly refuse to improve. The structure of NHS finance—the fact that its budget is set from general taxation by finance ministers balancing other priorities—means that it is far less prone to the cost inflation that plagues other systems. That focuses the politics of the NHS on getting something for the money; the politics of the NHS are mostly about efficiency and (latterly) quality rather than cost constraint; while other countries grope for ways to rein in free-spending doctors, the NHS systems must seek ways to make them do more with their budgets. It is natural that politicians would want something for their money, and natural that taxpayers should want them to want something for their money. There is a fundamental mismatch in political and health service timetables, as a given—new doctors can take a decade to enter the services, but a decade is three general elections (or more) and politicians are unlikely to be able to wait or counsel their voters to wait. Savvy professionals and managers speak of the need to give politicians "quick wins," that is to give them short-term, identifiable benefits in order to give the services space to develop longer-term projects. The problem is that it is difficult to generate enough quick wins to persuade the politicians they have enough to justify a tax increase.

Politicians have a right/obligation to take interest in health care

The question is not whether democratically elected politicians have a right or obligation to take an interest in the way public money is being spent. The question is why their interventions take the form of micro-management and reorganizations whose justification is generally invisible to well-wishers and those in the health services. I suggest that the activities of politicians can be explained by a well-established theory found in political science, namely, the approach known as the "multiple-streams" approach. This theory argues that the policy process has a very substantial element of randomness but that the randomness is channeled in particular ways. It explains much of the peculiar and incessant variation in health policy. While the political system is predictable in the ways it will produce random outcomes, and the outcomes can be explained, it is largely disconnected from the health service it must run.

The multiple-streams approach

Like many good theories, the multiple-streams explanation of policy decision sounds very simple (its origins are the classic Kingdon 1995; for an improved formulation that works specifically in the UK, Zahariadis 1995, esp. 27-45). It begins with the ingredients of a policy. The most basic formula for a policy outcome is a combination of a problem (something that seems to demand a response); a politician (who can and might actually do something) and a policy (something to do). If one of the three is absent, it is unlikely anything will happen. When the three come together, a policy is likely to be the result. This fundamental indeterminacy—it is based on whatever and whoever happens to be in the right place at the right time—reflects the fact that the political system is what is known as an "organized anarchy," or a system in which there is no overall hierarchy among components or borders (Cohen, March and Olsen, 1972). Rather, in politics, groups move in and out and increase and decrease in importance and there is no ultimate locus of authority (those who fight in democratic politics almost invariably live on to fight again).

Politics is, in the UK, the ideology and strategy of governing parties (Zahariadis, 1995:34). That incorporates the line-up of interest groups, the number and kind of players in the game, and the politicians' sense of the overall mood in the country, whether impressionistic or based on survey data. All of these come together to give politicians a sense of the political costs and benefits, the feasibility and likely outcome of a policy. It also incorporates an important factor, namely, the individual ministers' need to make a mark at something. It flows in ways that are much studied by politics specialists, endlessly documented by journalists, and much discussed by politicians themselves: according to wavering public opinion and focus groups, internal party pressure, the makeup of the government and its advisors, and the shifting "conventional wisdom" that marks the political classes of any arena. In sum, it is the extent to which a party sees a reason to address a problem or proffer a solution. It is not directly governed by the events in the policy sector and it can cause governing politicians to seek out solutions. Problems, however are something different. Kingdon usefully distinguishes between "problems" and "conditions" (109). A problem is something seen as requiring attention and amenable to attention. A condition is something disagreeable that we can or must live with. Poverty is a condition—the poor are always with us—but child malnutrition or pensioners without heat are conditions that get treatments. Things travel back and forth between the two statuses; spotty quality in the NHS was a condition, from the point of view of politicians, until the scandal of incompetent pediatric heart surgery in Bristol made it a political problem. Problems typically gain their status through media attention and can often compel politicians to respond. Sometimes politicians or policy entrepreneurs can engineer a condition's transformation into a problem in order to have something to treat (as happened with quality improvement in Scotland before devolution or Bristol). Problems, however, tend to erupt unpredictably—a slow news day combined with an enterprising reporter can create a political problem where none saw one before. The policies, then, also have lives of their own. Rather than being devised as solutions to problems already identified, they exist relatively independently, sustained by a support structure of professionals, academics, and adherents in the health services, professions, and civil servants (which generally form broad-based advocacy coalitions). Policy "entrepreneurs" sell their ideas, proposing their chosen policies as the responses to any number of problems. The business metaphor of "entrepreneurs" is not an accident; they sell wares by identifying clients, creating or identifying needs, and modifying their pre-existing product appropriately. With luck, they are in the right place with a plausible policy just when a politician needs a solution to a problem. All their years of preparation, analysis, and argumentation have served to make their solution seem feasible and acceptable (rather than outlandish) and give it a better chance of being the outcome of this fundamentally indeterminate process.

Policy ideas; Christmas trees

The policy ideas therefore tend to become what are known as "Christmas trees," or policies laden with justifications, answers adorned with questions they are supposed to answer. A policy idea becomes decorated with new justifications as time passes and policy entrepreneurs try to sell it as the solution to an increasingly large number of new problems. Thus primary care commissioning, information technology, data collection, and general management have by now accumulated explanations of why they solve almost any problem. They interact; health care markets have been sold by the same person (Alain Enthoven) as the way to avoid requiring data collection (because markets are automatic) and as the way to require data collection (because markets build in incentives to do so) (Enthoven, 1979, 1989). The policy is often more important to these entrepreneurs than the problem; problems are temporary and come and go, while the policy is long-lived and carries conviction. The policy, problem, and politicians allow in their interdependent streams, but occasionally flow together. When they do, a policy decision can emerge. Plausible ideas ardently proposed (and a few implausible ones) couple with a problem, often media-generated or noticed because of a well-timed press release, a politician who must make a mark to thrive and survive enters—and a policy ensues. Policy emerges from this organised chaos of newspapers, think tanks, MPs, MSPs, radio programmes, AMs, civil servants, conferences, professors, scandals, parliamentary timetables and opportunism in a way that never necessarily suits anybody working in the health system.

Implications

At a minimum, this model suggests that "evidence-based policy" and similar appeals to technocratic expertise will have a difficult career. Policy entrepreneurs base their arguments and conclusions on social science and considerations of feasibility and data play a major role in debates, but they are still advocating fundamentally political ideas (Majone, 1989). Then, regardless of evidence, the conflicting agendas, unpredictability, the skepticism of politicians.

The government machine goes to work defending the political decision, and the result is jokes about "policy-based evidence" (Constitution Unit, Northern Ireland Monitoring Report, Spring, 2003). A multiple-streams approach is not compatible with a science-based model of policy development; at most, the appeals to evidence and science that have justified professionals' involvement in policy for decades winnow out some ideas by raising technical standards and oblige all policy entrepreneurs to argue and persuade in a language favourable to expert intervention (Zahariadis, 1995). At a maximum, this model suggests that the political system is structurally given to interventions that are difficult to justify; if the policy idea has suddenly been enacted because of a favourable conjunction with politics and problem, that is no guarantee that it is a good or appropriate idea. Each of the streams is subject to important distortions that are unrelated to what we might call the management or professional imperatives of the health systems. The political stream is subject to the many factors that govern a government's political success or failure; reshuffles, elections, polls, and individual ministers' decisions are all capable of changing the direction of the public mood. Politics is shaped by interactions with events remote from health policies or problems; a war with Iraq can spill over into labour relations, September 11's terror attacks in the United States provoked abrupt changes in England's public health regime; the Chief Medical Officer was present with his ideas for reorganization just when the government needed a visible response and the public was awake to the problem of massive terror attacks in the UK (Department of Health, 2002). Political journalist Andrew Rawnsley argues that the NHS in England shifted direction because Frank Dobson's services were required as Labour's candidate for the Mayor of London, and his replacement Alan Milburn was told to "modernize" the service (Rawnsley, 2001).

Institutional conditions of instability

If the political system—any democratic political system, any "organized anarchy"—produces policies that do not necessarily reflect the goals and imperatives of health policy as seen by those who work in the services, then there is a problem. Despite the strong sentiments of many managers, political intervention is of course appropriate and usually justified; the health services must serve the people who are their paymasters. But it tends not to work. The question is how to find the balance between political demands, formulated through a policy process that does not produce stable or "rational" outcomes, and the goals of those charged by profession or managerial responsibility with operating a health system. What, then, are the attributes of the NHS and the British political system that make it easy for governments to intervene in even small matters? To some extent intervention is universal and bad policy is universal (the problematic beautifully treated in Brunsson and Olsen, 1993). Other countries also have waves of intervention and reforms, often for no easily identifiable good reasons (for a systematic study of such reforms' tidal movements, Light, 1997) and political systems that make their public services disagreeable and ineffective (Wilson, 1989:113-15). Nevertheless, the structure of the UK state and institutional position of the NHS lower the political costs of interventions and the organization of the NHS lowers the organizational costs.

Political costs of change

In striking the balance between political accountability and organizational stability, institutions matter. The changeability of any policy varies with the number of veto points in the policy system as well as the strength and number of institutions. Veto points are opportunities for important groups to stop a policy idea; multiplying veto points decreases the odds of any policy change because they are each a hurdle it must clear (Immergut, 1992). These are not just "hard," legislative veto points either (such as those created by referenda, separation of powers, or judicial review); there are also softer veto points when a crucial group can threaten to withhold an important resource. Classically, the resources that matter are advice (comment on technical feasibility, which can diminish the appeal of a policy); acquiescence (or the group's role in implementation and ability to scuttle the change—, i.e. its ability to make a prediction of implementation failure a reality); and acceptance (the group's public legitimacy and ability to affect parties' strategies and perceptions) (Beer, 1965:320). First there are the "hard" political institutions. The Westminster system of parliamentary government makes it easy for governments to act and the NHS existence as a direct part of the state makes it easy for governments to act upon it. The Westminster system and the design of the NHS lower the political costs of managerial intervention. Westminster-system governments, even if increasingly constrained by law or government coalitions, concentrate tremendous power and autonomy in the executive and therefore allow it great freedom of action. As a result, the political costs of making a decision are lower than in most comparable health care systems.

The first reason is common to public policies anywhere in the UK. The Westminster system focuses power and accountability in the government. On the one hand, the doctrine of parliamentary sovereignty brooks few limits; local government and local autonomy in general, the traditional check on the center, has been progressively swept away over the last century (Harris, 1983) while judicial oversight, based in European human rights and EU law is new and yet to have its full impact. On the other hand, this unimpeded Westminster parliament, towering above its institutional landscape, also focuses power on the government rather than on the wider assembly. This means that the freedom of action of the government is enormous and checked mostly by periodic general elections. Other governments, more constrained by interpenetrated levels of territorial politics, judicial oversight, or weaker parties, lack such freedom of action and must usually work harder to mobilize political force for a policy change. The devolved governments (with the intermittently suspended exception of Northern Ireland) remain Westminster-style systems that concentrate power and accountability in the government (even if their proportional representation broadens the representation of parties in government). The ones that function—Scotland and Wales—have certainly continued re-organizing their health services (Greer, 2003). Devolution did not produce radically more constrained governments; the flexibility and lack of fiscal intervention or formal control by the center is remarkable in comparative territorial politics (Banting and Corbett, 2002; Bell and Christie, 2002; Simeon, 2003:222-223).

Health systems financed out of general taxation

The second reason is that the "softer" institutional veto points in the policy process are also rare. Part of this micromanagement and incessant change is possible because the NHS is a relative rarity in comparative health policy. It is more directly subjected to the state than other advanced industrial health systems. It is a single large organization subject to a government, with very few other players (employers, unions, multiple layers of government, or professions) directly involved. Internationally, this is rare because health systems financed out of general taxation and directly run by the state are rare (Spain's main system, whose creators studied different models and selected the NHS model when it set-up its health system in the 1980s, is the most similar; India and Italy also chose the NHS model after considerable comparative study). Crucially, this means that there are more countervailing powers in health service policy decisions in those countries—they have more veto points. Governments can occasionally mobilize tremendous will in many different systems and surmount the resistance of health care system insiders, but their ability to intervene in small-scale managerial decisions is limited. There are few comparable systems in Europe. Continental welfare states (in the categories of Esping-Andersen, 1990) tend to use corporatist committees and Scandinavian welfare states tend to work through local government and often local government finance. Both of these kinds of systems build in very important groups that can use veto points (unions, employers, and local governments) and disconnect the central state from much of the power over and much of the blame for health issues. Their health systems' dense institutionalization channels conflict over health policy through a number of key actors including the state, and this means that there are more restraints on minor policy change.

The liberal states whose political systems are institutionally comparable to the UK—such as Australia, Canada, and the Republic of Ireland—all have powerful parliaments and governments that can redesign policy fields almost at will. They also, however, have private operators with provider power that are more integrated into their systems than the UK, or the ability to benefit from the interplay of multiple levels of government to frustrate change, or both. This means that despite the strength of Westminster-style parliaments, there are strong veto players and the process of organizational transformation is drawn out. The result is that it is more costly in terms of time, political effort, and opportunity costs to try and change the organization or management of these countries' health systems. They are responsible ultimately to the state, but there are important actors that can slow changes and that defend their own organizational autonomy.

By contrast, the political structure of the NHS is akin to that of Westminster. It centralizes authority, blame, power, and accountability in the Government and its individual responsible ministers or the Secretary of State. Like Westminster democracy, countervailing powers are few and far between. The territorial level of the health services in Britain (like local government) is very weak—the management structures between the individual hospital and the Department are entirely pliable and have been reorganized almost without cease since 1983 (Klein, 2000). Even groups with real power—professionals above all—are more likely to be cited as the reason that a given reform did not work in practice than as an explanation for the origins or decision upon an idea.

Organizational costs of change

The political system lowers the political costs of micromanagement and reorganization; the design of the NHS lowers the organizational and implementation costs of micromanagement and reorganization. The direct dependence of the health services on their political masters is well documented and explains the shibboleth that the NHS (or NHS Scotland, or NHS Wales, or the NHS in Northern Ireland) are "Stalinist." They certainly are Stalinist in the sense that most large organizations are: jobs and activities exist at the discretion of the top leadership. The top leadership in the NHS happens to be the Secretary of State or the devolved health minister rather than a corporate chief executive. The main difference is that the last century of capitalism has seen managers become the leaders of most big companies, with other stakeholders (including shareholders) firmly in the background. As long as their share price is acceptably high, managers are free. This naturally gives big corporations more focus than public-sector organizations, which are subject to the conflicting demands of many well-represented groups, and gives their chief executives more freedom. Thus, the charge of Stalinism is half-right and qualified. The NHS, like any big organization, is a hierarchical organization from the point of view of organization charts or managers. But unlike them, the NHS lacks a dictator (i.e. a corporate chief executive). Instead, it directly subjects hierarchical health service organizations with a sizeable management corps to a conflictual, unpredictable, and often very vague political process. The combination of a health system that is formally directly responsible to politicians with a highly centralized and institutionally relatively unencumbered government drastically lowers the political and official costs of change. There are, however, other costs to micro-management and reorganization, costs that cannot be reduced by political institutions alone. They are well documented in academic literature on organizational theory and public policy; reorganization takes up time, it diverts organizations from their goals and people from their work to survival and moving; it damages the morale of those reorganized or micromanaged; it requires significant investment in new organizational startup costs; and it confuses organizations' goals and priorities. Furthermore, even if it is possible for the ministers of the UK governments to tread upon professional organizations and unions when formulating policy, it is far more difficult for them to change medical practice. That politicians would try to manage a health system is not intuitive. Health care should be, it seems, seen as an even more unrewarding and costly field for political intervention than most, in large part because intervention is difficult and implementation fiendishly difficult. It has a pronounced tendency to develop according to its own logics, subject only to occasional interventions from outside the health policy system that require massive mobilizations of political energy (Tuohy, 1999). First, this is because like any system it changes as a result of previous policies' interaction with its actors—policies shape politics, and health care is unlikely to evolve in the ways politicians expect (Schattschneider, 1935; Pierson, 1993). Second, it is particularly notable for its complexity, powerful interest groups, and unpredictable interactions of different factors.

Top-down controls over professionals

Third, in addition to these problems, health management and policy necessarily is unstable. It is about top-down controls over professionals. This entails two serious problems. On one hand, professionals themselves quite rightly resist interference by non-professionals; the whole functional justification for professionalism is that highly trained and ethically sensitive specialists are required for decisions that cannot be made according to simple rules. Entrusted with such roles and obliged to make crucial decisions, and then socialized to expect respect, professionals such as those in medicine tend to resist managerial or other impositions from outside. On the other hand, professionals ultimately hold the trump card in health policy and politics. They ration. Health care comes down to repeated asymmetric dyadic actions in which a professional, usually a doctor, diagnoses a patient and decides on a treatment in conditions that cannot be rationalized or even subjected to meaningful organizational interventions. These interactions are the basis of health care provision, and they are a nut un-cracked by managerial intervention. The countries where management of professional decisions (and information technology use) has been most seriously tried, and tried virtually without budgetary constraint, is the United States. There, the track record has not been good; there appears to be no number of managerial staff adequate to "control" medical professionals' decisions. So in addition to spiraling medical costs the American private sector now can add spiraling managerial and information technology costs (Levit *et al.*, 2003).

Health policy interventions

All of these factors mean that health policy interventions seem unusually costly and doomed to fail. Yet the UK political systems have demonstrated that constant intervention can go on for decades and continue to remain appealing to political leaders. Much of this is due to the presence of professional management in the NHS. They are the solution to the collision of an unstoppable force—politics—with an immovable object—health care professionals. Management, first seriously introduced in the NHS in 1983 as part of Margaret Thatcher's first waves of managerialist public service reforms, is the object of the vast majority of political intervention. In quotidian health politics, it is managers as heads of various organizations who are obliged to meet government targets and it is managers as heads of various organizations who suffer when the targets are not met. Board chairs serve at the pleasure of the government, and are quite susceptible to pressure; chief executives and their staff also are largely unable to stand up against political interventions and thus focus on damping down political pressure. One chief executive of a large hospital trust (theoretically several steps removed from politicians) put it simply, when I asked in an interview what a chief executive had to do. He replied that being a good chief executive meant making sure there were no surprise headlines for the minister; balancing the books; and keeping the professionals happy so they did not cause problems in the hospital or in politics. In other words, the good chief executive tries to prevent too much friction between politics and professionals. The job is about fire prevention and firefighting more than management. When reorganization comes, then, hospitals, clinical networks, and GPs stay but organizations come and go. In England since 1989 health authorities have been abolished and strategic health authorities created; trusts created and merged repeatedly; primary care groups created and turned into primary care trusts; NHS regions turned into parts of the NHS Management Executive, given new frontiers, and then abolished; the Management Executive (a managerial central organization) partially merged with the Department of Health; Health and Social Care districts created to replace them and slated to be abolished a little over a year later. In most of these cases, with the partial exception of the changes to primary care, the professionals have been left alone. The enabling condition for reorganization and micro-management is something that buffers politicians and professionals from each other; the management cadre of the health services perform this function. By contrast, in Spain, which had copied the NHS system, the government's efforts to change practice have typically collided directly with professionals and professional organizations, leading to highly charged political disputes throughout the 1980s and early 1990s. It does not improve the functioning of the health services as a whole and probably degrades them over time, but the presence of a constantly re-organizable managerial layer does provide the malleable target for political intervention that the professions would not be.

Political Intervention and the UK's health services

The problem, then, is that the NHS is a theoretically hierarchical system with a direct, unmediated relationship with the "organized chaos" of the political system. This means that the relatively unpredictable political system, with its three streams poorly connected to the health service, is constantly creating direct and often remarkably detailed interventions in health policy. It is this close connection between ministers as politicians and the management of the health service that is unusual in international comparison, and it is explained by the centralization of the Westminster systems of the UK and by the otherwise effective NHS design that links its organization, management, and finance directly to the central government. The question then is what might raise the political or organizational costs of political interventions, or make them less appealing?

One political solution is to not really have a government. This is the option in Northern Ireland, where the party system gives politicians little incentive to divert themselves from constitutional politics into health policy. When the Northern Ireland Assembly is operating (as it has, intermittently, from 1999 onward), politicians see few votes to be won in health policy and many to be lost. Unlike their peers in healthier political systems, Northern Irish politicians can immerse themselves in constitutional politics, pay little attention to policy, and pay little electoral price. This unhealthy political situation is matched by an unhealthy population and a troubled health system, but at least there is no strong tendency among Northern Irish politicians to interest themselves in the organization of the health system. The experience does at least make the point that no government means no public policy, for better or for worse (when Westminster directly runs Northern Ireland, some more policy does get made).

Margaret Thatcher's reforms increased state power

A second political solution would be to try to induce politicians to behave differently. There are a number of political patches that can be used to try to dissipate the connection between multiple streams of policy-making and actual organizational outcomes. Blame for problems can be shifted to a different territorial level (such as NHS regions, boards and districts, before Margaret Thatcher's reforms increased state power in the health system). More broadly, there is the possibility that there can be broadly based learning processes among politicians. It has only been twenty years since the advent of the Griffiths report created a significant managerial structure allowing politicians to intervene in decisions systematically and a cadre of managers available for easy reorganization. It has only been a little over a decade since the Thatcher government produced, as in so many other spheres, a dramatic expansion of state power and intervention in health services. More cynically, it is something of a mystery why the need to fill news cycles with health stories leads to meaningful policy activity such as the abolition of whole layers of organization. Diverting media events such as campaigns for fitness or against alcoholism should be able to simply decrease the amount of policy activity by dawdling until policy, politician, and problem have gone their separate ways again. More optimistically, there might be institutional learning. Politicians and their civil servants might, over time, work out the costs and benefits of constant intervention and cease to reorganize and set as many targets. A consensus could develop, for example, that reorganization is not a technically feasible way to improve health system outcomes. Such a learning process would be a remarkable event in a political system that since 1979 has constantly intervened more frequently and in more detail.

Increase the checks and balances

A third political solution is to abandon trust in the central government's self-restraint and instead increase the checks and balances among different parts of the health care system. The outside agencies created by Labour in England, Scotland, and Wales to provide stable, quality regulation could be seen as restraints. However, these organizations, such as the Commission for Health Improvement, the National Institute for Clinical Excellence, and the Health Technology Board for Scotland, have highly politicized work programs and turn out to be just as susceptible to reorganization as NHS management. In other words, if the government creates the structures, it is unlikely to create groups that can truly stand upto it. Pursuing the analogy between the NHS and Westminster, the few political organizations that can stand upto Westminster are the Scottish Parliament and National Assembly for Wales, and they are both backed up by broad, powerful social coalitions. In the NHS, only the professions and the unions have been able to exercise anything like a veto on small policy changes. In short, to create such a solution, the government would have to introduce new players with control over the process of policy-making and real power through financing or delivery responsibilities—groups with which it must contend and which can veto incessant small changes in the health system. Broadening the base of representation on a level of health service management such as Strategic Health Authorities in England or Health Boards in Scotland would introduce more players, such as local government, with a solid basis from which to challenge. Alternatively, regional government in England could take pressure and accountability from London, and by being closer to its professionals might be more inclined to listen. Scotland and Wales have continued reforming their health services, but their policies are far more predictable than Whitehall's. Those political solutions all try to limit a theoretically sovereign Westminster Parliament, legally and politically a difficult task. Raising the organizational costs of intervention, rather than the political costs, might work better. An organizational solution would try to build on the professions and tried formulas for autonomy as the basis for stable governance in the NHS. The United Kingdom has some important organisations that have successfully avoided political intervention while remaining politically responsive and which could serve as models (Futures Group, 2002). The successfuk model seems to be a combination of a high-profile appointed board with an organizational focus on professional decision-making. The BBC is the greatest example of an organization that responds to its environment but does not brook political meddling. The model of the BBC, or other institutions around the world that build their independence from professional self-government (such as the American

National Institutes of Health), seems to begin with strong internal domination of decision-making tied to the values of the professions at work. Thus, for example, the BBC has an appointed board subject to close political and media scrutiny but the rest of the organization governs itself; combined with stable, hypothecated funding (the TV license fee) the political costs of government intervention are high and the organizational costs higher yet. If, beneath the board level, the professionals of the organization allocate resources they will be reliably autonomous and resistant to intervention. The Scottish White Paper of 2003 makes significant progress in this respect by transferring increasing authority from managers and organizations such as trusts to "managed clinical networks," which would be allocative mechanisms dominated by doctors (SEHD, 2003). If they are implemented, they should be strongly resistant to subsequent managerial or political intervention. This kind of model, combining professional values and political insulation, both makes the professionals more responsible for how they spend the public's money and makes political intervention harder and more visible. It would do this by making the professionals and the appointed board clearly responsible for their activities, and presumptively de-legitimize any interest by the Secretary of State for Health in a fallen bedpan. All of these would carry a price. The same centralization of the UK state that made the NHS possible makes it vulnerable to the incessant reorganizations that undermine it. The power of a Westminster parliament allowed Bevan to nationalize a great swathe of British life without many concessions to others, and gifted Britain with a cheap, effective, and popular health service that comes closer than any other to integrating health and health services, that inspires devotion in many people, and that many other countries can envy. That same power of a Westminster parliament, however, allows whoever is Secretary of State for Health to make important, and wrenching, policy decisions so often that their merits dissolve into a blur of damaging, incessant reorganizations. The question for Britain's politicians how to make the NHS work, how to get something for the money—and how to juggle their own intentions, desires, and political problems. That is also the question of how to make sure the fit between the decisiveness of a Westminster government and the need for stability of giant organizations such health services becomes better than it is. British governments, unlike most of their peers, still have much more freedom to pursue comprehensive policy ideas, whether good or bad, and stand before the electorate with full responsibility for them. The problem is that the workings of a healthy democratic system that gives the government such power can also slowly destroy the health service that is one of its greatest achievements.

Sources

Banting, K.G., and S. Corbett. 2002. Health Policy and Federalism: An Introduction. In Health Policy and Federalism: A Comparative Perspective on Multi-Level

Governance, ed. K.G. Banting and S. Corbett, 1-37. Montreal and Kingston: McGill-Queens University Press.

Beer, S.H. 1965. Modern British Politics. London: Faber and Faber.

Bell, D., and A. Christie. 2002. Finance—The Barnett Formula: Nobody's Child? In The State of the Nations 2001: The Second Year of Devolution, ed. A. Trench, 135-52. Thoreverton: Imprint Academic.

Brunsson, N., and J.P. Olsen. 1993. The Reforming Organization. London: Routledge.

Cohen, M., J.G. March, and J.P. Olsen. 1972. A garbage can model of rational choice. *Administrative Science Quarterly* 1:1-25.

Department of Health. 2002. Getting Ahead of the Curve: A strategy for combating infectious diseases (including other aspects of health protection). London: HMSO.

Enthoven, A.C. 1979. Consumer-Centred *vs*. Job-Centred Health Insurance. Harvard Business Review 57:141-52.

———. 1989. What Europeans Can Learn from Americans. Health Care Financing Review Annual Supplement ex. series: 49-77.

Esping-Andersen, G. 1990. The Three Worlds of Welfare Capitalism. Princeton, NJ: Princeton University Press.

Futures Group. 2002. The Future of the NHS: A Framework for Debate. London: Kings Fund.

Greer, S.L. 2003. Policy Divergence: Will it Change Something in Greenock? In The State of the Nations 2003: The Third Year of Devolution in the United Kingdom, ed. R. Hazell, 195-214. Exeter: Imprint Academic.

Harris, J. 1983. The Transition to High Politics in English Social Policy 1880-1914. In High and Low Politics in Modern Britain, ed. M. Bentley and J. Stevenson, 58-79. Oxford: Oxford University Press.

Himmelstein, D.U., J.P. Lewontin, and S. Woolhandler. 1996. Who Administers? Who Cares? Medical Administrative and Clinical Employment in the United States and Canada. *American Journal of Public Health* 86:172-78.

Immergut, E.M. 1992. The rules of the game: The logic of health policy-making in France, Switzerland, and Sweden. In Structuring politics: Historical institutionalism in comparative analysis, ed. S. Steinmo, K. Thelen, and F. Longstreth, 57-89. Cambridge: Cambridge University Press.

Kingdon, J.W. 1995. Agendas, Alternatives, and Public Policies. New York: HarperCollins.

Klein, R. 2000. The New Politics of the NHS. 4th ed. London: Longman.

Light, P.C. 1997. The Tides of Reform: Making government work, 1945-95. New Haven: Yale University Press.

Levit, K., C. Smith, C. Cowan, H. Lazerby, A. Sensenig and A. Catlin. 2003. "Trends in U.S. Health Care Spending, 2001." In Health Affairs, January/February, 154-164.

Majone, G. 1989. Evidence, Argument, and Persuasion in the Policy Process. New Haven: Yale University Press.

Pierson, P. 1993. When effect becomes cause: policy feedback and political change. *World Politics* 45 (4):595-628.

Pollitt, C. 1993. Managerialism and the Public Services. 2nd ed. Oxford: Blackwell.

Rawnsley, A. 2001. Servants of the People: The Inside Story of New Labour. 2nd ed. London: Penguin.

Schattschneider, E.E. 1935. Politics, Pressures, and the Tariff. New York: Prentice Hall.

SEHD (Scottish Executive Health Department). 2003. Partnership for Care: Scotland's Health White Paper. Edinburgh: HMSO.

Simeon, R. 2003. The Long-term Care Decision: Social Rights and Democratic Diversity. In The State and the Nations: The Third Year of Devolution in the United Kingdom, ed. R. Hazell, 215-32. Exeter: Imprint Academic.

Tuohy, C.H. 1999. Accidental Logics: The Dynamics of Change in the Health Care Arena in the United States, Britain, and Canada. Oxford: Oxford University Press.

Wilson, J.Q. 1989. Bureaucracy: What Government Agencies Do and Why They Do It. New York: Basic Books.

Woolhandler, S., and D.U. Himmelstein. 1991. The Deteriorating Administrative Efficiency of the U.S. Health Care System. *New England Journal of Medicine*, 314:1253-58.

Zahariadis, N. 1995. Markets, States, and Public Policy: Privatization in Britain and France.

APPENDIX 2

TERTIARY HEALTH CARE CANNOT SUSTAIN IN ISOLATION

Let us have a look at a tertiary hospital, tertiary referral center or tertiary care center in the first instance. It is a term without a formal definition which generally refers to:

- a major hospital that usually has a full complement of services including pediatrics, general medicine, various branches of surgery and psychiatry, or
- a specialty hospital dedicated to specific sub specialty care (pediatric centers, Oncology centers, psychiatric hospitals). Patients will often be referred from smaller hospitals to a tertiary hospital for major operations, consultations with sub specialists and when sophisticated intensive care facilities are required.

In India (as well as in the United Kingdom and the United States), a tertiary referral hospital can also mean any hospital that provides tertiary care.

Some examples of tertiary referral center care are:

- Head and neck oncology
- Perinatology (High-risk pregnancies)
- Neonatology (High-risk newborn care)
- PET scans
- Organ transplantation
- Trauma surgery
- High-dose chemotherapy for cancer cases
- Growth and puberty disorders
- Neurology and Neurosurgery

Another function of Tertiary Hospitals is to write and disseminate state of the art medical procedures and policies. Tertiary Hospitals are major source of the latest medical technologies. While defining tertiary health care it would be in order to define comprehensive health care, which is the expectation of every community.

Comprehensive Health Care

It means the provision of integrated preventive, curative and promotive Health Care service from womb to tomb. This mainly comprise of:

1. Provide adequate preventive curative and promotive health services.
2. Be as close to the beneficiaries as possible.
3. Has the widest cooperation between the people, the services and the profession.
4. Look after specifically the vulnerable and weaker sections of the community.
5. Create and maintain a healthy environment both in homes as well as working places.
6. Accessibility and affordability of primary, secondary and tertiary health care to every citizen (universal).

Growing inequities of well-being and health

WHO issued a Report from the 'Commission on Social Determinants of Health' that cites the growing inequities of well-being and health between rich and poor countries on the one hand and rich and poor communities of the same country on the other. The report highlights the fact that the global health community continues to fail to frame strategies for long-term health systems development. They continue to implement disease specific approach to health care-aid that will only save some lives at a huge cost. (Geraldine Luongo). Primary care is one component of a comprehensive system of care. It is arguably less expensive than tertiary care. If done well, it should have tremendous, positive impact on a large percent of the population; and, if developed in isolation from or in lieu of a comprehensive health-care system will not be able to sustain itself. Primary, secondary and tertiary care must be developed simultaneously within emerging nations if such nations are to stabilize overtime and come into there own. The good examples are Thailand, Malaysia and Singapore. The tertiary care requires hospitals and regional centers of excellence comprised of physicians, surgeons, nurses with college degrees, researchers; highly skilled, highly educated professionals who serve as faculty and medical advocates besides advanced equipment. Hospitals are central to comprehensive health-care systems. Teaching hospitals provide with the life-saving pipeline of well-trained health-care professionals at all levels. Unfortunately, the champions of tertiary care are viewed as self-serving. The global health community has myopically embraced the philosophy that all resources must be directed toward the most people for the least amount of money. It is certainly not the intent to deny the value of community-based health-workers, traditional birth attendants or other first-line workers. They are vital. Nor it is the intent to imply that immunizations and/or other preventive care are unimportant. These initiatives are critical to survival of all nations/communities. Prevention is important but all morbidity is not preventable. Also, once the person reports in a critical condition, any preventive measures will not be effective. Developing nations are sorely lacking in their ability to produce higher level medical professionals. These nations also lack resources to invest in infra structure. However, if they can muster resources to set-up centers of excellence for the treatment of unpreventable ailments or critical conditions, it is laudable. It is also essential to compliment primary and secondary health care centers with tertiary hospitals/institutes.

Human Development Report (HDR)

The United Nations Development Programme's (UNDP) latest Human Development Report (HDR) puts India's public spending on health among the lowest in the world—$4 a person a year or 0.9 per cent of its gross domestic product (GDP). Of the 175 countries documented by the HDR, only four have a lower public spending on health than India. In sharp contrast, India ranks an impressive 18th in private health care spending (4.2 per cent of GDP). The contrast is so stark for very few countries.

India's health care system, comprising government and private sectors, barely covers half its population. The public sector health infrastructure has about five lakh doctors, 7.4 lakh nurses, 3.5 lakh chemists, 15,000 hospitals and 8,70,000 beds. It is a three-tier structure comprising some 23,000 primary health centres (PHCs), 1,37,000 sub-centres and 3,000 community health centres, serving the semi-urban and rural areas. But, according to Ravi Duggal of the Centre for Enquiry into Health and Allied Themes (CEHAT), private health care accounts for 70 per cent of primary medical care and 40 per cent of all hospital care in India. It employs 80 per cent of the country's medical personnel. In 2002, the outlay of the Ministry of Health and Family Welfare was Rs. 5,750 crores (Rs. 57.5 billion), while the private sector spent Rs. 69,000 crores.

China, with which India is often compared, spends 2 per cent of its GDP on health; even Nepal (1.5 per cent), Bangladesh (1.6 per cent) and Pakistan (1 per cent) spend more on public health than India in percentage point terms. In the matter of basic health care infrastructure and facilities, the country is far behind international standards. It has 94 beds per 100,000 people, compared to the World Health Organisation norm of 333. According to some estimates, there are only 43 doctors for 10,000 people in India; exclude the private sector and it becomes an abysmal 1:30,000. Government hospitals need at least 40,000 more doctors and a large number of paramedics.

The demand-supply gap for public health care delivery is large

The gap is increasingly being filled by private health care institutions. The urban health care industry is booming, with a host of private hospitals offering state-of-the-art services for the rich and the middle class. A 2002 study, "Health Care in India: The Road Ahead" by the Confederation of Indian Industry and McKinsey and Company, put the total value of the health sector in India at over Rs. 1,500 billion or 6 per cent of GDP. Of this, 15 per cent is publicly financed, 4 per cent is financed through social insurance, 1 per cent through private insurance and the remaining 80 per cent is out-of-pocket user-fees. Two-thirds of all users fall into the last category, and 90 per cent of them are from the poorest sections. National data reveal that 50 per cent of the bottom quintile sold assets or took loans to access private hospital care. An annual interest rate of 1,200 per cent on loans is not uncommon; hence many poor people end up in the vicious cycle of bondedness, from which they do not dream to escape during their lifetime—or even over generations.

Says Union Health Secretary J.V.R. Prasad Rao: "With health funding being so low, the government can either fund doctors or get medicines or provide support services. Not all of these." In its Common Minimum Programme, the United Progressive Alliance (UPA) government has promised to spend 2 per cent of GDP on health. So far, it has not indicated from where the funds would come or how they would be spent. But a Health Ministry spokesperson has said that the emphasis would be on enhancing public-private partnership to improve health care delivery. Says Dr. Rama Vaidyanathan Baru of the Jawaharlal National University's Centre for Social Medicine and Community Health: "In its 1947 resolution, the government proposed to spend 12 per cent of GDP on health every year. Even in the best of days, it has never been anywhere close to this figure."

The quality of public health care delivery is woeful

The health care system is not only cash-strapped but also fraught with inefficiency; it is prone to misuse, even abuse. According to Dr. K. Nagaraj, Senior Professor, Madras Institute of Development Studies, Chennai, comprehensive public health care system is to be provided with PHCs at the base and referrals to provide secondary and tertiary care. But the system is hardly effective, making comprehensive health care delivery impossible. First, the system of primary health care is only an infrastructural intervention that does not take into consideration the local needs. Second, the referral system almost never works owing to infrastructural problems such as lack of medical professionals, medicines, transport and so on. According to him, the situation is only worsening with the government's privatization drive.

Health care delivery is dismal

In a survey of 100 Rajasthan villages, researchers from the Massachusetts Institute of Technology and Princeton University found an absenteeism rate of 44 per cent among medical professionals in public clinics. The absenteeism was cited to be because of meetings and other work-related problems. Apart from that, the PHCs remained closed half the time. Most rural PHCs did not have running water, electricity or emergency medicines, leave alone phones or vehicles. Some did not even have routine medicines to treat children for fever, cough and the common cold. The survey showed that 65 per cent of households in India go to private hospitals for treatment while only 29 per cent use the public medical sector. Even among poor households, only 34 per cent used PHCs. They are increasingly turning to amateur private "doctors" and faith healers, even to treat such infectious diseases as tuberculosis (TB) and malaria.

According to Nirupam Bajpai, Senior Development Adviser and Director, South Asia Programme Centre on Globalisation and Sustainable Development, Columbia University, the resurgence of communicable diseases such as malaria and TB in India is partly because of the low levels of public expenditure on health care and the commercialisation of medical care. The country accounts for a third of the TB incidence globally and has the largest number of active TB patients. An estimated 20-30 million episodes of malaria occur in India each year; mortality on account of malaria is the highest in India. Profit-oriented curative care is therefore on the rise, 80 per cent of which is in the private sphere. This has resulted in spiralling medical care costs and rural indebtedness. Tuberculosis is the big killer, claiming nearly 500,000 lives in India every year. This costs the country $300 million (about Rs. 1,350 crores) a year of which more than $100 million (about Rs. 450 crores) is debt incurred by patients and their families. Says Mira Shiva of the Voluntary Health Association of India: "Medical care has emerged as the second major cause of indebtedness in the country next to dowry."

Climate change threatens health care

It is projected that the health status of millions will be affected through increases in malnutrition, increased risk of deaths, diseases and injuries due to extreme weather events. There would also be increased burden of diarrheal disease, increased cardio-respiratory and infectious diseases due to higher concentration of ground level ozone in urban areas related to climate change and the altered spatial distribution of some infectious diseases. Climate change will also result in higher frequencies and intensities of floods, droughts, heat waves and extreme precipitation events. All of these also have serious health implications."

Can some people change the health care scene?

"Indian villages are filthy, people do not have any sense of public hygiene and children, who are most vulnerable die of infections, which can easily be prevented if only one could improve sanitary conditions in our villages", said Dr. Naresh Trehan at a function. How by just improving village sanitation and building a proper school in a village in North India, he and his team has been able to cut down disease and infection in the village. This he said was accomplished with financial support from a few large business houses who generously donated for this cause. One would reckon that this can just as easily be done with funds from the government. After all this is an investment in health care and education of the future citizens of the country and is bound to pay healthy (no pun intended) dividends.

Dr. Trehan acknowledged that no self-respecting doctor wishes to practice medicine in the hinterlands of the country. The quality of life that he expects for himself and for his family, just does not exist in Indian villages as yet. Thus, it makes no sense to have Primary Health Care

Centres in every village simply because it would be impossible to have qualified doctors functioning at these centres. Dr. Trehan instead suggested mobile clinics located in district headquarters and small towns, which can visit nearby villages on fixed schedules and offer Primary Health Care services in remote villages.

The government has a fairly vast health care infrastructure at the district level. The district hospitals can easily serve as good secondary care hospitals, provided they are managed efficiently and are held accountable for the quality of care they deliver. Dr. Trehan mooted a model based on a Private Public Partnership (PPP), which would allow efficient utilization of these resources and also generate a decent profit, which can be used to further strengthen these hospitals.

As far as the Tertiary Health care is concerned, Dr. Trehan indicated access and pricing as the big issues. He felt that low-cost universal health insurance as a possible answer. Dr. Trehan also believes that tertiary health care costs can be significantly brought down if a hospital has a high throughput of patients. Thus, a tertiary hospital can amortize its fixed costs over a large number of patients, bringing the overall costs down.

Trauma services are rudimentary

One example of the failure to build hospital based capacity in the emerging world is the dramatic and steadily growing rate of death by trauma and injury. While some injuries are indeed preventable, many are simply unavoidable. What is absolutely preventable is a life long disability due to lack of access to surgical care needed to appropriately respond to the injury. The likelihood of dying from an injury is twice as high as the risk of maternal death in developing nations. WHO estimates that injuries reflect 12 percent of the burden of disease: twice that of HIV and greater than TB, diarrhea and malaria combined. The leading cause of death for people ages 5-45 is injury or more precisely, the injury leads to death from a lack of even the most basic hospital and surgical care. Poor surgical care is a major public health threat in the developing world. The lack of qualified surgeons and hospital care contributes to the burden of disease and death at a rate greater than that of communicable diseases.

The Strategies of tertiary care

As mentioned elsewhere, three men are redefining India's tertiary care in the private sector. That first honor goes to Prathap C. Reddy, who set-up Apollo Hospitals in 1983. In fact, Wockhardt, Fortis and Max have been built somewhat along Apollo's lines. But what is significant is that they have taken the game to another level. In less than a decade, Wockhardt, Fortis and Max have added close to 5,000 beds, something that took Apollo 20 years. (It is another matter that India still needs an additional 80,000 hospital beds each year.) Their revenues have grown briskly—about 30 per cent annualized for the past five years for each, according to Vivek Desai, managing director, Hosmac, a hospital consultancy.

There aren't any precise estimates of how big the hospital industry is. Apollo's hospitals group has a turnover of Rs. 719 crore over 8,000 beds. That translates into revenues of Rs. 2,460 per bed per day. According to some approximations, there are around 875,000 hospital beds in India. So that translates into an industry worth Rs. 78,630 crore. However, that would perhaps be on the higher side as majority of the beds wouldn't fetch Apollo rates. According to a CII McKinsey report, the entire health care industry is worth $18.7 billion, with the private sector controlling 65 per cent of it. But this figure includes the pharma industry as well as other health care related businesses like pharmaceuticals, diagnostics, etc.

Also, traditionally health care is a recession-proof industry. This means hospitals can flourish pretty much, as long as they get two things right-managing doctors and understanding the psyche of Indian patients. A quick insight: unlike in the west, where people go to GPs for everyday illnesses, Indians tend to go to specialists. Max Health Care tried changing this, but failed. Indeed, Max bore the brunt of public scrutiny far more than any other given that it came up in Delhi, and was the first private player of any significance after Apollo. The original Max plan was simple. Have local primary care centres, which would feed into secondary care centers, which would converge at a tertiary care centre. This model is established abroad, but was being tried for the first time here. It did not work-though Analjit still defends this original plan. "A pilot does not start with a 737; he begins with a turbo jet so that he does not take a large number of people with him." Doctors and patients differed. The former felt that the primary clinics were competing with their private practice and, therefore, were reluctant to join up. The absence of a full fledged hospital within Max was another disincentive for doctors who were usually attached to big hospitals for tertiary care treatment, which is the big ticket spend. Primary care is like a filter. The absence of a tertiary care hospital also meant that Max's clinics were used as referral centres to other hospitals. Also, Max had started its centers at up-market Delhi localities, assuming correctly that the resident had more spending power and would be willing to afford better medical care. But this turned out to be a bit of a liability, since those patients were used to visiting marquee doctors, whom Max did not have. Though Max had consultants trained internationally, they were unknown names in Delhi. Analjit Singh describes those days as "his struggle to understand the Indian health care market". Worse was to follow. By 2003, Max's CEO and the chief medical officer quit. Also, a tie-up with Harvard Medical International (HMI) was terminated in 2004. (Wockhardt would sign up with them later.) Many blamed Singh for his unwillingness to delegate. He took the criticism in his stride and continued to be closely involved. What he learnt has shaped the Max Health Care of today. It has adapted the original primary-secondary-tertiary model to a roughly secondary-tertiary model. The secondary care clinics have been upgraded to smaller hospitals (a 20-bed outfit is now a 60-100 bed outfit); simultaneously, the practice of the primary centers has moved to the secondary and main hospital and all primary centers have been closed down.

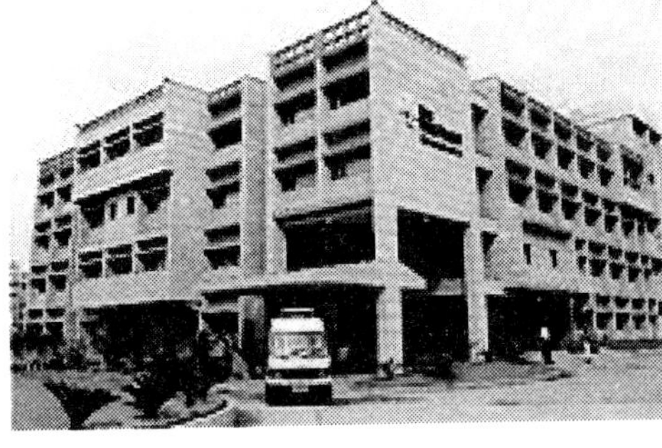

Max today has four secondary care centers—two at Panchsheel in south Delhi and one each at Noida and Pitampura (north-west Delhi). Plus, it has a general hospital (half- way between a secondary and tertiary care) in Patparganj in east Delhi. It also has as a massive tertiary care unit at Saket (south Delhi), which comprises a general hospital (Institute of Allied Medical Sciences), plus five super specialty institutes. "Our strategy to meet the demand has been to create five institutes—cardiac, orthopedics and joint replacement, neurosciences, pediatrics and one for obstetric and gynecology," says Max executive director and CEO Mukesh Shivdasani. Work is on for another super specialty hospital in Gurgaon, which will focus on transplant surgery and another one in Patparganj with oncology as the super specialty. Analjit Singh feels he now has the critical mass to expand. But his advice to all who want to get into hospitals: "The business is capital-intensive, it has long gestation, and the viability comes when you have played that out."

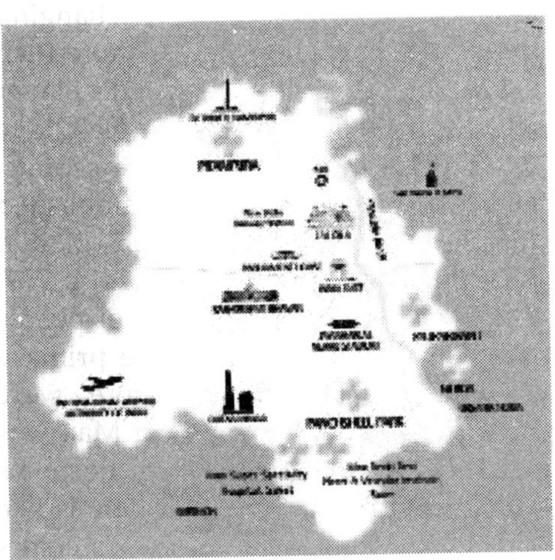

Nephew Shivinder's experience was different. Fortis decided to set-up its first hospital at Mohali, Chandigarh, a market that didn't have any other large, tertiary care private hospital. The idea was to attract patients from Himachal Pradesh, Haryana and Punjab. Simultaneously, it planned secondary care centers in other locations, which would be linked to the big Mohali hospital. It was a classic hub and spoke model.

Max health care model

When it started in 2001, Max Health Care was a two-clinic set-up. The metamorphosis from Dr Max Clinic to superspecialty Max Health Care hospitals shows sharp marketing acumen and patient-centric approach. Max Health Care, a venture by Analjit Singh, was established in 2001 to provide primary, secondary and tertiary care hospitals across the National Capital Region (NCR). The aim was to offer patient care that combines medical and service excellence. When they started, Dr Max clinics used to be conveniently located neighbourhood clinics with services designed to

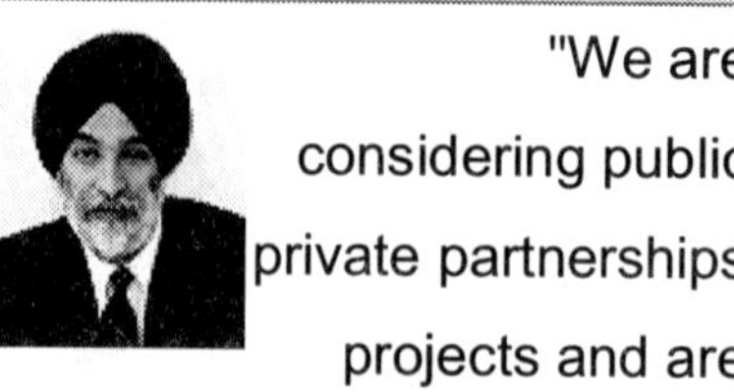

"We are considering public private partnerships projects and are open to green-field projects, brown-field projects and also management of hospitals"

- **Analjit Singh**
CMD
Max Healthcare

support and supplement the service of the regular family physician. Today, Max is a name associated with superspecialty health care.

The Group has seven centers within Delhi and is now looking at expanding to other cities, including Dehradun. It was announced recently that the company will raise between Rs. 350 crore and Rs. 400 crore to expand its hospital chain. "The funding has been a combination of equity and debt," says Analjit Singh, CMD, Max Health Care. With venture capitalist firm Warburg Pincus investing Rs. 200 crore in Max India, some of the funds are expected to flow into health care too. There's a perceptible flurry of activity at Max Health Care as management looks at strengthening existing facilities and scouts for locations to set-up new hospitals. In the next two years, the Group plans to double its bed capacity from the existing 765 to 1,500. Plans include expanding the Patparganj facility to 268 beds by October-November, 2008. The upcoming 100-bed Max Hospital in Gurgaon is also likely to be commissioned soon.

Max Health Care has seven centers in and around Delhi. These offer services in over 30 medical disciplines with super-specialized services in cardiac care, neurosciences, orthopedics, pediatrics, obstetrics and gynecology.

- Max Devki Devi Heart and Vascular Institute, Saket, is an internationally-recognized center of excellence for cardiac care.
- Max Super Specialty Hospital, Saket has an advanced brain tumor centre, minimally invasive spine centre, stroke centre.

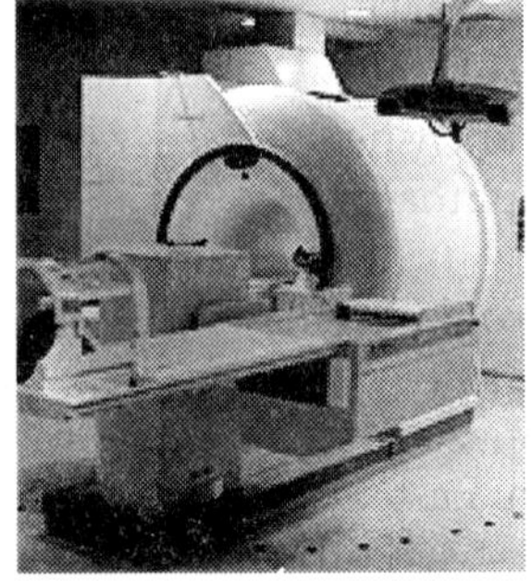

- Max Balaji Hospital, Patparganj is a world-class tertiary health care facility. It is equipped with high-end equipment and infrastructure, has systems and processes that rival the very best in the world.
- Max Hospital, Pitampura provides excellent health care over a range of services. Well-equipped OTs, dialysis services and facilities for advanced laparoscopic surgery are some of the services available.

- Max Hospital, Noida offers specialty treatment for a wide range of ailments including chronic care programmes in diabetes, asthma, arthritis and hypertension.
- Max Medcentre, Panchsheel Park is mainly an outpatient centre.
- Max Eye and Dental Care Centre, Panchsheel Park has latest facilities for eye surgeries and offers comprehensive eye examination.

Max Hospital, Gurgaon: Starting in 2007, this hospital will offer services in ophthalmology, health checks, nephrology and urology, reconstructive surgeries, neurosurgery, orthopaedics, and general and minimally-invasive surgeries.

Image Makeover

What was unique with the initial growth model for Max was the fact that while most health care institutions first build the hub and later expand, Max expanded the other way round. The management first built Dr Max Clinics and other secondary care hospitals in and around Delhi and then established a tertiary care hospital. This model was emulated from the US health care system on the advice of Harvard Medical School and also equally determined by the lack of immediate availability of large tracts of land to build a tertiary care hospital.

But soon, the business model had to be changed. "The hub and spoke model works well in the US, but is not suitable for India. It gave rise to the perception that Max clinics were primary care centers meant for non-serious ailments," explains Dr Narottam Puri, Executive Director, Medical Services, Max Health Care. Patients from Dr Max clinics were going to other hospitals and the secondary clinics like the one in Panchsheel, New Delhi were being used for simple surgical procedures.

The process of revamping and re-invention required immense marketing effort and unique brand positioning. As part of the business strategy, the management also brought on board some of the best doctors and renowned specialists.

The Group focused its expansion activities in the NCR region of Delhi in the first phase. Along with Dr Max clinics, the Max Medcentre in Panchsheel Park in South Delhi was developed as a speciality clinic for ophthalmology and dentistry.

Likewise, secondary care hospitals in Pitampura in North Delhi and Noida were set-up. This was followed by the state-of-the-art tertiary care facilities at Saket (Max Heart and Vascular Institute and Max Super Speciality Hospital) in South Delhi and Balaji Max Hospital at Patparganj in East Delhi.

Internal focus

At present, Max Health Care has a base of over 1,000 leading doctors, 2,400 employees, and 3,60,000 patients with the number of beds growing to over 900 by next year. "We strongly believe in the dictum that leadership should have high expectations while maintaining the value systems and hence fulfil the needs of all stakeholders, including patients," asserts Dr Sanjiv Malik, Chief Executive, NCR-II, Max Health Care.

According to Malik, what makes the Group unique is its leadership, which has helped align and integrate the clinical requirements and business needs. "As a result, Max has grown to be known as a patient-focused brand that offers excellent services," he says. Patients are made a part of decision-making process at Max Hospitals, which has helped it become popular.

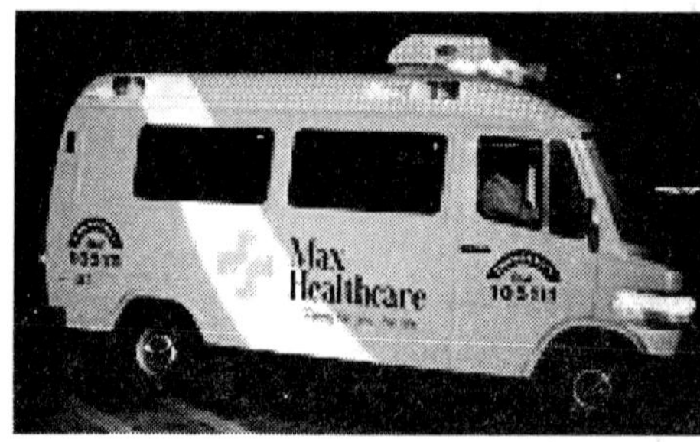

To improve service, feedback from employees is encouraged. Max Health Care also stands out because of getting the latest cutting-edge technology. A case in point is its brain suite, which is the first of its kind in Asia.

"Most importantly, this organization is receptive to the dynamics of change. People's ideas are listened to, which brings in creativity and positivity," avers Dr Malik. Additional factors responsible for Max Health Care's stupendous success and unbridled growth, are training and development, customer satisfaction, quality and continuity, he adds.

Continuous learning

Great emphasis is laid on training and development of employees. A dedicated centre called Max Institute of Medical Excellence (MIME) offers customised training programmes for doctors, nurses, paramedical staff and even non-medicos. MIME offers about 50 courses that are critical for the medical fraternity and also provides high-quality education material including online clinical information and access to medical journals, guidelines, etc.

Education is yet another initiative. Max wants to enter the league of institutes which have a tie-up with Diplomate of National Board of Examination (DNB), and recently it has received approval for cardiology, cardiac anaesthesia and interventional cardiology. Now, it has applied in four other specialities.

MIME has a state-of-the-art clinical skill laboratory equipped with the latest range of simulators, which are used by the trainees to learn and practise clinical skills and procedures in a safe and controlled environment.

The lab simulates a hospital setting which facilitates innovative teaching strategies by means of computer-assisted learning. MIME also offers specially-designed modules for those from a non-medical background including executives and school students. The courses offered include first aid, stress management, CPR, etc. MIME also publishes patient education booklets for patients to learn about diseases, drug usage and procedures.

Quality Control

Continuous improvement in quality is mandatory for retaining quality. According to Dr Puri, "Reaching the acme of quality excellence can only happen through right education, right training and right credentials (choosing the right people for the job).

Max Health Care has introduced Six Sigma Methodology to improve the processes and quality and reduce costs. All the institutions of Max have ISO 9000:2001 certification or are undergoing it.

"Our laboratory at Saket is undergoing NABL accreditation. Max Heart and Vascular Institute and Max Super Speciality Hospital at Saket are expected to be NABH accredited very shortly," says Singh. Internal medical audits and medical governing councils viz. ethics, medico-legal, infection control, pharmacy and therapeutics ensure excellent quality checks and controls.

Service is the best reward

Max doesn't believe in advertising. "Through our onsite and off-site camps, people experience our service and end up becoming our brand ambassadors," says Dr Malik.

At Max Health Care, management believes that the best way to market services is through CMEs and workshops, "Because they help us showcase our work that is morally, scientifically and ethically correct," avers Dr Puri. These programmes expose the medical fraternity to their world-class facilities and that results in increased popularity.

Tele-medicine

Over 600 million Indians live in rural areas. Access to medical specialists operating in urban areas is a distant dream for them. Statistics show that there is only one hospital bed for about 1,300 Indians, and one doctor per 15,500 people. Less than 9 per cent of the country's billion plus population is covered under health insurance schemes. So, what could be an ideal solution to reach the 600 million plus Indians in rural areas in terms of medical help? Tele-medicine could be a very possible answer, say experts in the health care and IT industries. In the last few years, a lot has been talked about tele-medicine. However, despite the awareness, it is yet to take-off in a big way. The concept is still restricted to some of the large corporate, considering the cost involved in creating the necessary infrastructure, feel sources in the health care and IT industry.

Tele-medicine remains effective. Yet at best it connects only tertiary-care hospitals to the selected primary-care centers. Unless there is a national initiative and government support, tele-medicine will not be effective in providing specialized care to distant satellite centres. Tertiary hospitals in the private and public sector would continue to be overcrowded, says Prashanth Prakash, Founder and Chief Strategy Officer, Netkraft Private Ltd, a Bangalore-based firm and provider of IT solutions in health care.

Says Dr Sunil Shroff, Professor and head of department, Urology and Renal Transplantation, Sri Ramachandra Medical College and Research Institute, Chennai, "Tele-medicine is going to entirely change the way we practice medicine. The day is not far away when a patient in Chennai is likely to have his general practitioner in Mumbai or London, or a specialist in Australia may help a surgeon in Aurangabad to perform a difficult surgery. However, Indian IT companies need to create cost-effective applications suited for the domestic sector."

The Indian Space Research Organisation (ISRO) used its INSAT (Indian National Satellite) and IRS (Indian remote Sensing) satellites for various applications, including tele-medicine. A recent application of space technology initiated by ISRO was in tele-medicine to provide expert medical services to rural areas. Under the tele-medicine project, hospitals/health centres in remote locations are linked through INSAT satellites with super specialty hospitals at major towns/cities, bringing in connectivity between patients at remote ends with specialist doctors for medical consultations and treatment.

There are over 30 tele-medicine centres in the country linked with ISRO's INSAT, including the Andaman Islands, says Dr Shroff, who is also the President, Medical Computer Society of India.

Tele-medicine helps patients in distant and rural areas to avail timely consultations of specialist doctors without travelling long distances. The facility caters normally for transmission of patient's medical images, records, output from medical devices and sound files, besides live two-way audio. With the help of these, a specialist doctor could advise a doctor or a paramedic at the patient's end, online, on medical care or even guide the doctor during a surgery.

Tele-medicine systems consists of customised medical software integrated with computer hardware, along with medical diagnostic instruments connected to the commercial VSAT (Very Small Aperture Terminal) at each location. Generally, the medical record/history of the patient is sent to the specialist doctors, who in turn, study and provide diagnosis and treatment during videoconference with the patient's end.

ISRO's facility serves the tele-medicine project at a larger scale. However, deploying it at a smaller scale and at smaller hospitals could be costly. Only large hospitals can afford to spend a few lakh rupees, feel experts in the IT and health care industries.

For instance, using ISRO's satellite, the Apollo Hospitals provides expert opinion from its tertiary level hospitals in bigger cities to those in the far-flung towns of India on various medical issues. Similarly, Sankara Nethralaya has spent about Rs. 1 crore on tele-medicine, of which Rs. 75 lakh has been provided by ISRO for a mobile van and equipment.

Says an official of a large IT firm, tele-medicine need not necessarily need large investments. With just a personal computer, a modem, a scanner, a Web camera and a telephone line, all costing less than Rs. 50,000, a tele-medicine project can be up and running.

For instance, using a 64 kbps line, a patient's reports can be sent through text, voice, images or even video, and medical advice can be offered from a remote location. Using this solution, successful pilot tests have been conducted at various places in Tami Nadu, the official says. "Cost-effective tele-medicine solutions could be spread across the country. We are not looking at conducting surgeries through tele-medicine. We are only looking at diagnosing patients' disease and advising them accordingly," he says.

Says Dr Praveen Soti, Consultant, Health Care Practice, Domain Competency Group, Infosys Technologies, there have been pilot projects on tele-medicine by some large corporate hospital groups and the response has been mixed. Though some projects have been successful, success has been seen in larger tertiary-care settings for focused disease conditions. This has helped doctors understand the patient condition better and plan treatment accordingly. Considering the patient load on doctors, it would be too early to comment on possibilities of tele-medicine in primary care settings in India. Improvements in infrastructure and systems for capture of complete patient details (History and Investigations) and standardised referral mechanisms will help needy patients to benefit from tele-medicine.

For better utilisation of tele-medicine services, awareness needs to be spread at the end-user level, says Mohan Narayanan, Vice-President, Health Care and Life Sciences Practice, of Cognizant Technology Solutions. Tele-medicine in India is still in the embryonic stages and will soon catch up. There are success stories where tele-medicine has played a major role in saving lives in instances of natural disasters, he says.

Better medical education

The area of improving skill of the trainers and medical teachers is crucial to better physicians and surgeons. Basic medical education and training should be tailored to (i) develop appropriate manpower to meet common health needs, (ii) recognise and manage common health problems, (iii) teach critical appraisal of new information to keep abreast of advances, and (iv) ensure ethical practice. The current system falls far short of these objectives. The medical training continues to be inappropriate and inadequate for meeting the health needs of the country. The referral patterns of tertiary hospitals make uncommon conditions presenting at these centres appear common with the exotic seeming standard. Since medical colleges in India operate at the level of tertiary care centres, such uncommon conditions are used for educating India's basic physicians. The curriculum: In India, the medical college setting, with its different specialities, drives the medical curriculum. Systems and areas of expertise are organised into separate departments, each with a narrow focus and circumscribed field. The demands of the specialty, the teachers and the settings are the factors that tailor medical education rather than the needs of the population they are meant to serve. The failure to develop simple and relevant guidelines for the management of common local medical problems implies a reliance on strategies meant for developed countries. While the need for clinically relevant basic science education is often discussed, in reality, the curriculum continues to be loaded with inconsequential detail.

The development of tertiary health care; Improving medical education

The pyramid of health-seeking has its base in informal household remedies, traditional medicine and primary care, and moves through secondary hospitals with tertiary care facilities at its apex. The vast majority of patients seek outpatient services in clinics and small hospitals. A small proportion visits—and an even smaller fraction is admitted to—tertiary care centres. The medical colleges, modelled on European-American institutions, retain their colonial inappropriateness. A model, with its focus on local reality (for example, as used in Cuba), is probably more suitable.

The examination system

In practice, the systems of examinations have a greater impact on the approach of students to education than the curriculum. The tertiary care focus results in the use of uncommon conditions for assessment during clinical examinations. For example, mitral valve stenosis, an uncommon condition, is a standard case for the final clinical examination, while common conditions (diabetes mellitus, hypertension) are never used for assessment. A medical graduate can pass this examination without ever having been assessed on the diagnosis and management of malaria, endemic in many parts of the country.

Knowledge, skill and confidence

Most medical colleges focus on the transmission of information to students. Many new subjects have been added to the curriculum at the cost of basic clinical medicine and surgery. The acquisition of skills and the confidence to apply them are limited. The emphasis is on arriving at a clinical diagnosis, while a hands-on approach to the management of patients is not stressed. Clerkships during the course and exposure to secondary hospital settings are the exception than the rule and, even when present, occur for short periods. Internship is fragmented with brief periods spent in many specialties. The superficial and theoretical approach to patient care makes students less competent doctors. The general population realizes this lack of skill and shops for specialist care. Young graduates also quickly appreciate this deficiency and seek postgraduate qualifications in order to acquire clinical expertise. Seeking a postgraduate qualification is a survival strategy for most doctors, rather than a choice based on aptitude or one based on need. The long periods of training, investment and specialization in urban-based tertiary centres make doctors reluctant and less suited to work in rural primary and secondary health facilities.

Role models and mentors

Young medical students see their seniors as role models and their teachers as mentors. However, even good medical teachers, while emphasizing clinical skills and focusing on common conditions that affect the health of the majority of the general population, are seen to pay lip service to these goals by actually practicing in tertiary care facilities. Their actions speak louder than their words and their message of clinical care and service to the underprivileged sounds hollow. In fact, the resistance of the majority of the faculty to change the *status quo* was one of the major reasons for the failure of the re-orientation of the system.

The way forward

Solutions for the absence of skill-based training during undergraduate medical education are postgraduate courses, including family medicine and the master's course in medicine and surgery. The compulsory posting of new physicians to rural health centers will also have a limited impact on health care delivery. The insufficient skill and confidence of these doctors will result in the continuation of second class health care for the rural poor, the underprivileged and the marginalized. There is a need to revamp basic medical education. There is a need for patient and community-centered medicine and for the dismantling of disciplinary and specialist boundaries during undergraduate medical education. Training should be set in primary care and secondary hospital facilities, which is crucial to learn about common health problems in the community and to manage them without expensive technological input. Testing of skills required for working in primary care and in secondary hospitals, rather than the practice of assessing theoretical knowledge of uncommon disorders, is mandatory for success.

There is no doubt that medical education in India is not equipping doctors with skills to manage the common medical conditions. But doctors learn those basic skills by working as an apprentice with some practising doctors. The real problem in India is the urbanisation and industrialisation. When there are so many ways you can spend the money in modern India, any common man will aspire to earn more (Except people like Gandhi and Buddha). To earn money in developing country like India is to practise as superspecialist in Corporate hospitals. The only way you can practise in this corporate hospital is you should not have any ethical conscience. So whatever the country does it won't be able to solve the current menace until the common man (doctors are part of common man, he is not someone came directly from heaven) change his attitude towards material and money. Certainly among 1.2 billion population there will be a few thousand educated people with good cause and will be able to become the doctors what our country needs (Such as Chhattisgarh-based human rights activist and few other doctors. So the admission into medical college should be given at least 50% of the seats to those people who would certainly be practicing ethically and in rural area. How to identify those people, certainly not by their final year marks, but the way they have so far been living as a citizen, their interest to serve the community without expecting any rewards. I am certain if the medical admission is given to rural students, they are more likely to go and work in rural areas with less corruption than that to an affluent city student whose English is so good that he won't stay in India. Until we change the policy of admission to medical school any kind of reforms will only result in more chaos, with less reward.

For a strong health care system it is necessary to get down to the field and study the climatic, environmental, and lifestyle factors of people and their vulnerability to any diseases. With these facts and information, the medical and other health education curriculum should be periodically revised. It should also enable provisions for continued research on the factors affecting the health of the people and its interdependency with the lifestyle. The health education departments or association should actively try to promote continued education programs seriously with a focus not just on finding a cure but to implement the preventive and protective measures.

Anomalies in health care delivery to employees

Various PSU's adopt administrative procedures that are convenient to their employees and there are no proper guidelines/rules or reimbursement for different medical/surgical/investigative procedures and this results in different amount of payment that is reimbursed to different Nursing Homes/Hospitals. This is not the problem with the CGHS wherein the minimum rates are fixed for practically all the procedures and the reimbursement is done accordingly to the employee (regardless of the amount the employee spends). (CGHS has a list pertaining to admissible reimbursement for various procedures that is circulated from time to time). The problems that are being faced by the present system are two-fold. One aspect is huge amount of reimbursement claims and the other aspect is expenses for the Scrutinising systems in the Accounts Department of the medical claims. (The employees of the account section, Medical doctors and the time and effort of the employees that goes in for getting the advance, reimbursement claim, etc.) It is difficult to determine the genuineness of the medial claim of the employee and very often false claims are submitted by certain employees and the PSU's have to reimburse the claim as the panel doctors are not under their administrative control. This problem is faced by most of the PSU's.

It is one of the observations that patients are kept in the Nursing Home/Hospital even after the illness does not warrant admission/observation by the Nursing Homes/Hospitals. This practice results in inflating the claims and at times the employees are kept as hostages till such time that bills of the hospital are settled, which inflates the bill further, since most of the employees depend upon their organization for making payment directly to the hospital or advance the payment in the form of reimbursement to such an employee. This may often be a hidden motive of the Nursing Home to extract more money from organization. The employee in such circumstances also suffers, even though innocent.

The data on the expenditure on the Health Care of the PSU employees is not systematically available. In many of PSU's it appears that the expenditure on the Health Care is included under the Welfare Head. The statistics on desegregated amount spent on the different aspect of the Medical expenses, i.e., Manpower, Medicines, expense on the internal set-ups, Secondary/Tertiary Care Set-ups and disease patterns which require exceedingly high reimbursement claims are not available.

The Medical personnel may rise upto the rank of General Manager maximum in the couple of PSU's. Even on they attain only the grade and perks of the post. Usually they would not have any say in the administrative matters in regard to their divisions. Mostly these medical personnel are also not interested in asserting themselves to insist upon their administrating superiors. The administrative superiors though well meaning and interested in improving the organizational set-up, usually, would not be able to do so due to lack of specific knowledge in the field of Health Administration.

Financial aspects of concept

The analysis of the financial aspects could be done by examining the current expenditure pattern of Medical claims, Medical advances, Credit scheme or other mechanisms of the payment to the Panel Nursing Homes, Hospitals by all the participating organizations.

The financial analysis also would require to be done by the participating organizations, i.e., Cost per employee (Per capita cost being spent by each of the participating organization), Number of instances of hospitalization per year per organization, Average cost per hospitalization, etc. Certain percentage of the amount of the per capita cost could be levied as an Health insurance deposit from the employees (on the lines of the CGHS and ESI schemes). The involvement of the employees of the PSU's in contribution towards the Health insurance expenses probably varies from one PSU to the other. A uniform/graded approach could be developed amongst the participating PSU's (number of the employees per PSU) so that the generation of funds is also there and a sense of ownership also is generated amongst the employees.

As the Health insurance multinationals are also coming in for providing the Health Care Services in the country and the aspect of operationalisation could include their participation in the financial aspects of the Health Care of the employees of the participating organizations. This also would depend on the results of the analysis stated above.

The financial sharing equation between the PSU's could be developed to the extent of the shared resources, the employee strength of each participating PSU and involvement of the Health insurance and the contribution from the employees as it is in the case of the CGHS and ESIC.

The initial capital expenses for creation of the facilities could be done by the participating PSU's according to the number of the employees, the financial standing of a PSU and possibly generating funds from other financial institutions/participation of employees in the ownership of the scheme.

Human resource aspects of the scheme

The existing manpower in the Medical units serving the PSU's could be utilized by doing the manpower analysis and matching with the needs at the work place and at the other levels of treatment (Secondary/Tertiary) to be created. The skill enhancement techniques, i.e., rotation of manpower, redeployment in areas where special skills could be developed in certain occupation, retraining (need-based and work on hand experience) would result in diversification of the services for the organization and experience of different work areas would enrich the Medical and Para-medical personnel by avoiding the problems that arise from stagnation of the person on the same job.

The available GPs in the area can be given a platform to practice in the facilities created/Existing facilities and their timings suited to the convenience of the employees (in case of shift duties). Certain amount of monetary package, and/remuneration commensurate with the amount of time spent could be given to the GPs in the local area.

The Human resources for the administration of the scheme should be drawn mainly from the fields of Health/Hospital Administration for providing effective leadership to the Independent Board of experts proposed to be created.

The Specialists/super specialists could be drawn from the reputed hospitals in the vicinity and can work in these facilities and can be given remuneration according to the time spent in the Clinic/Number of operations performed, etc.

The paramedical staff for the scheme could be appointed separately or the existing/available could be redeployed.

Primary Medical care and Primary Health Care!

Primary medical care, whilst often used as synonymous with primary health care, should be clearly distinguished. Primary health care includes the provision of primary medical care, therefore, a selective component of primary health care. Primary health care is the first point of contact a person encounters with the health care system. In mainstream health primary health care is normally provided by general practitioners, community health nurses, pharmacists, environmental health officers, etc. although the term usually means medical care.

World Health Organization definition: "Primary Health Care" means "...essential health care based on practical, scientifically sound and socially acceptable methods and technology made universally accessible to individual and families in the community through their full participation and at a cost that the community and country can afford to maintain at every stage of their development in the spirit of self-reliance and self-determination. It forms an integral part both of the country's overall health system, of which it is the central function and main focus, and the overall social and economic development of the community. It is the first level of contact of individuals, the family and community with the national health system bringing care as close as possible to where people live and work, and constitutes the first elements of a continuing health care process."

Primary/coordinated health care will naturally involve liaison with other forms of primary health care agencies such as general practitioners, community health services, pharmacists and local government. It will also include such services as referral and/or transportation to secondary health care (hospitals) or tertiary health care (specialists). The diverse provision of services includes counselling; health education; preventative medicine; provision for supporting people with disabilities; liaison with families and school children; family health strategies; sexual health programs; counselling for bereavement and illness; funeral arrangements; integration with other pertinent social and economic services; liaison with other health and social agencies; the implementation of health programs; health promotions; data collection and other public health services.

Core Functions of Primary Health Care

Medical Care

Clinical Health Services: Clinical Health Services may include, but not be restricted to, the following services provided by medical practitioners and/or appropriately qualified allied health professionals, trained Health Workers or qualified nursing staff using standard treatment procedures:

Diagnostic and clinical care

Treatment of illness/disease

Management of chronic illness

Referral to secondary health care (inpatient hospital and other health residential facility) and tertiary health care (specialist services and care)

Dialysis services and endocrinology referral

Collections for pathology testing and/or referral

Radiology services or referral

Sterilization of equipment meeting standards

Respiratory disease testing, services and referral

Cardiovascular testing, services and referral

Outreach clinical health services to satellite clinics or communities

(i) Domiciliary health care

(ii) Pharmaceutical Services

Prescription of medication and drugs

Pharmaceutical supplies, (subject to State and Federal legislation and mindful of the W.H.O. Alma Ata Declaration advocating provision of essential drugs)

Pharmaceutical supply arrangements with hospital pharmacies or local pharmacists

(iii) Preventative Care

Population health promotional program

Early intervention

Otitis Media examination and testing

Immunisation

Health education and promotion

Socially communicable disease control, manuals and education programs

Health protection supplies and distribution

Antenatal instruction and classes

Maternal and child care (0-5 years)

Diabetic screening, testing and counselling

Screening, individual and mass screening programs

Vaccinations

Infection control

Injury/accident prevention education

Outreach health promotional programs

Dietary and nutrition education

Medical Records and Health Information System

Up-to-date comprehensive Medical Record System

Monitoring sheets and Follow-up Files

Health registers

Health Information Data system

Immunization and vaccination registers

Dental Health Services

Dental Health Services may include, but not be restricted to, the following services provided by dental practitioners and/or appropriately qualified dental health workers or trained dental technicians using standard treatment procedures.

Dental Clinical Services

Diagnostic and dental care

Treatment of tooth decay/extraction

Provision of dentures

Orthodontic and specialist services

Orthodontic and specialist services referral

Sterilization equipment meeting standards

Outreach dental services to satellite clinics or communities without dental services

Preventative Dental Care

Dental health promotional program

Early intervention

Dental health education

Dental health supplies and distribution
Dental Records and Information System
Up-to-date comprehensive Dental Record System
Monitoring sheets and Follow up Files
Dental Health registers
Health Information Data system
Health-related Services and Community Support Services

Psychiatric services and care

Counselling and group activities
Cultural promotion activities
traditional methods of healing
Clinic usage as venue for visiting specialists
Aged care services
Pediatric services
Client follow-up and support
Home and community care
Assistance with surgical aids
ENT services
Ophthalmology services
Optometry services
Advocacy work e.g. support letters for public housing issues
Homelessness support and temporary shelter services

Submission writing for community organizations

Advocacy/interpreting services
Community development work
School-based activities
Transportation health services and Community bus activities
Accommodation or assistance for visiting rural and remote patients
Meeting of patients travelling long distance by public transport
Deceased transportation and arrangements
Funeral assistance
Youth activities and counselling
Satellite primary health services to remote outlying communities or towns without services
Support services for people in custody

Prison advocacy services

Welfare services and food assistance
Affordable and wholesome food provision
Financial assistance for medical supplies or prescriptions
Environmental health services
Substance misuse counselling, education and promotions
Detoxification services
Needle exchange services

Services for people with disabilities
Men's and women's business services
Family counselling services
Crisis intervention services
Audiometry services
Audiology services

The Public Health Sector

The public sector provides health services through the Central and State Governments, municipal corporations and other local bodies. The private health sector consists of the 'not-for-profit' and the 'for-profit' organizations. Individual practitioners from various systems of medicine provide the bulk of medical care in the for-profit health sector. The not-for-profit sector is heterogeneous, with varying objectives, sizes and the areas they cater to. Their activities could be multifunctional and include welfare programmes such as health, education, nutrition, family planning, water supply and housing, agriculture-related development programmes, livelihood programmes, etc.

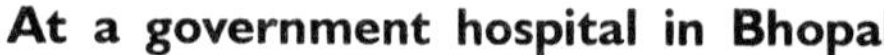

At a government hospital in Bhopal

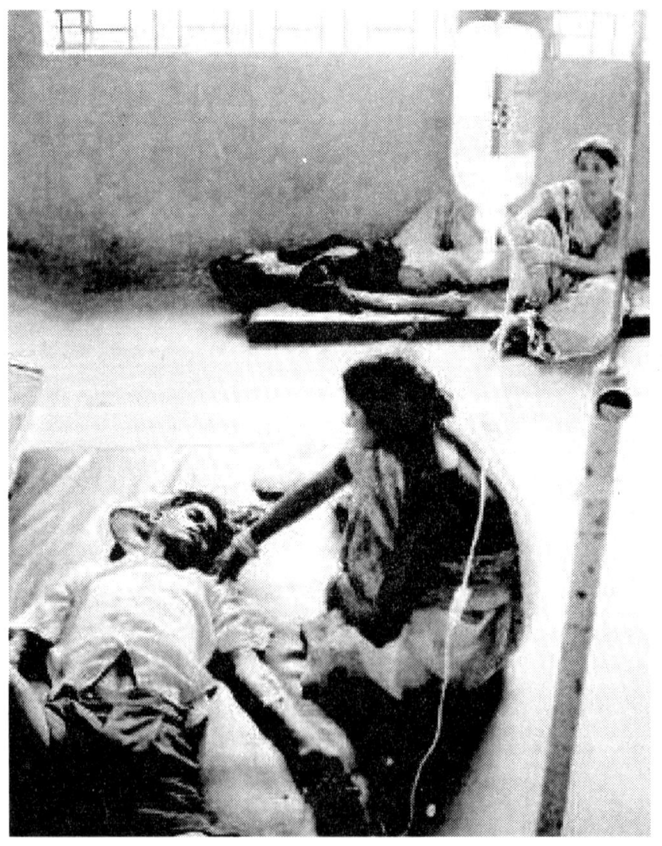

The quality of public health care delivery in India remains woeful while the private health care sector attains impressive heights thanks to the government's privatization drive. But can we all afford the private care?

What is 'not-for-profit'

The not-for-profit sector is generally said to comprise non-governmental organizations (NGOs), the third sector, and the voluntary or charitable sector. There is no clear definition as to what precisely constitutes a not-for-profit organization. However, it is important for the purpose of setting internal government policy that at least within a country a workable definition is adhered to. In India, one of the criteria for a not-for-profit organization/NGO given in the Seventh Plan document is that the organization should have a legal entity. The Planning Commission considers societies, associations, trusts or companies registered under the Societies Registration Act, 1860; Indian Trust Act, 1882; the Charitable and Religious Trusts Act, 1920 or Section 25 of the Companies Act, 1956 as NGOs (Planning Commission, 2002). Religious trusts and missionaries are usually governed by the Charitable and Religious Trusts Act, 1920. 'Charitable purpose' includes relief for the poor, education, medical relief and the advancement of any other object of general public utility but does not include a purpose that relates exclusively to religious teaching or worship. The Societies Registration Act, 1860 defines society as any seven or more persons associated for any literary, scientific or charitable purpose. Both trusts and societies are exempted from income tax. At present, almost every State has adapted its own Societies Act and Charitable Trust Act. For example, Maharashtra registers not-for-profit medical care providers under the Bombay Public Trust Act, 1950. Some States have retained the original Act. Public Trusts are constituted for the benefit of the public at large but the author of a Public Trust may restrict the benefit to a particular group or section of society, on the basis of caste, class, creed, sex, age, etc.

Ideologically, the development potential of the not-for-profit sector originates from the currently dominant neo-liberal perception that State organizations are inefficient. It is commonly argued that non-profit organizations constitute the 'third sector' located between the State and the market. Organizations grouped in the third sector are bound by an appeal to voluntarism. According to the proponents of the 'third sector', the organizations in this sector share distinct characteristics: they possess an internal organizational structure, they are structurally separate from the Government, and they do not generate profits that are distributed to members (Robinson and White, 1997).

Private health sector

Private providers which include qualified and alternative private practitioners account for a large share of all Health care delivered in India. (80%) This share which is increasing rapidly, is more evident in tertiary health care services. This is because of the perception of better quality of services. The private health care providers also account for the largest share of India's health expenditure. (G.K. Lath; Role of Private Sector in Health Care in India).

80% of world population relies on traditional medicine. More then 1/3rd of populations in developing countries lack access to essential medicine. Global market for Alternative and complimentary therapies is currently pegged at 60 million $ by WHO. Even in wealthy countries growing numbers of patients rely on alternative medicine (France—75%; Germany—77%).

Rise of private health care—a bane or boon

The last decade has seen a significant increase in private sector participation in health care delivery. Existing players such as Apollo, Wockhardt, Manipal, Care Hospitals and Narayan Hrudalaya have expanded aggressively. New players such as Fortis, Max, Sterling, Global Hospitals, AMRI, Ruby Hall and Reliance ADAG have entered the sector with plans to establish national and regional presence. International players such as Elbit, Columbia Asia and Parkway have also entered India with plans of establishing a network of hospitals. These corporate players together operate around 25,000 beds across the country. Health care providers have also attracted investments from private equity players such as IDFC, Apax Partners, Actis, Indivision, ICICI Ventures, and Trinity Capital.

Health care delivery can be segmented into primary, secondary and tertiary care. Primary care constitutes treatment on an out-patient basis. Secondary care refers to hospitalisation for "non-critical" ailments. Tertiary care relates to treatment of critical ailments and requires high-tech and expensive facilities and equipment. As of now the corporate sector is focused on tertiary care. The opportunity exists because of the lack of adequate facilities, high investment requirement (which becomes an entry barrier for smaller players), higher revenue realization per patient, less competition from doctor-entrepreneur led facilities as well as an ability to differentiate product offerings.

Five key factors are currently driving private participation in "for profit" health care delivery.

Increasing population base—Population growth of 1.7 per cent per annum for the next five years will result in a need for approximately 30,000 new beds every year.

Increasing income—The number of households with income greater than Rs. 2,00,000 per annum is likely to increase from 95 million (8 per cent of population) to 404 million (32 per cent of population) by 2015.

Rising insurance penetration—Private medical insurance penetration has increased from 0.4 per cent of population in 2001 to 1.5 per cent of population in 2006.

Increasing incidence of "lifestyle" diseases—Cardiac ailments, diabetes, and the like result in an increased requirement of tertiary care beds.

Increase in the number of senior citizens—Driven by higher life expectancy, from 59 to 63 in the last decade, senior citizens (around 4 per cent of population) constitute around 20 per cent of in-patients at hospitals.

The above drivers are likely to result in an annual increase of 10-12 per cent in the size of the health care delivery market over the next five years. However, the financial performance of players has not been very encouraging. Average operating margins have been less than 18 per cent (and declining), and Return on Capital Employed has been less than 15 per cent. This is a key area of concern.

This rather lacklustre financial performance has been due to:

High capital expenditure per bed: Capital expenditure of Rs. 50-75 lakh (Rs. 5-7.5 million) per bed for tertiary care and Rs. 25-30 lakh (Rs. 2.5-3 million) for secondary care, is essentially driven by high cost of land as well as high cost of medical equipment. Given the importance of location while establishing a new facility, providers are forced to pay a high cost for acquiring land especially in the metros and Tier I cities. Medical equipment typically comprises 30-40 per cent of project cost. State-of-the-art medical equipment is being deployed to attract "star" physicians as well as being used as a marketing tool. Given the large share of imported equipment, providers have to pay dollar prices on par with international players thus increasing capital costs. Increasing customer expectations have also resulted in an increased spend on hospital interiors and services.

Ongoing capital expenditure: Significant investment is required on an ongoing basis given the high obsolescence of medical equipment.

Limitations on revenue realization per bed-night: Revenue realization per bed-night has been limited by increasing competition especially in metros and Tier I cities. For example, the average price increase in competitive markets over the last five years has been only around 5 per cent per annum. The large share (greater than 40 per cent) of secondary care patients at most tertiary care hospitals also results in low realization per bed-night. Thus, while the facility has been created for tertiary care (high capex), it is being sub-optimally utilized to offer secondary care (low realization).

Increasing share of bulk buyers (insurance, corporates, etc.) also limits the ability to increase realization significantly. The limited size of the population that can afford high-end tertiary care also restricts revenue growth.

Increasing operating costs: While most players in competitive markets have not been able to increase prices significantly, their operating costs have gone up disproportionately. This increase has been driven essentially by increasing human resource costs due to a shortage of trained personnel and increasing competition for talent. At a key tertiary care hospital in Delhi while the revenue has increased by 5 per cent per annum over the last five years, personnel costs have increased by 14 per cent per annum. High costs associated with attracting and retaining "star" physicians (since they continue to be key drivers of patient volumes) have resulted in high fixed operating costs, especially for new players. High costs incurred on marketing the facility over and above developing a referral network have also increased operating costs for most players.

High gestation period: High fixed operating costs and slow build-up of occupancy results in operating losses in the first few years. Patients have shown a preference for established facilities and physicians and are reluctant to try new facilities especially for critical ailments, thus increasing the gestation period for a new facility.

High capital expenditure, constrained revenue realization per bed-night and increasing operating costs have resulted in shrinking operating margins (average range 10-18 per cent) and low asset turnover ratios.

Clearly, innovative measures are the order of the day to improve financial performance. Such measures would include:

- Better planning at the time of conceptualization: Reducing capital expenditure through innovative hospital design, "optimal" selection of medical equipment, phased rollout, right choice of location, specialty-mix, etc.
- Leveraging scale to reduce procurement price—for capital equipment as well as consumables.
- Having the "right" doctor engagement model and building an "institutional" brand.
- Focus on untapped opportunities—geographic locations as well as undeserved segments.

The burgeoning Indian market, if handled smartly, offers a challenging opportunity for value creation. Health care, then, would definitely turn out to be a healthy business!

Indian Health Industry

In the Health Care segment, stagnant public spending on health (less than 1 percent of GDP) places India among the bottom 20 percent of countries. Most low-income countries spend more than India, where current levels are far below what is needed to provide basic health care to the population. The bulk of public spending on primary health care has been spread too thinly to be fully effective, while the referral linkages to secondary care have been suffered. As in other countries, preventive health services take a back seat to curative care.

Over the last five decades, India has built up a vast health infrastructure and manpower at primary, secondary and tertiary care in government, voluntary and private sectors. These institutions are manned by professionals and para-professionals trained in the medical colleges. Currently, private sector health services range from those provided by large corporate hospitals, smaller hospitals/nursing homes to clinics/ dispensaries run by qualified personnel.

As on June 2001, there were 181 medical colleges out of which 155 (46 of them private) were recognized and 26 (19 of then private) were permitted under the section 10A of the Indian Medical Council Act. A total 5,39,00 MBBS doctors were registered with the Medical council number of Physicians and specialists available is more than the estimated requirements. The current doctor population ratio is 1:1800.

Tertiary hospitals in major cities are in many cases, run by business houses and use corporate business strategies and hi-tech specialization to create demand and attract those with effective demand or the critically vulnerable at increasing costs. Standards in some of them are truly world class and some who work there are outstanding leaders in their areas. Public health spending accounts for 25% of aggregate expenditure, the balance being out of pocket expenditure incurred by patients to private practitioners of various hues.

Public spending on health in India has itself declined after liberalization from 1.3% of GDP in 1990 to 0.9% in 1999. Consider the contrast with the Bhore Committee recommendation of 15% committed to health from the revenue expenditure budget, against the WHO, which recommended 55% of GDP for health. The current annual per capita public health expenditure is no more than Rs. 160 and a recent World Bank review showed that over all primary health services account for 58% of public expenditure mostly but on salaries, and the secondary/tertiary sector for about 38%, perhaps the greater part going to tertiary sector, including government funded medical education.

Hub and spoke model: Making India health care hub of the world.

'Hubs' are tertiary health care providers that deliver specialized health care services including same-day surgery, endoscopy, dialysis, chemotherapy, pulmonary functions, ultrasound, radiology, mammography, CT scan, specialist consulting suites, diagnostic service, pre-admission and post-discharge services. These services require high technology and specialist doctors. (Jyoti Singh and Sugandha Bhandari)

Greater incentive for original drug discovery will create opportunities for Indian companies to develop new competencies through collaborative research and global alliances.

The increase in the population share of the elderly is also causing a change in the pattern of demand for health care services. Such change is opening up both preventive and curative care opportunities, which the existing and new players are exploiting. For instance, in-patient capacity in cardiac care is close to the point of reaching excess supply in certain cities.

Major corporates like the Tatas, Apollo Group, Fortis, Max, Wockhardt, Piramal, Duncan, Ispat and Escorts have made significant investments in setting up state-of-the-art private hospitals in cities like Mumbai, New Delhi, Chennai and Hyderabad.

Comparative Costs Advantage of India

A huge number of International patients are traveling to India to seek quality health care at a fraction of the cost back home. They are admitted at private hospitals with state-of-the-art equipment and medical practitioners trained abroad, these 'five-star' hospitals now attract a new breed of international traveler—the 'medical tourist'.

Hospitals on Wheels

- State-of-the-art ultra-sound, X-ray Machine CG 202.
- Computerized lab and three channels ECG machine available on road equipped to impart health education through audio visual facilities.

Open-Heart Surgery—Open-Heart Surgery in the UK can cost more than $20,000 and double that in the United States. In India, leading hospitals can perform that surgery for less than $5,000.

US ($) India ($)
Bone Marrow Transplant 400,000 30,000
Liver Transplant 500,000 40,000
Open Heart Surgery (CABG) 50,000 4,400
Neuro Surgery 29,000 8000
Knee Surgery 16,000 4,500

Value Added Services

Growing awareness levels on health conditions, urban lifestyles, higher paying power of the population and the emergence of concentrated posh neighbourhoods of the upwardly mobile population in most top cities of the country offer scope for a standardized, quality offering in the form of fitness centers.

These could typically include certain indoor sports like squash and badminton, running tracks (could be indoor), and gymnasium and other facilities like aerobics, yoga and meditation. Various forms of health counselling including nutrition advice, exercising, non-medicinal cure to certain diseases would also form revenue streams for such setups.

Sources

Baru, R. Inter-regional variations in health services in Andhra Pradesh. *Economic and Political Weekly*.

Baru, R. Missionaries in health care. Economic and Jesani, A., Duggal, R., Gupte, M. NGOs in rural health care; http://www.epw.org.in/showArticles.php?root=1999&leaf= Bombay: FRCH; 1986.

Baru, R. Private and voluntary health services: An analysis of inter-regional variations. Report submitted to UNDP. Governance, decentralisation and reform in China, India and Russia. London: Kluwer Academic Publishers; 2000.

Baru, R. Privatisation and corporatisation. Seminar 2000. Available from URL: http://www.india-seminar.com/sem-

Baru, R. Structural adjustment and health: Changing role of NGOs. Paper presented

at International Seminar on Global Governance and Social Policy, Baltic Sea Centre

Berman, P. and Dave, P. Experiences in paying for health care in India's voluntary sector. In: Pachauri, S. (ed).

Duggal, R. Do charitable hospitals deserve tax benefits?

Express Health Care Management, 16-30 September 2003. JNU, New Delhi: Centre of Social Medicine and Community Health; 2003.

Government of India. Directory of Hospitals. New Delhi:

Government of India. Five-Year Plans (First to Tenth Plan). New Delhi: Planning Commission of India. 1951-2002.

Government of India. Health Information of India. New Delhi: Central Bureau of Health Intelligence, Ministry of Government of India. National Health Policy. New Delhi: Ministry of Health and Family Welfare; 2002.

Government of India. National Health Policy. New Delhi: Ministry of Health and Family Welfare; 1983 37:1342-52.

Government of India. NSSO. Fifty-seventh round on unorganised sector, 2000-2001; 2002.

ICSSR/ICMR. Health for all: An alternative strategy. Report of a Study Group. New Delhi: ICSSR 1980.

Locost. Impoverishing the poor: Pharmaceuticals and drug pricing in India; Vadodra: Locost; 2004.

Mahal, A., Srivastava, V., Sanan, D. Decentralisation and its impact on public service provision in the health and education sectors: The case of India. In: Dethier, J. (ed).

Misra, R., Rao, S, Chatterjee, R. India Health Report Delhi: Oxford University Press; 2003.

Pachauri, S. (ed.). Reaching India's poor: Non-governmental approaches to community health. New Delhi: Sage Publications; 1994.

Reaching India's poor: Non-governmental approaches to community health. New Delhi: Sage Publications; 1994.

Robinson, M., White, G. The role of civic organisations in the provision of social services. New York: United Nations Catholic Bishops Conference of India (CBCI), Directory of University, World Institute for Development Economics catholic health facilities in India. New Delhi: CBCI Research; 1997.

Sarkar, A.K. Non-governmental organisations in health care: A study of West Bengal. Unpublished PhD Thesis.

Sen, G., Iyer, A., George, A. Structural reforms and health equity: A comparison of NSS Surveys, 1986-87 and 1995-96 in *Economic and Political Weekly*; 2002;

Sundar, P. NGO experience in health: An overview. In: Pachauri, S. (ed.) Reaching India's poor: Non-governmental approaches to community health. New Delhi: Sage Publications; 1994.

Valhans, M. The new popularity of NGOs. Development and Corporation; 1990; 3:20-2.

Voluntary Health Association of India (VHAI). Report of the Independent Commission on Health in India. Government of India. National Sample Survey Delhi: VHAI; 1997.

Appendix 3

SUMMARY OF HEALTH SYSTEM, HEALTH INSURANCE SCHEME, AND PHARMACEUTICAL SYSTEM IN THAILAND

Chaoncin Sooksriwong (Faculty of Pharmacy, Mahidol University)

Health System

The administrative structure of the MoPH is divided into two levels: central administration and provincial administration.

1. The Central Administration is composed of 10 agencies: (1) the Office of the Minister, (2) the Office of the Permanent Secretary for Public Health, and (3) eight departments in major clusters comprising the Department of Medical Services, the Department for Development of Thai Traditional and Alternative Medicine, the Department of Mental Health, the Department of Disease Control, the Department of Health, the Department of Health Service Support, the Department of Medical Sciences, and the Food and Drug Administration.
2. The Provincial Administration Public health agencies under the provincial administration are Provincial Public Health Offices, hospitals under the MoPH, District Health Offices, and health centers.

The present government has had a policy to restructure the management system of all health facilities so that they will be more independent and flexible like a public organization, but still under the government system. The details of such systems are still under the development process.

Basic Information on Human Resources

Previously 70% of MoPH personnel were civil servants and 30% were permanent employees. Nearly all MoPH personnel (particularly of the Office of the Permanent secretary) are working in the rural areas. In the year 2003, there were 2,877 medical doctors, 979 dentists, 2,173 pharmacists and 10,927 professional nurses.

Health services

Health services in Thailand are classified into five levels according to the level of care as follows:

1. *Self-care at Family Level.* Services at this level include the enhancement of people's capacity to provide self-care and make decisions about health.
2. *Primary Health Care Level.* The primary health care services include those organized by the community in providing services related to health promotion, disease prevention, curative care and rehabilitative care. The medical and health technologies applied at this level are generally not so high, in response to community's needs and culture. Service providers are the people themselves, village health volunteers (VHVs) or other non-governmental volunteers.
3. *Primary Care Level.* Primary care is provided by health personnel and general practitioners (GPs). The universal coverage of health care policy of the present government aims to develop a holistic primary care system for all families across the country. In the near future, the entire holistic primary care system will be more effective and stronger. The components of the primary care system are as follows:
   (1) *Community Health Posts.* A community health post is a village level health service unit established specifically in remote areas, covering a population of 500 to 1,000, and staffed by only one community health worker (a permanent employee of MoPH). Services provided at this level include health promotion, disease prevention and simple curative care.
   (2) *Health Centers.* A health center is a subdistrict or village level health service unit—a first-line unit, covering a population of about 1,000-5,000, with health staff including a health worker, a midwife and a technical nurse. Services provided at this level include health promotion, disease prevention, and curative care. Health centre staff run health programes according to the standard operational procedures established by the MoPH, under the technical supervision and support of the community hospital.
   (3) *Health Centers of Municipalities, Outpatient Departments of Public and Private Hospitals at All Levels, and Private Clinics.* At these facilities, outpatient care is provided by physicians and other health professionals.
   (4) *Drugstores.* A drugstore is a health care unit at the primary care level that is operated by a pharmacist or someone who has been trained in basic pharmacy.
4. *Secondary Care Level.* Medical and health care at this level is managed by medical and health personnel with intermediate level of specialization. General and specialized medical facilities include the following:
   (1) *Community hospitals.* A community hospital is located in a

district or minor-district with 10 to 150 inpatient beds, covering a population of 10,000 or more, and staffed by doctors and other health professionals. Generally, services provided are mostly curative care, compared to those at primary care facilities.

(2) *General or regional hospitals and other large public hospitals.* A general hospital in this category is located in a provincial city or a large district town, equipped with 200 to 500 beds, while a regional hospital located in a provincial city has over 500 beds and medical specialists in all fields.

(3) *Private hospitals.* Most private hospitals are operated as a business entity with both full-time and part-time staff, and clients are required to pay for services.

5. *Tertiary Care.* Medical and health services at this level are provided by medical specialists and health professionals. Tertiary care facilities include:
   (1) General hospitals
   (2) Regional hospitals
   (3) University hospitals and large public hospitals belonging to other ministries or local administrative organizations.
   (4) Large private hospitals have medical specialists in all specialties, mostly with over 100 beds.

The tertiary care facilities also provide primary care services

During 1964-2000, Thais, life expectancy at birth substantially increased from 55.9 years to 69.4 years for males and 62.0 years to 74.1 years for females.

In 2025, it is expected that the life expectancy of Thai citizens will reach 74.8 years for males and 80.3 years for females.

Causes of Death

For all age groups, the study revealed that the leading cause of death was the diseases of circulatory system (18.6% of all causes), more than half of which were due to cerebro-vascular diseases; the second leading cause was cancer and tumors (16.2%), nearly half of which were liver/bile-duct and lung cancers; the third leading cause was infectious diseases (15.5%), most of which were HIV infection particularly among teenage and young adult males, followed by tuberculosis; and the fourth leading cause was external causes among children and youths (12.4%), i.e. accidental drowning among school-age children and road traffic accidents among teenagers and adults, most of which were associated with motorcycles.

An analysis of the differences in causes of death in males and females revealed a proportion of 21.4% for the diseases of circulatory system and 16.5% for cancer/tumors in females and 18.2% for infectious diseases and 16.6% for the diseases of circulatory system in males, whereas external causes ranked third for males and fifth for females.

Health Insurance Scheme

There are three major health and welfare schemes in Thailand:

(1) *The Civil Servant Medical Benefit Scheme (CSMBS)* is a package of welfare and health care benefits for active and retired government employees and public sector workers, as well as their dependents including spouse, parents and children. In 2004, regarding the Health and Welfare Survey (HWS, 2004) report, the number of government and public sector workers is reported at 2.86 million, estimated to be 6.5 million or 10.0 percent of total population including their dependents.
The CSMBS is totally financed via general taxes. Expenditure per beneficiary is estimated to be as high as 3,800 baht. The rapid escalation of health expenditure is the result of problems with cost-containment, especially incentives for providers to over-prescribe due to the use of the "fee for service" payment method. However, a first step in cost containment was taken in April 2002 with the introduction of the Diagnosis Related Groups (DRGs) system within a global budget for the payment of inpatient services. The system was, nevertheless, revoked after four months due to the proof of objection to the enactment of the CSMBS's financing.

(2) *The Social Security Scheme (SSS)* provides social health insurance benefits and is compulsory for employees in private enterprises with more than one worker. However, compliance with it is not yet complete. In 2004, the number of workers covered stands at around 7.83 million, out of 14.71 million workers in the private sector, representing about 11 to 12 percent of the total population. The Social Security Office (SSO) manages the SSS. Contributions into the SSS fund are from three parties: employee, employer and the government each contributed 1 percent of the employee's salary during the period 1998-2003 but 1.5 percent each from 2004 on. Providers those have a contract with the SSO are paid on a capitation basis; the average per capita amount was about 1,830 baht in 2003.

(3) *The 30 Baht Scheme was introduced* in 2001 to cover the citizens who were neither covered by the CSMBS nor by the SSS. This particular group also included those formerly assisted by the Medical Welfare Scheme (MWS), or covered by the Voluntary Health Card Scheme (VHCS). The 30 Baht Scheme derives its name from the amount patients have to pay themselves, the co-payment, for each visit at the contracted health facility. The bulk of financing, however, comes via general tax revenue under the supervision of National Health Security Office (NHSO), Ministry of Public Health (MOPH). Health care is paid for with the per capita method, the capitation, where the amount is calculated in

the basis of the number of people covered, the utilization rates, and the unit costs for both outpatient and inpatient care. In 2004, with the use of utilisation rates and unit costs data of 2002, the capitation amount was assessed by the MOPH's International Health Policy Programme (IHPP) to be 1,447 baht, but in reality even less allocated at 1,308.5 baht. In spite of intentions to achieve equitable service provisions at affordable prices, situations of the 30 Baht Scheme are encountered with the problems of under-financed capitation amounts and budget limitations. Some have been concerning about the qualities of care provided, as well as sustainability and financing feasibility of the scheme in the long-run.

Pharmaceutical System

The pharmaceutical sector is regulated by the Office of Food and Drug Administration, the Ministry of Public Health. In 1981 the National Drug Policy started and was revised in 1993 which added policy in self-support in pharmaceutical by local manufacturing and promotion of National Essential Drug List utilization.

Classification of drugs

According to the Drug Act of B.E. 2530 (1987), medicines are classified into two major groups: modern and traditional drugs.

Modern Drugs are further divided into four categories, namely, (1) household remedies whose sales require no license; (2) ready-packed drugs that can be sold in drugstores by nurses or other medical professionals; (3) dangerous drugs; and (4) specially controlled drugs. Dangerous drugs can be bought without a prescription but must be dispensed by pharmacists. Drugs which may possess a potentially harmful effect on health, if misused, will be listed in the last category whose sales require a prescription.

Traditional drugs are those intended to be used in indigenous or traditional medical care as monographed in the official pharmacopoeia of traditional medicines or those declared by the Minister of Public Health as traditional medicines or those permitted to be registered as traditional medicines. The control and registration of drugs in this group are less stringent than those for modern drugs.

Laws and Regulations

The Drug Act of B.E. 2510 (1967) is currently stilled in effect, whereas the new Drug Act of B.E. 2546 (2003) is in the final stage of promulgation. Attempts to revise the Drug Act of B.E. 2530 (1987) are painstaking and time-consuming. When it becomes effective, many features will be changed accordingly, for example:

1. Types of medicines will be reclassified into 3 new categories:

prescription-only, pharmacy-dispensing and household remedies.

2. Physicians will no longer be allowed to compound medicines for their patients.
3. Manufacturers who are unable to comply with the good manufacturing practices (GMP) principles can no longer proceed with the drug business.
4. The new law provides more flexibility for revising the GMP requirements. Under the new law, the GMP requirements may be revised and approved by the Drug Committee and declared by the Minister of Public Health; no need to get approval from the Parliament as required in the 1987 law.
5. Government-owned enterprises or agencies will no longer be exempted from the requirements of licensing and product registration.
6. Pharmaceutical products may be registered in either of the two channels: one for general medicines and the other for Thai traditional medicines.
7. Product Licenses must be renewed every five years.
8. The Drug Committee will be authorized to withdraw any drug products if later evidence proves that the products are not scientifically efficacious.
9. The Food and Drug Administration will be able to declare certain charges for its services related to licensing, registration, dossier evaluation and approval processes, including expenses for testing the products.
10. Product liability will be implemented for the first time. Consumers may directly sue and get compensation from drug manufacturers if there is any serious harm occurring to them after consumption, provided that product indications are strictly followed.
11. The deviation of statements in advertisement from those permitted will have to be made known to the public through further apology advertisement along with the correct statements.
12. The amounts of fines will be increased upto ten-fold, compared to the previous ones.
13. A pharmacist will be allowed to work in as many drugstores as he/she can.

Drug selection system

Drug selection system in Thailand is approached at multi-level:

1. National drug selection
   a. Drug registration and revision of registered drugs by Thai FDA

   b. Drug selection by pharmaceutical entrepreneurs for registered in Thailand
   c. Selection of Orphan drugs
   d. Control of pharmaceutical chemicals
   e. Production or importing of non-registered drugs
2. Drug selection for the National Essential Drug List
3. Drug selection for health care institution
   a. Drug selection for public hospitals
   b. Drug selection for private hospitals

Both are performed by the Pharmacy and Therapeutic Committee at each hospital. All public hospitals employ the group purchasing program for drug procurement. This program started in 1987 and enlarged the program to all public hospitals in 1995.

Drug distribution channels

The patients at the hospitals will receive prescribed medicines through the hospital pharmacy department located within the hospitals. They rarely fill prescriptions at the pharmacies or drug stores. So the pharmacies or drug stores will serve only self-medication.

In 2005, the total local pharmaceutical production was approximately 808 M US$ (29,686 M Bht.) which in 2003 was 723.5 M US$ (26,587 M Bht.). The amount of imported pharmaceutical products in 2005 was approximately 1,041 M US$ (38,255 M Bht.) while in 2003 was 630 M US$ (23,137 M Bht.) In comparison, in the year 2003 the percentage of local pharmaceutical production was 53.45% while imported pharmaceutical products was 46.53%, and in the year 2005 the percentage of local pharmaceutical production was reduced to 43.7% while imported pharmaceutical products was increased to 56.3%.

In 2005 there were:

1. Drug store
   a. 8801 Modern pharmacies
   b. 4528 OTC drug stores
   c. 640 Veterinary drug stores
2. Pharmaceutical manufacturer
   a. 166 Modern pharmaceutical manufacturers
   b. 879 Traditional pharmaceutical manufacturers
3. Pharmaceutical Importer
   a. 600 Importers for modern drug
   b. 172 Importers for traditional drug

Drug controlling system

The system for controlling drug is composed of Pre-marketing Control (Licensing, Drug Registration), Control of Drug Advertisement, Post-marketing Control, and Re-evaluation of Pharmaceutical Products.

Pre-marketing Control

Licensing

The Drug Act requires that any person who wishes to sell, manufacture or import drugs into the Kingdom must obtain a license from the licensing authorities. The Drug Control Division is the licensing and registration authority for manufacturing, import and sale of drugs within Bangkok metropolis and its territories. Provincial Public Health Offices are the licensing authorities for manufacture and import of traditional drugs and sale of drugs in other provinces.

Applications for licenses must be submitted to the licensing authority. Their buildings and facilities will then be inspected. A License will be issued after the inspection has confirmed that the applicant has adequate capabilities of doing such business, and he/she can secure appropriate facilities and personnel for that purpose.

Licenses are issued, according to the business of the applicant, in nine different categories:

- License to manufacture modern medicines
- License to import modern medicines
- License to sell modern medicines
- License as a wholesaler of modern medicines
- License to sell modern medicines in sealed packages which are classified as neither dangerous nor specially-controlled medicines
- License to sell modern veterinary medicines in sealed packages
- License to manufacture traditional medicines
- License to sell traditional medicines
- License to import traditional medicines

Drug Registration

The registration process is necessary to ensure quality, safety and efficacy of the drugs being marketed in the country. Only authorized licensees are qualified to apply for product registration. Manufacturing plants, in which drug products are manufactured, are subject to inspection for GMP compliance.

According to the new Drug Act (expected to be enacted within 2003), a certificate of product registration is valid for five years as from the date of issuance. The process of drug registration will be carried out in 2 channels, which differ in degrees of control and dossier submission:

1. Registration of general medicines
2. Registration of Thai traditional medicines

Due to some differences in the requirements for dossiers to be submitted for product approvals, the general medicines will have to be further defined as:

- Generics whose registrations require only dossiers on product manufacturing and quality control along with product information;
- New medicines whose registrations require a complete set of product dossiers; and
- New generics whose registrations require dossiers of bioequivalence studies in addition to the required dossiers for generics submission.

Generics mean pharmaceutical products with the same active ingredients and the same dosage forms as those of the original products, but manufactured by different manufacturers.

New medicines include products of new chemicals, new indications, new combinations or new delivery systems and new dosage forms.

New generics are medicines with the same active ingredients, doses and dosage forms as those of the new compounds registered after 1992.

The amended registration procedure for new drug products, adopted in August 1989, involves a two-year period of safety monitoring program. This means that new drug products will be firstly approved for use only in hospitals or clinics for at least two years. Then safety reports must be submitted for consideration as to whether general marketing should be allowed. Meanwhile, new generic products have to pass bioequivalence studies to assure comparatively therapeutic outcomes. The bioequivalence data must be submitted to the authorities as proofs of the product bioavailability along with product information and quality dossiers.

Quality assurance of drug safety and efficacy before marketing can undoubtedly be achieved through good manufacturing practices. Inspection of drug manufacturers and sampling of drug samples from manufacturers, importers or retail pharmacies for analyses by the regulatory authorities cannot effectively solve the problems encountered. Drug manufacturers, importers and distributors must establish their quality assurance systems according to the GMP guidelines to ensure that the drug products have and continue to have the quality as claimed.

The Thai FDA has begun campaigning on GMP compliance since 1984. Projects on development of local pharmaceutical industry upto internationally acceptable standards were part of the Sixth National Economic and Social Development Plan (1987-91) and also of the Seventh Plan (1992-96). The projects aimed to promote and support local drug manufacturers in implementing good manufacturing practices. The first guidelines of Thai Good Manufacturing Practices were published in 1987. Since then numerous workshops, seminars and conferences as well as consultative visits have been held or carried out to promote the guidelines adoption.

Control of Drug Advertisement

Drug information available to health-care professionals and consumers is as important as drug quality for the safe use of drugs. Drug advertisements and other promotional materials need to ensure truthfulness and non-exaggeration. Advertisements through any means must be approved by the authorities before actually being disseminated. Advertisements of prescription or pharmacy-dispensed medicines are permitted only to professionals but prohibited to the general public. Drugs in the household remedy category may be advertised directly to consumers or the general public.

The control of drug advertisements is presently focused on the increasing advertisements on the Internet. A majority (>85%) of such advertisements are being run without FDA permission. Due to the fast growing number of and difficulties in catching up with these advertisements, the monitoring of violation as well as guidelines and measures for the violation control must therefore be comprehensive and updated periodically.

Post-marketing Control

To further ensure quality, safety and efficacy of the approved drug products, the marketed products are regularly sampled for testing at the drug analysis laboratory of the Medical Sciences Department, Ministry of Public Health. In addition, contracts have been signed with some qualified laboratories of local universities to assist in solving the problems of drug quality. The surveillance tasks involve the following:

- Inspection of GMP compliance at manufacturing sites;
- Monitoring of manufacturing process changes to ensure no adverse effects on the safety or efficacy of the medicines;
- Monitoring of the use of marketed drugs for unexpected health risks, taking action if risks are detected by informing the public, investigating the cause and removing the drugs from the market;
- Receiving and handling of complaints;
- Safety monitoring program for new drugs; and
- Re-evaluation of pharmaceutical products.

Re-evaluation of Pharmaceutical Products

Even though drugs have been strictly examined for their quality, efficacy and safety before being approved for marketing, chronological consumption data in a large population, new findings and pharmaceutical progress may later reveal very serious side effects that were not previously seen. A balance between efficacy/benefit and potential risks or serious adverse reactions is frequently questioned, especially those in combination. The Drug Committee in 1991 appointed a sub-committee to evaluate the registered products. Some criteria have been set and the evaluation process has been ongoing.

Index